Ovarian Cancer – Challenges and Innovations

Edited by

Tamara L. Kalir
The Icahn School of Medicine at Mount Sinai, USA

Ovarian Cancer – Challenges and Innovations

Authors: Tamara L. Kalir

ISBN (Online): 978-981-14-2186-0

ISBN (Print): 978-981-14-2185-3

© 2019, Bentham eBooks imprint.

Published by Bentham Science Publishers Pte. Ltd. Singapore. All Rights Reserved.

First published in 2019.

need for a court order if at any point you breach any terms of this License Agreement. In no event will any delay or failure by Bentham Science Publishers in enforcing your compliance with this License Agreement constitute a waiver of any of its rights.

3. You acknowledge that you have read this License Agreement, and agree to be bound by its terms and conditions. To the extent that any other terms and conditions presented on any website of Bentham Science Publishers conflict with, or are inconsistent with, the terms and conditions set out in this License Agreement, you acknowledge that the terms and conditions set out in this License Agreement shall prevail.

Bentham Science Publishers Pte. Ltd.
80 Robinson Road #02-00
Singapore 068898
Singapore
Email: subscriptions@benthamscience.net

BENTHAM SCIENCE

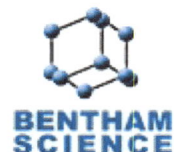

CONTENTS

FOREWORD

I was delighted when I received a request by Dr. Tamara Kalir to write a foreword for this e-book because of my admiration of the leading research conducted by her and her colleagues in ovarian cancers at Mount Sinai Hospital in the past two decades. This book covers a range of topics with a novel juxtapositioning of topics as diverse as: conventional oncology approaches, psychiatric considerations, and the role of belief in healing with commentaries by alternative practitioners.

This book starts with an in-depth overview by Dr. Jamal Rahaman, a leading gynecologic oncologist, on the current management of ovarian cancer, including surgery and chemotherapy that additionally discusses the prospects of emerging therapies inclusive of such entities as immune-modulation and cancer vaccines. Both the clinicians and pathologists would find informative the second chapter by Jessica Beyda, M.D., and Sedef Everest, M.D. on the pathology of ovarian cancer: detailing the various histologic types of epithelial ovarian cancer including low- and high-grade serous carcinoma, mucinous carcinoma, clear cell carcinoma, endometrioid carcinoma; their symptoms, gross pathologic findings, tumor histology, immunohistochemical features available for arriving at the diagnosis, molecular features and prognosis. Also, a discussion on pathogenesis of ovarian cancer with details of key genes and serous tubal intraepithelial carcinoma is presented. Each entity is illustrated by digital photomicrographs, for a total of sixty-nine labeled full-color pictures. Chapter 3 written by Stave Kohtz, Ph.D., further details the molecular pathogenesis of the various ovarian epithelial cancers per the dualistic model (Type I and Type II cancers), including discussion of: TP53, BRACA 1 and 2, PTEN, KRAS,CTNNB1, ARID1A, SWI/SNF, KLF5, CCNE1 and others, microRNAs, and concludes with mention of future pathways for targeted therapy. Gonzalo Carrasco-Avino, M.D. gives a step-by-step demonstration in Chapter 4, on how to utilize Public Gene Expression Omnibus (GEO) datasets and apply a Functional Genomics approach to study gene interactions of high-grade serous carcinoma in canonical pathways, in silico analysis activation of these pathways, and how chemotherapeutic drugs potentially affect them. Chapter 5 written by Jacob Appel, M.D., J.D., M.P.H., discusses the psychological aspects of healing in ovarian cancer, including psychiatric conditions such as depression and anxiety, demoralization, delirium; complicating factors such as loss of fertility, pain, fatigue; cosmetic issues; burnout in caregivers, treatments, and end-of-life considerations. The closing chapter written by Tamara Kalir, M.D., Ph.D., gives an historic overview of practitioners and their practices to explore the role of belief in the healing process, citing experiments on the placebo and nocebo effects, and mind-body interaction, with quotes from a diverse range of healers ranging from medical doctors to medical intuitive.

The material presented herein is current and is helpful, informative and inspiring. Clinicians, researchers and laypersons will find the information in this book invaluable to their work, research, and care for their patients and loved ones.

Linus Chuang MD
Professor and Network Chair
Department of Obstetrics and Gynecology
Western Connecticut Health Network
University of Vermont Larner College of Medicine
USA

PREFACE

Significant research has been carried out on ovarian cancer, inclusive of clinicians' and patients' points of view. My goal was to add something new. Currently ovarian cancer is, for many women a chronic disease which resists cure. The allure of personalized medicine is that we may one day identify biomarkers unique to a patient's ovarian tumor - the 'Achilles heel' of the tumor - that when targeted, results in complete remission of the disease. Today, we are at the beginning this journey. A new book on ovarian cancer would include a discussion on current medical practices and treatments, along with pathogenesis and pathological classifications. The authors (respectively Dr. Jamal Rahaman, and Drs. Jessica Beyda & Sedef Everest) have given excellent and thorough overviews of these subjects. The novelty of this book is threefold: i) commentary on future directions in treatment (respectively Drs. Jamal Rahaman and Stave Kohtz), ii) the use of *in silico* analysis/other computer programs to identify candidate genes for targeted therapy and likelihood of success (Dr. Gonzalo Carrasco-Avino), and iii) discussions on the psycho-spiritual aspects of healing. Dr. Jacob Appel has given a sensitive and comprehensive overview of psychological factors affecting patients with ovarian cancer and, finally, I have included a chapter on the role of belief in healing, with discussions on the placebo and nocebo effects, and the potent influence of our thoughts on our body's ability to heal.

This book is intended for a wide audience including: medical students, house staff, attending physicians, physician assistants, medical researchers, assistants, patients and other interested individuals. My hope is that readers will gain greater knowledge and understanding of ovarian cancer, and will gain their own inspirations and insights into healing and well being.

Tamara L. Kalir, M.D., Ph.D.
Associate Professor of Pathology
The Icahn School of Medicine at Mount Sinai
USA

DEDICATION

In loving memory of Anat Kalir, M.D., promoter of women's and children's health at home and abroad, who had the courage to personally confront both the Holocaust and ovarian cancer.

List of Contributors

Jamal Rahaman	Division of Gynecologic Oncology, Icahn School of Medicine at Mount Sinai New York, New York, USA
Lorene M. Yoxtheimer	Tulane Medical Center, New Orleans, LA, USA
Jessica Beyda	St. Francis Hospital Roslyn., New York, USA
Sedef Everest	Fellow in Pathology, The Mount Sinai Health, New York, USA
Stave Kohtz	Pathology Foundational Sciences, Central Michigan University College of Medicine, USA
Gonzalo Carrasco-Avino	Pathologist, Clinica las Condes, Pontificia Universidad Catolica de Chile, and Adjunct Assistant Professor of Pathology, The Icahn School of Medicine at Mount Sinai, New York, USA
Benjamin Greenbaum	Medicine and Pathology, The Icahn School of Medicine at Mount Sinai, New York, USA
Mireia Castillo-Martin	Molecular and Experimental Pathology Laboratory, Champalimaud Centre for the Unknown, Lisbon, Portugal; and Assistant Professor of Research, Department of Pathology, The Icahn School of Medicine at Mount Sinai, New York, USA
Adolof Firpo	The Icahn School of Medicine at Mount Sinai, New York, USA
Carlos Cordon-Cardo	The Icahn School of Medicine at Mount Sinai, New York, USA
Tamara Kalir	The Icahn School of Medicine at Mount Sinai, New York, USA
Jacob M. Appel	Psychiatry and Medical Education, Director of Ethics Education in Psychiatry, Icahn School of Medicine at Mount Sinai, New York, USA

Surgical Principles for the Management of Epithelial Ovarian Cancer and A Review of Seminal Theraputic Clinical Trials and Emerging Therapies

Jamal Rahaman[1,*] and **Lorene M. Yoxtheimer**[2]

[1] *Division of Gynecologic Oncology Icahn School of Medicine at Mount Sinai, New York, USA*

[2] *Division of Gynecologic Pathology, Icahn School of Medicine at Mount Sinai, New York, USA*

Abstract: Epithelial ovarian cancer (EOC) is the leading cause of gynecologic cancer death in the United States and is the fifth most common cause of US cancer mortality in women. It is estimated that 22,440 women are diagnosed with EOC and 14,080 die from the disease in the United States each year [1]. Using the Surveillance, Epidemiology and End Results 1995-2007 database, stage I,II, III, and IV EOC have 5-year survival rates that are 89%, 70%, 36%, and 17%, respectively while the 10-year survival rates are 84%, 59%, 23%, and 8%, respectively [2]. EOC is most commonly diagnosed in women in their sixth and seventh decades. The median age at diagnosis is 63. Incidence is directly proportional to age and more than 70% of patients have advanced disease at initial presentation [3].

In this chapter, we will explore the foundational principles of surgical management of EOC and highlight critical adjuvant therapeutic trials (mostly Level I data) including chemotherapy, biologic therapy, endocrine therapy, and targeted therapy. We will also evaluate the prospects of emerging therapies including immune-modulation and vaccine therapy.

Keywords: Bevacizumab, BRCA mutation, Carboplatin, Dose-Dense Chemotherapy, Epithelial Ovarian Cancer, Endocrine Therapy, Emerging Therapies, HIPEC, Immunotherapy, Intraperitoneal Chemotherapy, Minimally Invasive Surgery, Maintenance Therapy, Neoadjuvant Chemotherapy, Primary Cytoreduction, Prophylactic Salpingo-oophorectomy, Paclitaxel, PARP Inhibitor, Staging Operation, Secondary Cytoreduction, Vaccine Therapy.

* **Corresponding author Jamal Rahaman:** Division of Gynecologic Oncology, Icahn School of Medicine at Mount Sinai New York, New York, USA; Tel: 212-427-1415; E-mail: jamal.rahaman@ssm.edu

Tamara L. Kalir (Ed.)

SURGERY FOR EPITHELIAL OVARIAN CANCER

Surgical assessment and histologic evaluation are the only means by which a neoplasm can be classified as benign or malignant, primary or metastatic. When an early primary EOC is diagnosed, the next goal is determining the extent of disease or stage. Surgical staging is required to define those patients in whom surgery alone may be curative and those who will require adjuvant therapy, and to determine the modality, intensity, and duration of such treatment. Accurate surgical staging also permits assignment of prognosis, allows comparison of cure rates and defines subsequent surveillance. In the 70 to 75% of patients who present with advanced EOC, the goal of a laparotomy is also to remove as much tumor as possible through a process of surgical "cytoreduction" to maximize response to chemotherapy and improve survival. This method can also be used to treat ovarian germ cell tumors, sex cord stromal tumors, and other less common primary ovarian non-epithelial tumors [3].

PREOPERATIVE PREPARATION

A thorough medical history is important and should cover pregnancy outcomes, medications (especially oral contraception pills and drugs used to induce ovulation), polycystic ovarian disease, and endometriosis [3].

Inquiring about personal and family history of ovarian, breast, or colon cancer is useful because these patients are more likely to develop EOC. However, only 5-10% of patients with EOC have this personal or family history. Women over 40 in the general population have a 1 in 70 risk of developing EOC. Half of women with two or more first-degree relatives with a history of EOC may go on to develop the disease [4, 5]. Testing for BRCA1 and BRCA2 helps to further risk stratify patients [6]. Approximately 13 percent of women with ovarian carcinoma have a BRCA1 or BRCA2 mutation [7]. Patients with Lynch syndrome have an increased risk of possessing a synchronous primary cancer (*e.g.,* endometrial, colon) at the time of surgery for staging.

A thorough physical examination factors into clearance for extensive surgery and may expose the extent of disease. A fixed pelvic mass, nodules in the cul-de-sac or tumor in the upper abdomen may require bowel resection and this should be considered pre-operatively. Patients over 40 years of age and diagnosed with ovarian cancer should undergo a colonoscopy prior to treatment [3].

These women should also have a full medical examination prior to surgery complete with a complete blood count (CBC) and a comprehensive metabolic panel (CMP), which would cover electrolytes, liver, and renal function. Any abnormalities should be addressed before treating the ovarian cancer. Cancer serum markers should be assessed including CA-125, CA 19-9, CEA, alpha-fetoprotein, and inhibin A/B [3, 81].

Preoperative computerized tomography (CT) scanning of the chest, abdomen, and pelvis demonstrates disease spread to the chest and retroperitoneum, especially the lymph nodes. Ureters should be visualized because tumor spread can distort anatomy. CT also allows for the evaluation of the epigastrium to determine the likelihood of achieving optimal cytoreduction in this area. Neoadjuvant chemotherapy before cytoreduction should be considered in patients who are either poor surgical candidates or deemed unlikely to be successful in cytoreduction [8 - 10]. The CT scan criteria to predict poor response to cytoreduction have been documented [11]. PET scans have greater sensitivity than CT or MRI for smaller lesions and are sometimes useful in assessing other primary cancers with ovarian metastasis and also detecting occult metastatic and recurrent lesions [12].

Bowel resection is often required in patients with advanced ovarian cancer; therefore, when there is a high likelihood of extensive disease, the patient should undergo a complete bowel preparation prior to surgery [13]. Failure to adequately prep the patient can lead to increased infectious morbidity [14]. Preoperative hospitalization is not necessary as patients can drink clear liquids and use enemas with or without antibiotics [15].

Patients should understand the basics of the surgical procedure, possible complications, and the likelihood of a malignant diagnosis based on preoperative findings. Patients desiring future fertility should have expectations in line with the type and stage of cancer. Artificial Reproductive Technologies, such as oocyte cryopreservation, should be introduced to patients who are candidates. Even if there is low suspicion of ovarian cancer prior to surgery, all patients should understand that conversion to a laparotomy is a possibility if cancer is found. Discovering a malignancy intraoperatively in a patient who was not appropriately consented for surgery can have a number of ramifications.

EARLY EPITHELIAL OVARIAN CANCER STAGING LAPAROTOMY

The International Federation of Gynecology and Obstetrics (FIGO) is the standard in staging ovarian cancer (Table **1**). Staging of ovarian cancers is better understood when the three mechanisms of spread are appreciated [3]. First: Tumor may advance by direct extension to surrounding pelvic structures. Likewise, abdominal structures may become involved with disease by direct spread. Second: After the tumor breaks through the ovarian capsule, tumor cells can exfoliate into the peritoneal cavity, course through the abdominal cavity, implanting in the omentum, diaphragmatic surfaces, and large and small bowel mesentery. The third modality of tumor spread is through endo-lymphatic channels. The lymphatic channels in the broad ligament allow tumor cells to access the iliac vessels and then the paraaortic lymph nodes. Paraaortic lymph nodes could also be involved by direct lymphatic spread *via* the infundibulopelvic ligaments [16]. A thorough examination of all peritoneal and retroperitoneal surfaces in addition to other at risk structures in the peritoneal and abdominal cavities is required for proper staging.

Table 1. Ovary, fallopian tube, and primary peritoneal carcinoma TNM staging AJCC UICC 2017.

Primary Tumor (T)		
T Category	**FIGO Stage**	**T Criteria**
TX		Primary tumor cannot be assessed
T0		No evidence of primary tumor
T1	I	Tumor limited to ovaries (one or both) or fallopian tube(s)
T1a	IA	Tumor limited to one ovary (capsule intact) or fallopian tube surface; no malignant cells in ascites or peritoneal washings
T1b	IB	Tumor limited to one or both ovaries (capsules intact) or fallopian tubes; no tumor on ovarian or fallopian tube surface; no malignant cells in ascites or peritoneal washings
T1c	IC	Tumor limited to one or both ovaries or fallopian tubes, with any of the following:
T1c1	IC1	Surgical spill
T1c2	IC2	Capsule ruptured before surgery or tumor on ovarian or fallopian tube surface
T1c3	IC3	Malignant cells in ascites or peritoneal washings
T2	II	Tumor involves one or both ovaries or fallopian tubes with pelvic extension below pelvic brim or primary peritoneal cancer
T2a	IIA	Extension and/or implants on the uterus and/or fallopian tube(s) and/or ovaries
T2b	IIB	Extension to and/or implants on other pelvic tissues
T3	III	Tumor involves one or both ovaries or fallopian tubes, or primary peritoneal cancer, with microscopically confirmed peritoneal metastasis outside the pelvis and/or metastasis to the retroperitoneal (pelvic and/or para-aortic) lymph nodes
T3a	IIIA2	Microscopic extra pelvic (above the pelvic brim) peritoneal involvement with or without positive retroperitoneal lymph nodes
T3b	IIIB	Macroscopic peritoneal metastasis beyond pelvis 2 cm or less in greatest dimension with or without metastasis to the retroperitoneal lymph nodes
T3c	IIIC	Macroscopic peritoneal metastasis beyond the pelvis more than 2 cm in greatest dimension with or without metastasis to the retroperitoneal lymph nodes (includes extension of tumor to capsule of liver and spleen without parenchymal involvement of either organ)

(Table 1) cont.....

Primary Tumor (T)		
T Category	**FIGO Stage**	**T Criteria**
Regional lymph nodes (N)		
N Category	**FIGO Stage**	**N Criteria**
NX		Regional lymph nodes cannot be assessed
N0		No regional lymph node metastasis
N0(i+)		Isolated tumor cells in regional lymph node(s) no greater than 0.2 mm
N1	IIIA1	Positive retroperitoneal lymph nodes only (histologically confirmed)
N1a	IIIA1i	Metastasis up to 10 mm in greatest dimension
N1b	IIIB1ii	Metastasis more than 10 mm in greatest dimension
Distant metastasis (M)		
M Category	**FIGO Stage**	**M Criteria**
M0		No distant metastasis
M1	IV	Distant metastasis, including pleural effusion with positive cytology; liver or splenic parenchymal metastasis; metastasis to extra-abdominal organs (including inguinal lymph nodes and lymph nodes outside the abdominal cavity); and transmural involvement of intestine
M1a	IVA	Pleural effusion with positive cytology
M1b	IVB	Liver or splenic parenchymal metastases; metastases to extra-abdominal organs (including inguinal lymph nodes and lymph nodes outside the abdominal cavity); transmural involvement of intestine
Prognostic stage groups		
When T is...	**And N is...**	**And M is...**	**Then the Stage Group is...**
T1	N0	M0	I
T1a	N0	M0	IA
T1b	N0	M0	IB
T1c	N0	M0	IC
T2	N0	M0	II
T2a	N0	M0	IIA
T2b	N0	M0	IIB
T1/T2	N1	M0	IIIA1
T3a	N0, N1	M0	IIIA2
T3b	N0, N1	M0	IIIB
T3c	N0, N1	M0	IIIC
Any T	Any N	M1	IV
Any T	Any N	M1a	IVA
Any T	Any N	M1b	IVB

We prefer using a vertical midline incision with adequate length to ensure easy removal of large tumors in addition to inspecting and possibly treating the upper abdomen. Pelvic fluid should be collected when entering the peritoneal cavity for cytologic evaluation. Perform pelvic washings if no fluid is present. Take a moment to evaluate the pelvis. Document the sizes of the tumors, ovarian surface involvement of the tumor, presence of adhesions, extension of the tumor to surrounding structures, and whether a cystic lesion was ruptured preoperatively or intraoperatively. All these elements are factors in staging the tumor. Run the bowel, palpate the upper abdomen, the mesentery, and retroperitoneal structures, assessing these areas for tumor. A hysterectomy and bilateral salpingo-oophoroectomy should be performed unless it is an early stage cancer and future fertility is a possibility [19]. We suggest bilateral lymph node sampling, even in patients with early-stage disease. Both sides should be sampled because contralateral nodal involvement is unlikely, but not impossible, when ipsilateral nodes are negative [20, 21]. Paraaortic lymph node sampling should include the renal vessels as illustrated.

Inadequate staging with inappropriate incisions is relatively common [22, 23]. Young *et al*. reported that 31% of patients presumed to have stage I or II disease were upstaged after initial surgery, which was deemed inadequate. After proper staging, 77% of these upstaged patients had stage III disease [24]. Women with stage I disease have an almost 89% 5-year survival; however, once the tumor spreads beyond the pelvis, 5-year survival rates decrease to below 36% [2]. Patients who are incorrectly diagnosed with an early stage disease when, in fact, it is advanced disease have a decreased likelihood of being cured of disease.

Low-grade tumors confined to the ovary (stage IA, 1B) require no further treatment after removal because it does not affect survival [25, 26]. High-grade stage I tumors with poor prognosis, on the other hand, have longer disease-free intervals and improved survival after comprehensive staging and platinum-based chemotherapy [25]. Platinum-based therapy is important when treating advanced stage disease [27 - 30]. A taxane/platinum combination is the current standard of care [31 - 33]. An inadequate staging operation can have negative prognostic implications. This is a serious problem, reflected in one study using the NCI/SEER database. Only 10% of US women with early stage ovarian cancer underwent adequate staging procedures [34]. Increased intraoperative consultation with gynecologic oncologists for remedy of this deficiency after intraoperative histologic analysis of the removed specimen is recommended [3].

OVARIAN TUMORS OF BORDERLINE OR LOW MALIGNANT POTENTIAL

Atypical proliferative, also known as "borderline," tumors have histologic features that are more complex than benign entities but simpler than cancer and do not display extensive evidence of invasion (<5mm). 80% of borderline tumors are confined to the pelvis at the time of diagnosis. If the tumor is isolated to the ovaries, fertility conservation procedures are still viable options. Patients with borderline tumors will have long disease-free intervals if no residual tumor is left in the patient [3]. Most studies have concluded that adjuvant chemotherapy and radiotherapy do not increase disease-free intervals or survival [35, 36]. Invasive implants, found in 22% of cases, are the most important indicator of poor prognosis. These patients should be treated with adjuvant chemotherapy. In a study following women for 7.4 years, patients with non-invasive implants had a survival rate of 95.3% *vs.* 66% in patients with invasive implants [3, 37]. Stage I patients had a survival rate approaching 100%.

ADVANCED EPITHELIAL OVARIAN CANCER ROLE OF CYTOREDUCTION

Staging is the primary goal of the first surgery in the treatment of early epithelial ovarian cancer (stage I & II). In advanced disease (stage III & IV), the key is cytoreduction, which entails removing all visible tumor seen intraoperatively. This optimizes the patient's response to adjuvant chemotherapy and increases survival rates [3]. Even removing tumors that are larger than 1 cm improves survival after adjuvant therapy [38]. Between 1985 and 1994, 230 stage III primary ovarian cancer patients underwent primary cytoreductive surgery and platinum-based chemotherapy at Mt. Sinai. Optimal primary cytoreduction to < 1 cm (64.2%) significantly increased survival (p<.0001). Kaplan-Meier 2-year survival was 82.5% in those with optimal cytoreduction *vs.* 59.8% of patients with sub-optimal primary cytoreduction. At 3 years, the survival rates were 73.6% for optimal and 38.8% for suboptimal cytoreduction. The survival rates dropped to 59.2% for primary optimal cytoreduction and 18.8% for suboptimal at 5 years [39]. The impact of cytoreduction on survival was illustrated in a systematic review of 11 retrospective studies that found that optimal (<1 cm) *versus* suboptimal (>1 cm) cytoreduction was associated with a significant improvement in overall survival (hazard ratio [HR] 1.36, 95% CI 1.10-1.68). There was a greater improvement in survival with complete cytoreduction (no gross residual) compared with optimal cytoreduction (<1 cm; HR 2.20, 95% CI 1.90-2.54) [40].

The survival benefit of complete cytoreduction was also found in a meta-analysis of 18 studies (both retrospective and prospective studies) of women with stage IIB or higher ovarian, tubal, or peritoneal cancer who underwent cytoreduction and platinum/taxane chemotherapy. For each 10 percent increase in the proportion of patients undergoing complete cytoreduction to no gross residual disease, a 2.3-month increase in median survival compared with a 1.8-month increase for optimal cytoreduction (defined as residual disease ≤1 cm) is seen [41].

Optimal cytoreduction is, therefore, imperative. Previous studies have shown, and our research corroborates the fact that older patients with advanced disease who achieve optimal cytoreduction have survival rates similar to younger patients. Therefore, advanced age should not hinder the introduction of treatment options like cytoreduction [42 - 45].

While the actual cytoreductive surgery increases survival, whether a tumor achieves optimal cytoreduction could be a function of biological differences between cancers. Tumors with small-volume disease or tumors that are cytoreduced to small-volume may be intrinsically different from ones that cannot [46]. Although cytoreduction may increase overall survival, the survival benefit is not equal to that of small-volume abdominal disease at presentation. These differences may reflect variations in biologic activity or different durations of disease. Regardless of the skill a surgeon has in removing cancer, tumors that have been growing for a long period of time or showing aggressive behavior demonstrate a poorer prognosis. More research is required on these theories [3].

CYTOREDUCTION TECHNIQUES

Clinically, primary cancer of the pancreas, colon, and stomach may be indistinguishable from ovarian cancer. Cytoreduction effectiveness has not been proven in non-ovarian cancer. Accurate frozen section diagnosis during surgery may avoid an unnecessary and lengthy staging procedure when a palliative procedure is more appropriate. Accurate intraoperative frozen section analysis is important [3].

An initial assessment should determine whether the tumor is a candidate for resection. Tumor is deemed unresectable when the porta hepatis, the base of the small bowel mesentery or multiple liver parenchymal lesions are involved [47]. Cytoreduction of solitary intraparenchymal liver lesions is feasible and should only be attempted if the patient would be surgically disease-free as a result. In fact, the optimal cytoreduction of the liver lesions has an independent prognostic value in improving survival [48, 49]. Upper abdominal disease should be addressed and deemed resectable prior to the evaluation of pelvic disease. Pelvic organs are frequently involved when the cancer is advanced in stage. Persistent cytoreduction can be achieved in "frozen pelvis," which is often thought of as inoperable [47]. Patients, therefore, need clinicians with expertise in cytoreduction [3].

Large tumors on peritoneal surfaces can be removed by identifying retroperitoneal structures and accessing avascular retroperitoneal planes. Precision and an intricate understanding of retroperitoneal anatomy is essential for this approach to work successfully. Access the retroperitoneum by making an incision in the peritoneum lateral to the external iliac vessels and psoas. Locate, ligate, and cut the round ligament in the retroperitoneum. Continue the peritoneal incision to include bladder peritoneum and remove as many peritoneal implants as possible. Perform an "anterior culdectomy," which entails removing all anterior cul-de-sac involved by tumor. This is achieved by dissecting the peritoneum of the anterior cul-de-sac away from the bladder with a scalpel until it is only attached to the uterine serosa. Use a scalpel to detach the bladder from the lower uterine segment, anterior cervix, and vagina. Continue the lateral peritoneal incision up to the level of the infundibulopelvic (IP) ligament. Locate the ureter on the medial aspect of the pelvic peritoneum before cutting the IP ligament. Use the ureter as a guide to find the uterine artery, which will be divided. If no rectosigmoid involvement is identified, a subtotal or total hysterectomy completes the necessary surgery [3].

If the rectosigmoid colon is involved, it can be removed en bloc through the presacral space, which is avascular. If the sigmoid colon is involved, simply resect proximal to tumor with a stapler. Preserve as much colon as possible to increase the likelihood of a tension-free anastomosis. Individual mesenteric vessels should be ligated. Identify the base of the sigmoid mesentery to access the presacral space. Perforating veins on the anterior surface of the sacrum can cause significant blood loss if traumatized. The distal margin of the sigmoid colon is isolated following the ligation of the rectal pillars and the lateral rectosigmoid attachments [3].

Perform a subtotal hysterectomy or total hysterectomy. Mobilize the posterior cul-de-sac and access the rectovaginal space. Use a stapler to transect the distal resection margin of the rectum. An end-to-end stapler enables low-rectal reanastomosis without requiring a colostomy [50 - 52].

The omentum frequently harbors metastatic disease [53]. A total (supracolic) or partial (infracolic) omentectomy should remove gross residual tumor. Routine lymphadenectomy is not necessary when there is advanced disease. However, if pelvic and paraaortic retroperitoneal lymph nodes are palpable, they should be removed, especially if it enables complete cytoreduction [3].

Gynecologic surgeons have been more aggressive in removing tumor from adjacent pelvic structures because research has shown that cytoreduction ("debulking") increases survival [54]. Mechanical stapling devices are preferred to suture anastomosis when performing bowel resections and reanastamosis because complication rates and blood loss are lower, and hospital length of stay is shorter [50 - 52].

Although it is debatable whether these procedures to remove bulky tumor impact overall survival, most gynecologic oncologists will perform them [10, 55]. Randomized trials to evaluate the effect of surgeries such as optimal cytoreduction with bowel resection and other debulking procedures are not possible to perform. Additionally, malignancies that extend to the bowel may display different tumor biology [3].

Resecting organs that have metastatic ovarian cancer to achieve optimal cytoreduction is now commonly performed to achieve no visible disease. Splenectomy [56, 57], resection of the lower urinary tract [58, 62], liver, and diaphragm [49, 59 - 61] are now more frequently performed to optimize patient response to postoperative chemotherapy [3].

SECONDARY CYTOREDUCTION

In patients with disease that recurs more than 6-12 months after completion of initial chemotherapy, a second cytoreduction could be considered if the disease has the following criteria: small amount of tumor that can be completely resected and absence of ascites [62 - 65]. Current trials are evaluating the benefit of secondary cytoreduction. Selected cases may be amenable to minimally invasive surgery including robotic surgery [66].

PROPHYLACTIC SALPINGO-OOPHORECTOMY

Approximately 10-13% of all patients with ovarian cancer harbor a BRCA1 or BRCA2 mutation [7]. These mutations are more common in certain ethnic groups. For example, in a population-based series of 1342 patients with invasive ovarian cancer in Ontario, Canada, the prevalence of BRCA mutations was particularly high among women of Italian (43.5%), Jewish (30.0%) or Indo-Pakistani origin (29.4%) [7].

Women with BRCA mutations have an increased lifetime risk of developing ovarian or breast cancer. Carriers of BRCA1 mutation have an estimated 65-85% risk of developing breast cancer and a 39-46% risk of developing ovarian cancer by age 70. Similarly, BRCA2 mutation carriers have an estimated 45-85% risk of breast cancer and a 10-27% risk of ovarian cancer by age 70 [67]. Since genetic counseling and testing has become widely available for high risk patients, preventive measures are a choice for many of these women.

The proportion of women who tested positive for a BRCA mutation and opted for a risk-reducing salpingo-oophorectomy (RRSO), which addresses the risk of not only developing ovarian cancer but also hormone receptor-positive breast cancer, is as high as 49% [67]. No current screening techniques, including frequent pelvic examinations, pelvic ultrasound, or other imaging, and serum CA-125 level, have been shown to decrease the risk of death from ovarian cancer in women who are carriers of BRCA1 or BRCA2 mutation. A consensus panel of the National Institute of Health (NIH) recommended prophylactic oophorectomy for women considered high-risk at age 35 or later if the patient does not desires more children [68]. Risk-reducing salpingo-oophorectomy has been shown to effectively reduce the risk of ovarian cancer by 71-96% [69] and reduces the risk of breast cancer by 50% [70]. Moreover, RRSO decreases breast cancer-specific mortality by 90%, ovarian cancer-specific mortality by 95%, and overall mortality by 76% [71]. Considering this data, RRSO is highly recommended to all patients who are carriers of BRCA1 or BRCA2 mutation [3, 67].

After completing the RRSO, there is still some risk of developing primary peritoneal cancer. In a large international study by Finch, 5783 known carriers of BRCA1 or BRCA2 mutation underwent RRSO and were found to have an estimated cumulative incidence of peritoneal cancer of 3.9% for BRCA1 and 1.9% for BRCA2 at 20 years after oophorectomy [72].

RRSO is performed laparoscopically in the majority of the cases unless a laparotomy is performed for other indications. At the beginning of the procedure, all peritoneal surfaces and the upper abdomen should be carefully evaluated for any evidence of nodularity or implants. Pelvic washings need to be obtained for cytological evaluation. Any suspicious lesions should be biopsied and sent for pathologic examination. The surgeon should make an effort to avoid contact with the surface of the ovary and the fimbriated end of the fallopian tube, so that the delicate surface epithelium is not abraded. Microscopic occult carcinomas have been identified in RRSO specimens in approximately 2% of the BRCA mutation carriers [69, 73]. Patients who are undergoing a laparoscopic RRSO should be counseled on the probability of discovering cancer at the time of the surgery. If this occurs, the appropriate staging procedures need to be performed [3].

In addition to well-described familial syndromes associated with an increased risk of breast and/or ovarian cancer, other gene mutations appear to at least moderately increase the risk of these cancers. Lynch syndrome, also known as hereditary nonpolyposis colon cancer (HNPCC), is associated with mismatch repair (MMR) gene mutations (MSH2, MLH1, MSH6, and PMS2) and a mutation in the epithelial cell adhesion molecule (EPCAM) gene. Women with Lynch syndrome have a life-time risk of ovarian cancer between 4-12% [74, 75].

About 3 to 8 percent of women presenting for hereditary breast/ovarian cancer risk assessment have mutations in other moderate-risk genes recently described including BARD1, BRIP1, RAD51 paralogs, RAD51C and RAD51D, PALB2. However, the exact risk of cancer associated with mutations in these genes is not clear. Commercial multigene panels include testing for the BRCA genes, the high-risk genes listed above, as well as mutations in several moderate-risk genes [74, 75]. Patients with these moderate-risk genes require individual counselling by a certified genetic counsellor as well as a gynecologic oncologist about the appropriate timing and risk *vs.* benefit of RRSO.

SALPINGECTOMY

A growing body of literature suggests that a large proportion of ovarian high-grade serous carcinoma may actually arise from fallopian tube secretory epithelial cells. Many young female carriers of BRCA1 or BRCA2 mutation are reluctant to undergo RRSO because of post-RRSO induced menopause. While the risk of hormone replacement is less than the risk of retaining the ovaries and fallopian tubes, bilateral salpingectomy with ovarian retention until menopause may be offered to patients who refuse oophorectomy before menopause [76].

Opportunistic salpingectomy is the removal of the fallopian tubes for primary prevention of epithelial carcinoma of the fallopian tube, ovary, or peritoneum in a woman undergoing pelvic surgery for another indication. This procedure would be indicated in women at average risk, rather than high risk, for these cancers. The preventive strategy of opportunistic salpingectomy was introduced in 2010 by the British Columbia Ovarian Cancer Research (OVCARE) team [77] and is now routinely discussed and offered to patients undergoing elective hysterectomies and sterilization procedures [78]. There is no evidence of compromise to ovarian function by the addition of a salpingectomy [79, 80].

GYNECOLOGIC ONCOLOGIST

Women with ovarian masses that are highly suspicious for malignancy pre-operatively should consult a gynecologic oncologist [68] [NIH Consensus Statement, 1995]. This is emphasized in the study by McGowan *et al.*, which evaluated 291 women with ovarian cancer. They found that 97% of patients staged by a gynecologic oncologist were properly staged. In contrast, only 52% of patients operated on by general obstetrician/gynecologists and 35% of patients who saw general surgeons were staged appropriately [81]. Surgeries performed by gynecologic oncologists have a better prognosis than those treated by other surgeons, especially when performed at a high-volume tertiary hospital [82 - 85].

LAPAROSCOPIC SURGERY

The new minimally-invasive technologies have shaped the surgical management of primary ovarian cancer. Staging of a stage I ovarian cancer using laparoscopic methods has been documented [86]. Since that time, laparoscopic paraaortic lymph node dissection has been reported along with its associated morbidity [87 - 91]. There have been few high-quality studies about use of laparoscopy for ovarian cancer staging. A meta-analysis of 11 observational studies of women with presumed stage I or II ovarian cancer found no difference between laparoscopy and laparotomy in operative duration, but laparoscopic surgery was associated with decreased blood loss (244 *versus* 467 mL) [92]. There was a low rate of conversion to laparotomy (3.7 percent). Many women were upstaged after laparoscopy (22 percent), but this did not differ significantly from laparotomy in three comparative studies. There are no long-term data on the effect on progression-free and overall survival between the two techniques for staging procedures. Data from small studies suggest that the stage assigned *via* laparoscopy does not differ from laparotomy [93 - 96].

At present, laparoscopic surgical staging of early ovarian cancer can be technically difficult and should be reserved for select cases performed by surgeons with the appropriate training [97]. With the recent randomized trials demonstrating the utility of neoadjuvant, chemotherapy, laparoscopy is now frequently utilized to assess the feasibility of cytoreductive surgery to triage patients to neoadjuvant chemotherapy [9, 10].

More recently, robotic-assisted laparoscopy has been increasingly employed for selected cases of early stage ovarian cancer staging [98 - 102]. There have also been reports of selective use of conventional laparoscopy or robotic surgery to achieve optimal cytoreduction in selected cases for primary or interval cytoreduction [103].

CHEMOTHERAPY FOR EPITHELIAL OVARIAN CANCER

EOC is known as one of the most chemo-sensitive malignancies. In the US, approximately 22,440 patients are diagnosed with EOC each year in the US and about 14,080 die from EOC [1]. Most patients who respond initially will experience recurrences and die of their disease. Roughly 70-80% of patients recently diagnosed with advanced disease will achieve complete clinical response to primary platinum plus taxane chemotherapy [31, 104]. The most commonly used platinum compound is carboplatin. It is a second-generation platinum compound which is less nephrotoxic, neurotoxic, and emetogenic but as effective as cisplatin [32]. Platinum and paclitaxel are considered the standard chemotherapy agents for initial treatment of EOC. However, there is debate regarding the best route, dose density, and intensity, and sequence of therapy for initial treatment. Additionally, the best chemotherapeutic therapy for patients with recurrence is still controversial. In this review, we will summarize the cardinal clinical trials (mostly level I data) that form the foundation for adjuvant therapy in EOC. The details of the individual trials can be found in the references as well as the incidence of side effects and adverse events.

EARLY STAGE DISEASE

Patients with low-risk, stage IA, grade 1 tumors are usually treated with surgery alone. These women have a 95% overall 5-year survival rate, thereby, making adjuvant chemotherapy unnecessary [26, 105]. Despite this excellent 5-year prognosis, 20-30% of women with early-stage EOC ultimately die from their disease. Patients with a high risk of recurrence should be identified because these women should receive chemotherapy. However, identifying which patients have a high risk of recurrence has been difficult. Trials with long term follow up (5-10+ years) have demonstrated that the overall survival of patients with high-risk early ovarian cancer improves when adjuvant chemotherapy is administered [25, 26, 106]. A combined analysis of two parallel randomized clinical trials in early ovarian cancer, ICON 1 and ACTION, comparing platinum-containing adjuvant chemotherapy to observation following surgery was performed. In a study enrolling 924 patients, an 8% increase in survival was noted in the cohort receiving adjuvant chemotherapy compared to those who were observed [106 - 108]. Based on recurrence rates and improvement in survival, stage IA, grade 2 and 3 and higher should be treated with chemotherapy.

Duration of treatment is one of the most controversial issues regarding treatment for early stage EOC. Traditionally, chemotherapy has been given over six to eight cycles in advanced ovarian cancer. GOG 157 [109] was a trial of adjuvant therapy randomizing 3 *versus* 6 rounds of paclitaxel ($175mg/m^2$) and carboplatin every 3 weeks in patients with stages stage IA grade 3, IB grade 3, clear cell, IC, and completely resected stage II EOC. The authors suggested that three cycles would be appropriate after surgical staging for patients with high-risk, early-stage endometrioid ovarian cancer (EOC). An additional three cycles would only produce a small reduction in recurrence and increase toxicity. This study did have several issues. The therapy used carboplatin at an area under the curve (AUC) of 7.5. This is in contrast to conventional therapy, which uses lower dose of an AUC of 5-6. The recurrence risk decreased from 25.4% on 3 cycles to 20.1% in 6 cycles; however, the power of the study was questioned due to the small number of subjects. Additionally, 127 out of 427 subjects were inadequately staged [109].

ADVANCED STAGE DISEASE CONVENTIONAL INTRAVENOUS CHEMOTHERAPY

Although platinum and taxane–based chemotherapy continues to be the standard treatment for the past 20 years, exciting new chemotherapeutic options have flourished in recent years. The gold standard for frontline chemotherapy in advanced disease is based on two non-inferiority randomized phase III trials by the GOG (158) and AGO utilizing 6 cycles carboplatin (at an AUC of 5-6) and paclitaxel (175 mg/m^2) every 3 weeks [32, 33, 182].

In 2017, the NCCN Panel added carboplatin/liposomal doxorubicin as a first-line postoperative intravenous option for stages II to IV ovarian cancer; this regimen has a category 2A recommendation. The regimen was added based on a Multi-center Italian Trials in Ovarian Cancer-2 (MITO-2), an academic multicenter phase III randomized trial in 820 patients with stages III and IV ovarian cancer [110], comparing carboplatin AUC 5 plus liposomal doxorubicin 30 mg/m^2, every 3 weeks *versus* standard carboplatin/paclitaxel in GOG 158. No significant difference was noted in the median overall survival with carboplatin/liposomal doxorubicin *versus* carboplatin/paclitaxel (61.6 and 53.2 months, respectively). Toxicity varied between the two groups. Less alopecia and neurotoxicity but more hematologic effects were observed with carboplatin/liposomal doxorubicin. This regimen could be used for those with a propensity for neurotoxicity or those patients who would like to avoid hair loss [182].

INTRAPERITONEAL CHEMOTHERAPY

The reintroduction of intraperitoneal (IP) chemotherapy has significantly modified the standard of care for those who have achieved optimal cytoreduction (<1 cm). Three randomized controlled studies have demonstrated survival benefit when administered IP therapy instead of intravenous (IV) conventional chemotherapy [111 - 113]. The GOG 172 reported a 16-month survival benefit in those patients receiving intraperitoneal (day 1 cisplatin 100 mg/m^2 and day 8 paclitaxel 60 mg/m^2) chemotherapy compared to patients who received intravenous therapy (IV) with paclitaxel (175 mg/m^2 over 24hrs) and cisplatin (75 mg/m^2). Cisplatin and paclitaxel are delivered as front-line therapy directly into the intraperitoneal cavity in patients after they have undergone optimal surgical cytoreduction (defined as residual tumor <1 cm in maximal diameter after initial surgical cytoreduction). This method has shown statistically significant improvement in progression-free and overall survival [111]. In 2006, The National Cancer Institute (NCI) endorsed the utilization of IP therapy in an NCI Consensus Statement shortly after the findings of this study were published. Unfortunately, this strategy is associated with a higher risk of side effects due to the use of cisplatin (rather than carboplatin) and the necessity of an intraperitoneal catheter for drug delivery [114]. Only 42% of patients in the GOG 172 trial completed all 6 cycles due to toxicity, and the trial did not use the standard therapy of paclitaxel and carboplatin (GOG 158) as a comparison. These concerns created resistance to the universal application of this protocol in front-line chemotherapy; however, some clinicians have adopted a modification of the IP protocol (with intraperitoneal cisplatin at 75 mg/m^2). Others continue to use carboplatin and paclitaxel intravenous chemotherapy, while many patients enroll in trials utilizing biologic therapy [183].

DOSE-DENSE INTRAVENOUS CHEMOTHERAPY

JGOG 3016 Trial – Dose-dense weekly administration of paclitaxel is another strategy to enhance anti-tumor activity and prolong survival. Preclinical studies have suggested that duration of exposure is an important determinant of the cytotoxic activity of paclitaxel. Adequate cytotoxicity can be achieved at fairly low concentrations of the drug provided that exposure is extended. In the Japanese Gynecologic Oncology Group 3016 (JGOG 3016), 631 women, approximately half of whom had optimal cytoreduction, were randomly assigned to treatment with carboplatin and paclitaxel (every three weeks) or to carboplatin (every three weeks) with **dose-dense weekly paclitaxel (80 mg/m^2)**. In both arms, the regimen was repeated every three weeks for up to nine cycles [115, 116]. With a median follow-up of 77 months, dose-dense therapy resulted in:

A significant improvement in PFS (median, 28 *versus* 17.5 months, respectively) and OS (median, 100.5 *versus* 62 months) compared with conventional treatment.

Women with at least 1 cm of residual disease following surgical cytoreduction appeared to benefit the most from dose-dense therapy. Compared with conventional treatment every three weeks, dose-dense treatment resulted in an improvement in PFS (median, 17.6 *versus* 12 months) and OS (median, 51 *versus* 33 months). There was no significant advantage to dose-dense treatment for patients with optimally cytoreduced disease. Subgroup analysis showed that the schedule of treatment did not influence survival outcomes for patients with clear cell or mucinous cancers [115]. However, for women with serous and other histologic types, dose-dense therapy improved both PFS (median, 28.7 *versus* 17.5 months) and OS (median, 100.5 *versus* 61.2 months) compared with conventional therapy.

Given these long-term outcomes, several clinicians often prefer dose-dense therapy to conventional (once every three weeks) treatment, especially in patients who had a suboptimal cytoreduction and whose tumors are not of clear cell or mucinous type [183].

DOSE-DENSE INTRAVENOUS *VS.* INTRAPERITONEAL CHEMOTHERAPY

How dose-dense intravenous therapy compares with conventional IV/IP treatment is the subject of active investigation. Preliminary data from one randomized study suggest that dose-dense IV therapy may result in similar progression-free survival as traditional IV/IP therapy with fewer adverse effects [117, 183].

In GOG 252, 1560 women with optimally cytoreduced stage II to III ovarian cancer were randomly assigned to one of several treatment arms, including a dose-dense IV therapy arm (weekly paclitaxel administration and carboplatin administered every three weeks) and an IV/IP arm with paclitaxel IV and cisplatin/paclitaxel IP (with cisplatin dosed at 75 mg/m^2 *versus* 100 mg/m^2, which was used in GOG 172). All treatment arms also received bevacizumab, in contrast to GOG 172. Those receiving dose-dense IV therapy experienced similar PFS (27 months) compared with those receiving IV/IP therapy (PFS 28 months). Patient symptoms included neurotoxicity, abdominal discomfort, and reported decrease in QOL among patients receiving IV/IP therapy with cisplatin [117].

Interpretation of this trial is limited by several factors. Firstly, 28 percent of patients crossed over from the IV/IP paclitaxel and cisplatin arm to the dose-dense IV therapy arm, which may have diluted any potential PFS benefit. Secondly, the effect of the addition of bevacizumab to all arms is unknown. Finally, we await data on patients who underwent a pathologically confirmed complete surgical resection, as this group of patients had historically derived greater PFS benefit with IV/IP therapy relative to what was reported in the overall population of GOG 252.

At this time and in light of the preliminary results of GOG 252, there is no consensus among ovarian cancer experts on whether IP therapy represents the standard treatment for women with optimally cytoreduced EOC. Additional reasons for this include increased toxicity associated with the IV/IP regimen, which frequently results in discontinuation of planned treatment compared with standard IV administration of chemotherapy [183] as in GOG 172, 42 and 83 percent completed planned IV/IP *versus* IV therapy, respectively [111].

NEOADJUVANT CHEMOTHERAPY (NACT)

Neoadjuvant chemotherapy (NACT) refers to the administration of systemic therapy before definitive surgery. The goal of NACT is to reduce perioperative morbidity and mortality and increase the likelihood of a complete resection of disease at the time of cytoreductive surgery [183].

EORTC 55971 trial — The European Organization for the Research and Treatment of Cancer (EORTC) 55971 trial enrolled 670 women with stage IIIC/IV epithelial ovarian cancer (EOC) who were randomly assigned to either primary debulking surgery (PDS) followed by six cycles of platinum-based chemotherapy or to NACT with carboplatin and paclitaxel for three cycles followed by interval surgical cytoreduction and adjuvant chemotherapy [118]. Compared with PDS, NACT resulted in the following:

1. A lower rate of complications as compared with initial surgery, including fewer postoperative deaths (0.7 *versus* 2.5 percent, respectively), infections (2 *versus* 8 percent), grade 3/4 hemorrhage (4 *versus* 7 percent), and thrombotic events (0 *versus* 2.6 percent).
2. A higher rate of optimal cytoreduction (defined as <10 mm of residual disease at the end of surgery) (81 *versus* 42 percent).
3. No difference in median progression-free survival (PFS, 12 months in each arm) or overall survival (OS, 29 *versus* 30 months). However, patients treated with primary surgery experienced a statistically nonsignificant improvement in overall survival (OS) compared with those who underwent NACT if there was no residual disease at the time of surgery (45 *versus* 38 months, respectively) or if there was microscopic residual disease only (*i.e.,* to less than 10 mm residual disease, 32 *versus* 27 months).

The Chemotherapy OR Upfront Surgery **(CHORUS) trial** was a non-inferiority trial that included 550 women with stage III to IV EOC (16 percent with stage IV disease) randomly assigned to primary surgery or NACT [119]. Among patients randomly assigned primary surgery, optimal cytoreduction to no residual disease were achieved in only 18 percent of patients. Compared with primary surgery, NACT resulted in:

1. Similar OS outcomes compared to primary surgery, including three-year OS rate (34 *versus* 32 percent, respectively) and median OS (24 *versus* 22.6 months).
2. Similar PFS (median, 12 *versus* 10 months, respectively). The HR for death was 0.87 in favor of NACT (95% CI, 0.72-1.05). The upper limit of the confidence interval was within the predefined non-inferiority boundary set at 1.18, which shows that NACT was deemed non- inferior to primary surgery. Surgical cytoreduction has determined survival outcomes [54]. However, optimal cytoreduction is achieved only in a low percentage of cases, reducing any potential survival benefit of this approach [183].

RECURRENT OVARIAN CANCER

The majority of patients with advanced EOC will have recurrences, despite an initial response to chemotherapy. Determining whether a patient is platinum-sensitive is the most important factor in management. Response to platinum is assessed by the patient's response to first-line platinum agents and length of disease-free (or platinum-free intervals) [120 - 122]. A patient is considered "platinum-sensitive" if there is no relapse for six months after the completion of first-line platinum agents. "Platinum resistance" refers to patients who have progression on treatment (refractory group) or who relapse within 6 months of completion of treatment. Although 6 months is given as a guide, there is no definite interval that completely separates these two categories of patients. The response rates for re-treatment with platinum increases as the disease-free interval increases: platinum-free interval <6 months-10%, 6- 12 months-27%, 13- 24 months 33%, >24 months- 59% [120, 122].

PLATINUM-SENSITIVE RECURRENT OVARIAN CANCER

Women with platinum-sensitive recurrent EOC should be considered for both secondary cytoreduction and second-line chemotherapy, with or without anti-angiogenesis therapy followed by maintenance therapy. The role of biologic therapy with bevacizumab and maintenance therapy with either bevacizumab or a PARP inhibitor will be discussed in a later section.

Each patient must be assessed to optimize treatment in terms of recurrence, sensitivity to platinum, toxicity, ease of administration, and patient preference. Patients who qualify should be offered the opportunity to participate in randomized trials, if available. Combination platinum-based chemotherapy could be a solution for patients with prior sensitivity to platinum-containing chemotherapy, barring any contraindications.

1. At least two large randomized clinical trials have demonstrated the superiority of a platinum-based doublet over platinum monotherapy in platinum-sensitive recurrent patients. The ICON- 4/AGO-OVAR 2.2 trial [123] demonstrated that the combination of paclitaxel-carboplatin (or cisplatin) is likely to provide a survival benefit compared with carboplatin monotherapy. This benefit was more apparent in patients with a treatment free-interval >12 months.
2. Moreover, the AGO-OVAR 2.5 trial, with the cooperation of National Cancer Institute of Canada Clinical Trials Group (NCIC CTG) and European Organization for Research and Treatment of Cancer Gynecological Cancer Group (EORTC GCG), has confirmed the advantage in response rate and progression free survival of the doublet carboplatin-gemcitabine compared to

carboplatin [124].

3. The Calypso trial [125] was a multicenter phase III study designed to compare efficacy and safety of arboplatin-pegylated liposomal doxorubicin (PLD) (C-D) and carboplatin-paclitaxel (C-P) in relapsed platinum-sensitive Ovarian Cancer patients. This trial showed significant superiority of PLD-carboplatin combination in terms of PFS (11.3 *vs.*. 9.4 months, HR 0.821, p= .005). In addition, compared to paclitaxel-carboplatin, PLD-carboplatin was well tolerated with lower rates of severe and long-lasting (neuropathy) toxicities. This was also confirmed in a Cochrane review of Gynecological Cancer Group (CGCG) trials register [126].

If combination platinum-based chemotherapy is not appropriate, either due to a history of a hypersensitivity reaction or persistent toxicities from first-line therapy, then a single platinum agent should be considered. Carboplatin has demonstrated efficacy across trials and has a manageable toxicity profile. If a single platinum agent is not appropriate, then monotherapy with the following agents are among the most active agents for women with platinum-sensitive recurrent EOC: pegylated liposomal doxorubicin [127], paclitaxel [128], docetaxel [129], nanoparticle albumin-bound paclitaxel, gemcitabine [130], topotecan [127, 131], or etoposide [132]. A choice among them should take into account patient preferences and toxicity profile [184].

PLATINUM-RESISTANT RECURRENT OVARIAN CANCER

Combination chemotherapy *versus* monotherapy is a clinically relevant dilemma for clinicians involved in the treatment of recurrent EOC patients. Combination chemotherapy has a higher toxicity profile without a clear benefit to patients with platinum-resistant relapse. Therefore, resistant patients should consider clinical trials or a monotherapy with less toxic side effects. The list of agents effective in ovarian cancer treatment includes paclitaxel [133, 134], docetaxel [135], nanoparticle albumin-bound paclitaxel [136], topotecan [137 - 139], doxorubicin, pegylated liposomal doxorubicin [138, 140], gemcitabine [140], cyclophos-phamide, etoposide [132], ifosfamide [141, 142], vinorelbine [143, 144], altretamine (hexamethylmelamine) and melphalan (alkeran). In addition, premetrexed [145] and trabectedin [146, 147] have recently been shown to have significant activity in ovarian cancer. There are multiple agents with activity in platinum-resistant EOC, but there is not one universally preferred agent for use in the first- or subsequent-line treatment. A Cochrane systematic review of trials (n = 1323) with platinum-resistant EOC concluded that topotecan, paclitaxel, and pegylated liposomal doxorubicin (PLD) have similar efficacy, but different patterns of side effects [137]. A choice among these agents depends upon the clinician's experience, the side effect profile, and prior therapy. In general, at our institution, we prefer single-agent treatment with PLD because of its schedule (*i.e.,* once every four weeks administration) and lack of typical side effects associated with chemotherapy (*e.g.,* little risk of myelosuppression, no risk of alopecia). The addition of biologic therapy with bevacizumab to single agent chemotherapy for platinum-resistant disease will be discussed below.

ANGIOGENESIS INHIBITORS BEVACIZUMAB

Bevacizumab hinders angiogenesis, thereby, decreasing the growth of new tumor. In patients with recurrent and resistant ovarian tumors, an objective response rate of 20% has been seen with single-agent bevacizumab [5, 16]. Garcia *et al.* demonstrated a 24% partial response and 44% stable disease rate in a heavily pretreated group of patients with recurrent ovarian cancer who received bevacizumab and metronomic oral cyclophosphamide [148].

BEVACIZUMAB IN FRONT LINE THERAPY

The incorporation of bevacizumab as part of a first-line treatment program for women with newly diagnosed EOC was evaluated in two trials conducted by GOG 218 and the International Collaborative on Ovarian Neoplasms (ICON 7):

GOG 218 – GOG 218 was a randomized placebo-controlled study involving almost 1900 women with stage III or IV EOC who had undergone surgical cytoreduction [149]. Women were randomly assigned to standard chemotherapy, bevacizumab (15 mg/kg every 3 weeks) concurrently with standard Taxol/carboplatin chemotherapy, or bevacizumab concurrently with standard chemotherapy and continuing as monotherapy until month 15. Standard chemotherapy consisted of six cycles of paclitaxel and carboplatin. Due to progressive disease, only 19 percent of patients completed all planned treatment. At a median follow-up of 17 months, compared with standard chemotherapy, there was no difference in PFS with the addition of concurrent bevacizumab (11 *versus* 10 months). However, PFS was longer among patients receiving bevacizumab both concurrently and after chemotherapy (14 months). This translated into a significant reduction in the risk of disease progression or death (HR 0.72, 95% CI 0.63-0.82). There was no improvement in OS with bevacizumab in either arm receiving the drug; median OS across all arms was approximately 39 months. An unplanned subgroup analysis demonstrated, however, that treatment with bevacizumab improved PFS and OS specifically in women with ascites but not in other women [150].

ICON7 – The Gynecologic Intergroup Trial (ICON7) randomly assigned 1528 previously untreated women with high-risk, early-stage (I or IIA clear cell or grade 3) or advanced EOC to standard chemotherapy (carboplatin AUC 5 or 6 and paclitaxel 175 mg/m² every 3 weeks) for six cycles with or without bevacizumab (7.5 mg/kg) during chemotherapy and, then, as maintenance treatment for 12 additional cycles. Unlike GOG 218, over 90 percent of patients completed assigned treatment. Of those assigned to treatment with bevacizumab, 62 percent completed the maintenance phase. Compared with standard chemotherapy, the incorporation of bevacizumab resulted in an increase in the overall response rate (ORR, 67 *versus* 48 percent), a longer median PFS at 42 months follow-up (24 *versus* 22 months), and more serious (grade 3/4) adverse events (66 *versus* 56 percent), including a higher rate of mild to serious (grade 2 or higher) hypertension (18 *versus* 2 percent) [151]. There was no difference in overall survival or global QOL. For women at high risk for progression (stage III with >1.0 cm residual disease at the end of surgery, inoperable stage III, or stage IV), bevacizumab was associated with improvement in PFS (16 *versus* 10.5 months, respectively) and OS (39.3 *versus* 34.5 months) [152]. However, this analysis was a post-hoc subgroup analysis and requires prospective validation before being accepted as a definitive result.

In summary, at our institution, we do not routinely recommend angiogenesis inhibitors in combination with initial chemotherapy for advanced EOC, largely because only modest benefits have been demonstrated in randomized first-line trials. However, it is worthy for consideration for patients at high risk for progression (stage III with >1.0 cm residual disease at the end of surgery, inoperable stage III, or stage IV) or with massive ascites [182, 183].

BEVACIZUMAB IN PLATINUM-SENSITIVE RECURRENT OVARIAN CANCER

The use of bevacizumab should be considered in combination with platinum-based chemotherapy and as single-agent maintenance treatment for women with platinum-sensitive recurrent EOC. The data regarding bevacizumab specifically for women with platinum-sensitive recurrent EOC come from two seminal randomized trials:

1. **OCEANS trial** – In the phase III study of carboplatin and gemcitabine plus bevacizumab in EOC (also referred to as the OCEANS study), 484 women with platinum-sensitive EOC were randomly assigned to carboplatin (AUC 4 on day 1) and gemcitabine (1000 mg/m² on days 1 and 8) with cycles repeated every 21 days with or without bevacizumab (15 mg/kg on day 1 every three weeks) concurrent with chemotherapy for 10 cycles maximum, followed by bevacizumab alone until disease progression or toxicity [153 - 155]. Bevacizumab with chemotherapy resulted in the following when compared with chemotherapy plus placebo:

1. An improvement in PFS (12 *versus* 8 months); however, OS was similar between the two arms (34 *versus* 33 months).
2. A higher objective response rate (79 versus 57 percent).
3. A higher rate of treatment discontinuation for adverse events (23 *versus* 5 percent), including higher rates of serious hypertension (17 *versus* <1 percent), proteinuria >grade 3 (9 *versus* 1 percent), and non-central nervous system bleeding (6 *versus* 1 percent). Of note, there were no cases of gastrointestinal perforation reported.

2. **GOG 213** – In the GOG 213 trial, women with platinum-sensitive recurrent EOC were randomly assigned to surgical treatment (secondary cytoreduction *versus* no secondary cytoreduction) and separately, to chemotherapy (carboplatin and paclitaxel) with or without bevacizumab [156]. For those patients treated with bevacizumab, it was administered with chemotherapy and then continued as a single agent until disease progression.

The results of the medical treatment randomization, which included almost 700 women, were presented at the 2015 Annual Meeting for Women's Cancers [156]. Compared with treatment with chemotherapy alone, the administration of bevacizumab resulted in:

1. An improvement in PFS (14 *versus* 10 months, respectively).
2. A trend towards improved OS, which was significant upon reanalysis using corrected data obtained from electronic case report forms (43 *versus* 37 months, respectively; HR 0.82, 95% CI 0.68-0.996).
3. Higher rates of serious (grade 3/4) gastrointestinal complications, such as perforation, necrosis, or fistula (6 *versus* 3 percent), and infections (13 *versus* 6 percent). In addition, combination treatment resulted in more reports of joint pain (15 *versus* 5 percent) and proteinuria (8 *versus* 0 percent).

The data consistently demonstrate that incorporating bevacizumab can improve PFS for women with a platinum-sensitive recurrent EOC and may also improve OS. Clinicians should discuss the potential benefits to those with platinum-sensitive disease in the context of patient preferences. For example, women with severe hypertension may opt against the use of bevacizumab [183].

BEVACIZUMAB IN PLATINUM-RESISTANT RECURRENT OVARIAN CANCER

For appropriately selected patients with platinum-resistant EOC, combining single-agent chemotherapy with bevacizumab, a vascular endothelial growth factor receptor (VEGFR), is indicated with the following caveats: that there is no history of bowel obstruction in the past six months or evidence of malignant bowel involvement [184].

This recommendation is based on the **AURELIA study**, which included 361 patients with platinum-resistant ovarian cancer (defined as progression ≤6 months after ≥4 platinum-based cycles) who were randomly assigned treatment with chemotherapy plus or minus bevacizumab (15 mg/kg every three weeks) [157]. All patients met specific eligibility criteria, including:

- No evidence of disease progression during platinum-based chemotherapy (*i.e.,* chemo refractory disease)
- No more than two prior lines of chemotherapy
- No prior treatment with bevacizumab
- No history of bowel obstruction (although as stated above, we administer the combination to patients with no history of bowel obstruction in the past six months or evidence of malignant bowel involvement)

Chemotherapy options were based on the investigator's choice of one of the following:

- Paclitaxel 80 mg/m^2 on days 1, 8, 15, and 22 every four weeks (n = 115)
- Topotecan 4 mg/m^2 on days 1, 8, and 15 every four weeks (or 1.25 mg/m^2 on days 1 through 5 every three weeks) (n = 120)
- Pegylated liposomal doxorubicin (PLD) 40 mg/m^2 on day 1 every four weeks (n = 126)

Of note, patients who received chemotherapy alone were allowed to cross over to single-agent bevacizumab at the time of disease progression. With a median follow-up of 13.5 months, compared with chemotherapy alone, chemotherapy plus bevacizumab resulted in:

1. A statistically significant improvement in the overall response rate (ORR, 31 *versus* 13 percent, respectively).
2. A reduction in the risk of disease progression (median duration 6.7 *versus* 3. 4 months), but no statistically significant improvement in overall survival (median 16.6 *versus* 13.3 months).
3. An increase in the rate of grade 2 or greater adverse events, including hypertension (20 *versus* 7 percent) and proteinuria (11 *versus* 0.6 percent). In addition, four patients (2.2 percent) treated with bevacizumab experienced a gastrointestinal perforation.

The results of a planned subset analysis of the AURELIA study evaluated the outcomes associated with the individual regimens [158]. The addition of bevacizumab to chemotherapy consistently resulted in better outcomes compared with treatment with chemotherapy alone:

1. Among those who received paclitaxel, the ORR was 53 *versus* 30 percent with or without bevacizumab, respectively; median progression-free survival (PFS) was 10 *versus* 4 months.
2. Among those who received topotecan, the ORR was 17 *versus* 0 percent; median PFS was 6 *versus* 2 months.
3. Among those who received PLD, the ORR was 14 *versus* 8 percent; median PFS was 5 *versus* 4 months.

Therefore, these results support the use of chemotherapy plus bevacizumab in the treatment of appropriately selected women with platinum-resistant ovarian cancer. Moreover, in November 2014, bevacizumab plus chemotherapy was approved for this specific indication by the US Food and Drug Administration (FDA) [184].

OTHER ANGIOGENESIS INHIBITORS

Cediranib

Cediranib is an investigational oral inhibitor of the vascular endothelial growth factor receptors (VEGFR1, 2, and 3). In the International Collaborative Ovarian Neoplasms trial (ICON6), over 450 patients were treated with platinum-based chemotherapy alone (reference arm) or with concurrent cediranib (concurrent arm); or with concurrent and maintenance cediranib for 18 months (maintenance arm) [159]. Due to drug shortages after the manufacturer discontinued production, the trial was redesigned to evaluate the reference and concurrent arms only, using PFS rather than OS as the primary outcome measure. At a median follow-up of 19.5 months, maintenance cediranib treatment improved PFS (11.0 *versus* 8.7 months) [159]. While there was also a trend towards improved OS (median, 26.3 months *versus* 21.0 months), data were immature given that approximately 50 percent of patients were still living at the time of data collection. Toxicity led to treatment discontinuation for 12 percent of patients on the reference arm and 39 percent of patients on the maintenance cediranib arm. Diarrhea, neutropenia, hypertension, voice changes, and hypothyroidism were more common with cediranib treatment.

Given that the reported survival advantage required that maintenance therapy continue for an additional 18 months, the benefit of treatment is not entirely clear, especially given the toxicities associated with this drug [183].

Pazopanib

Pazopanib is an orally administered tyrosine kinase inhibitor against the vascular endothelial growth factor (VEGF), platelet-derived growth factor (PDGF), and c-kit receptors. Its role in maintenance treatment was evaluated in a trial conducted by the Arbeitsgemeinschaft Gynaekologische Onkologie Studiengruppe Ovarialkarzinom group **(AGO-OVAR 16)** that included over 900 women who had surgery for EOC and subsequently completed standard first- line chemotherapy without evidence of disease progression [160]. Patients were randomly assigned to pazopanib (800 mg daily) for up to 24 months or placebo. Compared with placebo, maintenance treatment with pazopanib resulted in a significant improvement in PFS (18 *versus* 12 months, respectively). An interim survival analysis suggested that there was no corresponding improvement in overall survival. Treatment with pazopanib was associated with significant grade 2 or greater hypertension (52 *versus* 17 percent), grade 3 or 4 diarrhea (8 *versus* 1 percent), and grade 3 or 4 hepatotoxicities (9 *versus* <1 percent).

Unlike the bevacizumab trials, the AGO-OVAR16 was the only prospective trial to evaluate maintenance angiogenesis inhibition as a single agent at the completion of first-line chemotherapy. However, it provides more evidence that maintenance therapy using an angiogenesis inhibitor can prolong PFS. However, until this is shown to also improve OS, we do not administer angiogenesis inhibitors in this context as part of standard clinical practice [183].

ENDOCRINE THERAPY

For women with radiologic evidence of disease progression but with little or no symptoms associated with recurrent EOC, endocrine therapy can be a reasonable option. These studies illustrate the potential role for endocrine agents:

Tamoxifen – The efficacy of tamoxifen was explored in a Cochrane review that included 623 women with recurrent EOC who participated in 1 of 14 studies [161]. Overall, 60 women (10 percent) achieved an objective response to tamoxifen alone, although the range within individual studies was 0 to 56 percent. An additional 32 percent achieved stable disease for periods of longer than four weeks.

In a randomized trial of 138 patients with platinum-resistant ovarian cancer [162], randomly assigned in a 2:1 ratio to chemotherapy (paclitaxel or pegylated liposomal doxorubicin) *versus* tamoxifen, those receiving tamoxifen experienced a shorter median PFS (8.3 *versus* 12.7 weeks). However, overall survival and control of gastrointestinal symptoms were similar between the two groups. Both hematologic and nonhematologic side effects as well as worsened social functioning were more frequent with chemotherapy.

Letrozole – In a phase II trial of letrozole in 42 women with estrogen receptor-positive recurrent EOC based on cancer antigen (CA) 125 values, a serologic decrease in CA 125 >50 percent was seen in 17 percent. Radiologic response was noted in 3 of 33 women (9 percent) [163].

Fulvestrant – In a phase II trial, the selective estrogen receptor down-regulator, fulvestrant (500 mg IM on day 1 then 250 mg on days 15, 29, and then every 28 days), was administered to 26 women with estrogen receptor-positive recurrent EOC. While there were no objective responses, 50 percent had stable disease and one patient normalized a previously elevated serum CA-125. The median time to disease progression was 60 days, and treatment was well tolerated [163].

Although the studies with letrozole and fulvestrant selected patients with estrogen receptor- positive disease, we do not routinely perform estrogen receptor testing in women with recurrent EOC. We reserve the use of endocrine therapy for women with asymptomatic recurrent disease. In addition, we prefer observation to endocrine therapy in the setting of CA-125 relapse, given the results of a randomized trial showing no benefit to initiation of treatment solely defined by CA 125.

PARP INHIBITORS

Patients with a BRCA mutation — For patients with recurrent EOC and a known germline mutation involving the BRCA genes, and who have progressed on multiple prior lines of therapy, a poly-ADP ribose polymerase (PARP) inhibitor is now an option. For women with BRCA mutation-associated advanced ovarian cancer, rucaparib, a PARP inhibitor, is US Food and Drug Administration (FDA)-approved for those who have progressed after at least two prior lines of treatment, and olaparib, another PARP inhibitor, is approved after at least three prior lines.

Olaparib – Patients with advanced cancer and a germline BRCA mutation may respond to olaparib if they have experienced progression on multiple previous lines of chemotherapy [164, 165]. A meta-analysis of phase I and II trials including 273 patients with advanced ovarian cancer, in a cohort of 205 patients who had received ≥3 lines of showed chemotherapy [165]:

- The tumor response rate was 31 percent.
- The median duration of response was 7.8 months.
- The rate of serious (grade 3/4) toxicities was 54 percent with the most frequent toxicities being anemia and fatigue.

Rucaparib – Rucaparib is approved for use in the United States to treat patients with advanced ovarian cancer who harbor either a deleterious germline or somatic BRCA mutation who have undergone at least two chemotherapies. It may be used in either platinum-resistant or platinum-sensitive disease. A pooled analysis of two phase II studies in which 106 patients with BRCA-mutated, high-grade ovarian cancer who had received at least two chemotherapy regimens were treated with rucaparib [166], with an objective response rate (ORR) of 54 percent and duration of response of 9.2 months.

The safety of rucaparib was evaluated in 377 patients with advanced ovarian cancer. Common adverse reactions included nausea, fatigue, abdominal pain, dysgeusia, constipation, decreased appetite, diarrhea, thrombocytopenia, and dyspnea. Myelodysplastic syndrome/acute myeloid leukemia (MDS/AML) were reported in 2 of 377 patients (0.5 percent).

PARP INHIBITORS FOR MAINTENANCE

For patients with platinum-sensitive relapsed ovarian cancer with a partial or complete response to platinum-based chemotherapy, PARP inhibitors niraparib and olaparib are approved by the FDA for maintenance therapy [183].

Niraparib —Niraparib has shown efficacy as maintenance therapy in platinum-sensitive, relapsed disease, which appears independent of the presence of either BRCA mutation or homologous recombination deficiency (HRD). In the phase III **NOVA study**, 553 patients with platinum-sensitive, recurrent ovarian cancer were randomly assigned after completion of platinum-based chemotherapy in a 2:1 ratio to niraparib maintenance or placebo [167]. All patients were grouped according to BRCA germline mutation status (gBRCA cohort or non-gBRCA cohort); those in the non-gBRCA cohort were further classified by the presence or absence of a homologous recombination deficiency (HRD, using a central laboratory DNA-based test). Patients with a somatic mutation (sBRCA) were included in the non-gBRCA HRD cohort. Compared with placebo, niraparib increased PFS in all cohorts: in the gBRCA group, 21.0 *versus* 5.5 months; in the overall non-gBRCA cohort, 9.3 *versus* 3.9 months; and in the HRD-positive subgroup of the non-gBRCA cohort, 12.9 *versus* 3.8 months. The most common grade 3 or 4 toxicities associated with niraparib were hematologic: thrombocytopenia (34 percent), anemia (25 percent), and neutropenia (20 percent). Myelodysplastic syndrome occurred in 5 of 367 patients (1.4 percent).

Olaparib - Olaparib has also been studied as maintenance therapy for those with platinum- sensitive relapsed disease in both women regardless of a BRCA mutation (Study 19) [168] and specifically, in those with a BRCA mutation (SOLO2).

In the phase III **SOLO2/ENGOT-Ov21 trial**, in which 295 patients with relapsed, platinum-sensitive, germline BRCA- associated high-grade serous ovarian cancer or high-grade endometrioid cancer who had received at least two lines of previous chemotherapy were randomly assigned in a 2:1 ratio to olaparib maintenance or placebo [169]. Those receiving olaparib experienced improved PFS (19.1 *versus* 5.5 months). Grade 3 or higher adverse events occurred in 18 percent of those receiving olaparib *versus* 8 percent of those receiving placebo.

HEATED INTRAPERITONEAL CHEMOTHERAPY (HIPEC)

The administration of heated intraperitoneal chemotherapy (HIPEC) is indicated for mucinous carcinomas such as appendiceal carcinoma and pseudomyxoma peritonei. Given the tendency of recurrent ovarian cancer to present as abdominal disease, there is growing interest in the use of HIPEC for women with recurrent EOC following surgical cytoreduction. However, HIPEC is still considered an investigational modality for the treatment of patients with platinum-sensitive recurrent EOC [170 - 172].

The best prospective randomized data supporting HIPEC investigated whether the addition of HIPEC to interval cytoreductive surgery would improve outcomes among patients who were receiving neoadjuvant chemotherapy for primary stage III epithelial ovarian cancer [173]. Of the 245 patients, disease recurrence occurred in 110 of the 123 patients (89%) who underwent cytoreductive surgery without HIPEC (surgery group) and in 99 of the 122 patients (81%) who underwent cytoreductive surgery with HIPEC (surgery-plus-HIPEC group) (P=0.003). The median recurrence-free survival was 10.7 months in the surgery group and 14.2 months in the surgery-plus-HIPEC group. At a median follow-up of 4.7 years, 76 patients (62%) in the surgery group and 61 patients (50%) in the surgery-plus-HIPEC group had died (P=0.02). The median overall survival was 33.9 months in the surgery group and 45.7 months in the surgery-plus- HIPEC group. Rate of grade 3 or 4 adverse events was similar in the two groups (25% in the surgery group and 27% in the surgery-plus-HIPEC group, P=0.76).

IMMUNOTHERAPY

Immunomodulation

Immunomodulation with novel immune checkpoint inhibitors such as CTLA-4 inhibitors **(ipilimumab)**, PD-1 inhibitors **(nivolumab, pembrolizumab)**, and PDL-1 inhibitors (atezolizumab, avelumab, durvalumab) has produced a great deal of excitement in recent years, and some of these agents have been approved in a number of solid tumors including melanoma, kidney cancer, and lung cancer.

A small trial of **nivolumab** in 20 patients with platinum-resistant ovarian cancer demonstrated an overall response rate of 15%. Two of these responders had complete responses that lasted 17 and 14 months (nivolumab was given only for a year); one of these had a clear cell carcinoma [174]. The prolonged duration of the responses achieved has generated substantial excitement, and multiple trials are attempting to determine which ovarian cancer patients will benefit from such immunotherapies.

There remains interest in vaccine-type therapies, which have used a variety of antigens, including MUC 1 carbohydrate epitope [175], p53 peptide [176], HER2/neu peptides [177], and the cancer-testis antigen NY-ESO-1 [178, 179], which are sometimes directly injected, sometimes loaded onto dendritic cells, and sometimes expressed in recombinant viral vectors. However, there have been no randomized trials published showing clinical benefit. No immunotherapy has yet been approved for the therapy of ovarian cancer.

To test whether a diversified prime and boost regimen targeting NY-ESO-1 will result in clinical benefit, Odunsi and colleagues conducted two parallel **phase II clinical trials of recombinant vaccinia-NY-ESO-1 (rV-NY-ESO-1)**, followed by booster vaccinations with recombinant fowlpox-NY-ESO-1 (rF-NY-ESO-1) in 25 melanoma and 22 epithelial ovarian cancer (EOC) patients with advanced disease who were at high risk for recurrence/progression. Integrated NY- ESO-1-specific antibody and CD4(+) and CD8(+) T cells were induced in a high proportion of melanoma and EOC patients. The median PFS in the melanoma patients was 9 month (range, 0-84 months) and the median OS was 48 months (range, 3-106 months). In EOC patients, the median PFS was 21 months (95% CI, 16-29 months), and median OS was 48 months (CI, not estimable). CD8(+) T cells derived from vaccinated patients were shown to lyse NY-ESO-1-expressing tumor targets. These data provide preliminary evidence of clinically meaningful benefit for diversified prime and boost recombinant pox-viral-based vaccines in melanoma and ovarian cancer and support further evaluation of this approach in these patient populations [178].

As NY-ESO-1 is regulated by DNA methylation, Odunsi and colleagues hypothesized that DNA methyltransferase (DNMT) inhibitors may augment NY-ESO-1 vaccine therapy. In agreement, global DNA hypomethylation in EOC was associated with the presence of circulating antibodies to NY-ESO-1. Pre-clinical studies using EOC cell lines showed that decitabine treatment enhanced both NY-ESO-1 expression and NY-ESO-1-specific CTL-mediated responses. Based on these observations, they performed a **phase I dose-escalation trial of decitabine, as an addition to NY-ESO-1 vaccine and doxorubicin liposome (doxorubicin)**

chemotherapy, in 12 patients with relapsed EOC. The regimen was safe, with limited and clinically manageable toxicities. Both global and promoter-specific DNA hypomethylation occurred in blood and circulating DNAs, the latter of which may reflect tumor cell responses. Increased NY-ESO-1 serum antibodies and T cell responses were observed in the majority of patients, and antibody spreading to additional tumor antigens was also observed. Finally, disease stabilization or partial clinical response occurred in 6/10 evaluable patients. Based on these encouraging results, evaluation of similar combinatorial chemo-immunotherapy regimens in EOC and other tumor types was considered warranted.

OTHER NEW DIRECTIONS

The folate receptor is highly overexpressed in ovarian cancer, and a number of therapies have attempted to take advantage of this. IMGN853 (mirvetuximab soravtansine) is a **folate receptor alpha-targeting antibody drug conjugate** that comprises a folate receptor alpha-binding antibody conjugated with the potent maytansinoid, DM4. It is associated with some ocular toxicity. A preliminary report in 46 heavily pretreated platinum-resistant patients confirmed an objective response rate was 26%, including one complete and 11 partial responses, and the median PFS was 4.8 months. The median duration of response was 19.1 weeks. Notably, in the subset of patients who had received three or fewer prior lines of therapy (n = 23), an objective response rate of 39%, PFS of 6.7 months, and duration of response of 19.6 weeks were observed [180].

Other antibody–drug conjugates have also had promising preliminary results in the therapy of ovarian cancer, but remain early in development. DMOT4039A is an antibody–drug conjugate targeting mesothelin. Three of 10 ovarian cancer patients with platinum-resistant ovarian cancer and a mesothelin IHC score of 3+ treated on the q3 week schedule at the recommended phase 2 dose level had a confirmed partial response [181].

Aberrant DNA methylation is a frequent epigenetic event in ovarian cancer and represents an additional source of potential molecular markers. Hypomethylating agents and histone deacetylase inhibitors are currently being studied in combination with standard chemotherapies. Matei *et al.* tested low-dose deci-tabine administered before carboplatin in 17 patients with heavily pretreated and platinum-resistant ovarian cancer.

The regimen induced a 35% objective RR and a PFS of 10.2 months, with 9 patients (53%) free of progression at 6 months. Demethylation of MLH1, RASSF1A, HOXA10, and HOXA11 in tumor biopsies after treatment positively correlated with PFS, suggesting that low-dose decitabine altered DNA methylation of genes, restoring sensitivity to carboplatin [182].

CONSENT FOR PUBLICATION

Not applicable.

CONFLICT OF INTEREST

The author confirms that this chapter contents have no conflict of interest.

ACKNOWLEDGEMENTS

Declared none.

REFERENCES

[1]   Siegel RL, Miller KD, Jemal A. Cancer Statistics, 2017. CA Cancer J Clin 2017; 67(1): 7-30.
        [http://dx.doi.org/10.3322/caac.21387] [PMID: 28055103]

[2]   Baldwin LA, Huang B, Miller RW, *et al*. Ten-year relative survival for epithelial ovarian cancer.
        Obstet Gynecol 2012; 120(3): 612-8.
        [http://dx.doi.org/10.1097/AOG.0b013e318264f794] [PMID: 22914471]

[3]   Rahaman J, Kolev V, Cohen C. J Ovarian Cancer: The Initial Laparotomy. Altchek's Diagnosis and
        Management of Ovarian Disorders. Cambridge University Press 2013.
        [http://dx.doi.org/10.1017/CBO9781139003254.026]

[4]   Piver MS, Baker TR, Jishi MF, *et al*. Familial ovarian cancer. A report of 658 families from the Gilda
        Radner Familial Ovarian Cancer Registry 1981-1991. Cancer 1993; 71(2) (Suppl.): 582-8.
        [http://dx.doi.org/10.1002/cncr.2820710214] [PMID: 8420680]

[5]   Frank TS. Testing for Hereditary Risk of Ovarian Cancer. Cancer Control 1999; 6(4): 327-4.
        [http://dx.doi.org/10.1177/107327489900600401]

[6]   Struewing JP, Hartge P, Wacholder S, *et al*. The risk of cancer associated with specific mutations of
        BRCA1 and BRCA2 among Ashkenazi Jews. N Engl J Med 1997; 336(20): 1401-8.
        [http://dx.doi.org/10.1056/NEJM199705153362001] [PMID: 9145676]

[7]   Zhang S, Royer R, Li S, *et al*. Frequencies of BRCA1 and BRCA2 mutations among 1,342 unselected
        patients with invasive ovarian cancer. Gynecol Oncol 2011; 121(2): 353-7.
        [http://dx.doi.org/10.1016/j.ygyno.2011.01.020] [PMID: 21324516]

[8]   van der Burg ME, van Lent M, Buyse M, *et al*. Gynecological Cancer Cooperative Group of the
        European Organization for Research and Treatment of Cancer The effect of debulking surgery after
        induction chemotherapy on the prognosis in advanced epithelial ovarian cancer. N Engl J Med 1995;
        332(10): 629-34.
        [http://dx.doi.org/10.1056/NEJM199503093321002] [PMID: 7845426]

[9]   Vergote I, van Gorp T, Amant F, Neven P, Berteloot P. Neoadjuvant chemotherapy for ovarian cancer.
        Oncology (Williston Park) 2005; 19(12): 1615-22.
        [PMID: 16396153]

[10]   Vergote I, Amant F, Kristensen G, Ehlen T, Reed NS, Casado A. Primary surgery or neoadjuvant
        chemotherapy followed by interval debulking surgery in advanced ovarian cancer. Eur J Cancer 2011;
        47 (Suppl. 3): S88-92.
        [http://dx.doi.org/10.1016/S0959-8049(11)70152-6] [PMID: 21944035]

[11]   Bristow RE, Duska LR, Lambrou NC, *et al*. A model for predicting surgical outcome in patients with

advanced ovarian carcinoma using computed tomography. Cancer 2000; 89(7): 1532-40.
[http://dx.doi.org/10.1002/1097-0142(20001001)89:7<1532::AID-CNCR17>3.0.CO;2-A]   [PMID: 11013368]

[12]   Son H, Khan SM, Rahaman J, *et al.* Role of FDG PET/CT in staging of recurrent ovarian cancer. Radiographics: a review publication of the Radiol Soc N Am. Inc 2011; 31(2): 569-83.

[13]   Hammond RH, Houghton CR. The role of bowel surgery in the primary treatment of epithelial ovarian cancer. Aust N Z J Obstet Gynaecol 1990; 30(2): 166-9.
[http://dx.doi.org/10.1111/j.1479-828X.1990.tb03254.x] [PMID: 2400363]

[14]   Donato D, Angelides A, Irani H, Penalver M, Averette H. Infectious complications after gastrointestinal surgery in patients with ovarian carcinoma and malignant ascites. Gynecol Oncol 1992; 44(1): 40-7.
[http://dx.doi.org/10.1016/0090-8258(92)90009-8] [PMID: 1730424]

[15]   Handelsman JC, Zeiler S, Coleman J, Dooley W, Walrath JM. Experience with ambulatory preoperative bowel preparation at the Johns Hopkins Hospital. Arch Surg 1993; 128(4): 441-4.
[http://dx.doi.org/10.1001/archsurg.1993.01420160079013] [PMID: 8457157]

[16]   Feldman GB, Knapp RC. Lymphatic drainage of the peritoneal cavity and its significance in ovarian cancer. Am J Obstet Gynecol 1974; 119(7): 991-4.
[http://dx.doi.org/10.1016/0002-9378(74)90021-0] [PMID: 4276313]

[17]   Dembo AJ, Davy M, Stenwig AE, Berle EJ, Bush RS, Kjorstad K. Prognostic factors in patients with stage I epithelial ovarian cancer. Obstet Gynecol 1990; 75(2): 263-73.
[PMID: 2300355]

[18]   Vergote I, De Brabanter J, Fyles A, *et al.* Prognostic importance of degree of differentiation and cyst rupture in stage I invasive epithelial ovarian carcinoma. Lancet 2001; 357(9251): 176-82.
[http://dx.doi.org/10.1016/S0140-6736(00)03590-X] [PMID: 11213094]

[19]   Navot D, Fox JH, Williams M, Brodman M, Friedman F Jr, Cohen CJ. The concept of uterine preservation with ovarian malignancies. Obstet Gynecol 1991; 78(3 Pt 2): 566-8.
[PMID: 1870826]

[20]   Cass I, Li AJ, Runowicz CD, *et al.* Pattern of lymph node metastases in clinically unilateral stage I invasive epithelial ovarian carcinomas. Gynecol Oncol 2001; 80(1): 56-61.
[http://dx.doi.org/10.1006/gyno.2000.6027] [PMID: 11136570]

[21]   Pereira A, Magrina JF, Rey V, Cortes M, Magtibay PM. Pelvic and aortic lymph node metastasis in epithelial ovarian cancer. Gynecol Oncol 2007; 105(3): 604-8.
[http://dx.doi.org/10.1016/j.ygyno.2007.01.028] [PMID: 17321572]

[22]   Young RC, Decker DG, Wharton JT, *et al.* Staging laparotomy in early ovarian cancer. JAMA 1983; 250(22): 3072-6.
[http://dx.doi.org/10.1001/jama.1983.03340220040030] [PMID: 6358558]

[23]   Trimbos JB, Schueler JA, van Lent M, Hermans J, Fleuren GJ. Reasons for incomplete surgical staging in early ovarian carcinoma. Gynecol Oncol 1990; 37(3): 374-7.
[http://dx.doi.org/10.1016/0090-8258(90)90370-Z] [PMID: 2351322]

[24]   Morice P, Joulie F, Camatte S, *et al.* Lymph node involvement in epithelial ovarian cancer: analysis of 276 pelvic and paraaortic lymphadenectomies and surgical implications. J Am Coll Surg 2003; 197(2): 198-205.
[http://dx.doi.org/10.1016/S1072-7515(03)00234-5] [PMID: 12892797]

[25]   Bolis G, Colombo N, Pecorelli S, *et al.* Adjuvant treatment for early epithelial ovarian cancer: results of two randomised clinical trials comparing cisplatin to no further treatment or chromic phosphate (32P). G.I.C.O.G.: Gruppo Interregionale Collaborativo in Ginecologia Oncologica. Ann Oncol 1995; 6(9): 887-93.
[http://dx.doi.org/10.1093/oxfordjournals.annonc.a059355] [PMID: 8624291]

[26]   Young RC, Walton LA, Ellenberg SS, *et al.* Adjuvant therapy in stage I and stage II epithelial ovarian cancer. Results of two prospective randomized trials. N Engl J Med 1990; 322(15): 1021-7.
[http://dx.doi.org/10.1056/NEJM199004123221501] [PMID: 2181310]

[27]   Cohen CJ, Goldberg JD, Holland JF, *et al.* Improved therapy with cisplatin regimens for patients with ovarian carcinoma (FIGO Stages III and IV) as measured by surgical end-staging (second-look operation). Am J Obstet Gynecol 1983; 145(8): 955-67.
[http://dx.doi.org/10.1016/0002-9378(83)90849-9] [PMID: 6404174]

[28]   Bruckner HW, Cohen CJ, Goldberg JD, *et al.* Cisplatin regimens and improved prognosis of patients with poorly differentiated ovarian cancer. Am J Obstet Gynecol 1983; 145(6): 653-8.
[http://dx.doi.org/10.1016/0002-9378(83)90569-0] [PMID: 6402934]

[29]   Cohen CJ, Bruckner HW, Goldberg JD, Holland JF. Improved therapy with cisplatin regimens for patients with ovarian carcinoma (FIGO III and IV) as measured by surgical end-staging (second-look surgery)--the mount sinai experience. Clin Obstet Gynaecol 1983; 10(2): 307-24.
[PMID: 6413114]

[30]   Aabo K, Adams M, Adnitt P, *et al.* Chemotherapy in advanced ovarian cancer: four systematic meta-analyses of individual patient data from 37 randomized trials. Advanced Ovarian Cancer Trialists' Group. Br J Cancer 1998; 78(11): 1479-87.
[http://dx.doi.org/10.1038/bjc.1998.710] [PMID: 9836481]

[31]   McGuire WP, Hoskins WJ, Brady MF, *et al.* Cyclophosphamide and cisplatin compared with paclitaxel and cisplatin in patients with stage III and stage IV ovarian cancer. N Engl J Med 1996; 334(1): 1-6.
[http://dx.doi.org/10.1056/NEJM199601043340101] [PMID: 7494563]

[32]   Ozols RF, Bundy BN, Greer BE, *et al.* Gynecologic Oncology Group Phase III trial of carboplatin and paclitaxel compared with cisplatin and paclitaxel in patients with optimally resected stage III ovarian cancer: a Gynecologic Oncology Group study. J Clin Oncol 2003; 21(17): 3194-200.
[http://dx.doi.org/10.1200/JCO.2003.02.153] [PMID: 12860964]

[33]   du Bois A, Lück HJ, Meier W, *et al.* Arbeitsgemeinschaft Gynäkologische Onkologie Ovarian Cancer Study Group A randomized clinical trial of cisplatin/paclitaxel *versus* carboplatin/paclitaxel as first-line treatment of ovarian cancer. J Natl Cancer Inst 2003; 95(17): 1320-9.
[http://dx.doi.org/10.1093/jnci/djg036] [PMID: 12953086]

[34]   Muñoz KA, Harlan LC, Trimble EL. Patterns of care for women with ovarian cancer in the United States. J Clin Oncol 1997; 15(11): 3408-15.
[http://dx.doi.org/10.1200/JCO.1997.15.11.3408] [PMID: 9363873]

[35]   Kaern J, Tropé CG, Abeler VM. A retrospective study of 370 borderline tumors of the ovary treated at the Norwegian Radium Hospital from 1970 to 1982. A review of clinicopathologic features and treatment modalities. Cancer 1993; 71(5): 1810-20.
[http://dx.doi.org/10.1002/1097-0142(19930301)71:5<1810::AID-CNCR2820710516>3.0.CO;2-V] [PMID: 8383580]

[36]   Fort MG, Pierce VK, Saigo PE, Hoskins WJ, Lewis JL Jr. Evidence for the efficacy of adjuvant therapy in epithelial ovarian tumors of low malignant potential. Gynecol Oncol 1989; 32(3): 269-72.
[http://dx.doi.org/10.1016/0090-8258(89)90622-7] [PMID: 2920945]

[37]   Seidman JD, Kurman RJ. Ovarian serous borderline tumors: a critical review of the literature with emphasis on prognostic indicators. Hum Pathol 2000; 31(5): 539-57.
[http://dx.doi.org/10.1053/hp.2000.8048] [PMID: 10836293]

[38]   Griffiths CT. Surgical resection of tumor bulk in the primary treatment of ovarian carcinoma. Natl Cancer Inst Monogr 1975; 42: 101-4.
[PMID: 1234624]

[39]   Rahaman J, Dottino P, Jennings TS, Holland J, Cohen CJ. The second-look operation improves

survival in suboptimally debulked stage III ovarian cancer patients. Int J Gynecol Cancer 2005; 15(1): 19-25.
[http://dx.doi.org/10.1136/ijgc-00009577-200501000-00004] [PMID: 15670292]

[40]   Elattar A, Bryant A, Winter-Roach BA, Hatem M, Naik R. Optimal primary surgical treatment for advanced epithelial ovarian cancer. Cochrane Database Syst Rev 2011; (8): CD007565
[http://dx.doi.org/10.1002/14651858.CD007565.pub2] [PMID: 21833960]

[41]   Chang SJ, Hodeib M, Chang J, Bristow RE. Survival impact of complete cytoreduction to no gross residual disease for advanced-stage ovarian cancer: a meta-analysis. Gynecol Oncol 2013; 130(3): 493-8.
[http://dx.doi.org/10.1016/j.ygyno.2013.05.040] [PMID: 23747291]

[42]   Rahaman J, Jennings TS, Dottino P, *et al.* Impact of Age on Survival in Advanced Ovarian Cancer: a Re-examination J Clin Oncol, 2001; 20(1): 217 a.

[43]   Susini T, Amunni G, Busi E, *et al.* Ovarian cancer in the elderly: feasibility of surgery and chemotherapy in 89 geriatric patients. Int J Gynecol Cancer 2007; 17(3): 581-8.
[http://dx.doi.org/10.1111/j.1525-1438.2007.00836.x] [PMID: 17309560]

[44]   Sharma S, Driscoll D, Odunsi K, Venkatadri A, Lele S. Safety and efficacy of cytoreductive surgery for epithelial ovarian cancer in elderly and high-risk surgical patients. Am J Obstet Gynecol 2005; 193(6): 2077-82.
[http://dx.doi.org/10.1016/j.ajog.2005.06.074] [PMID: 16325619]

[45]   Cafa EV, Pecorino B, Scibilia G, *et al.* Role of Surgery in the Elderly Patients Affected from Advanced Stage Ovarian Cancer. J Cancer Ther 2015; 6(5): 428-33.
[http://dx.doi.org/10.4236/jct.2015.65046]

[46]   Hoskins WJ, Bundy BN, Thigpen JT, Omura GA. The influence of cytoreductive surgery on recurrence-free interval and survival in small-volume stage III epithelial ovarian cancer: a Gynecologic Oncology Group study. Gynecol Oncol 1992; 47(2): 159-66.
[http://dx.doi.org/10.1016/0090-8258(92)90100-W] [PMID: 1468693]

[47]   Heintz AP, Hacker NF, Berek JS, Rose TP, Munoz AK, Lagasse LD. Cytoreductive surgery in ovarian carcinoma: feasibility and morbidity. Obstet Gynecol 1986; 67(6): 783-8.
[http://dx.doi.org/10.1097/00006250-198606000-00007] [PMID: 3010203]

[48]   Bristow RE, Montz FJ, Lagasse LD, Leuchter RS, Karlan BY. Survival impact of surgical cytoreduction in stage IV epithelial ovarian cancer. Gynecol Oncol 1999; 72(3): 278-87.
[http://dx.doi.org/10.1006/gyno.1998.5145] [PMID: 10053096]

[49]   Kolev V, Pereira EB, Schwartz M, *et al.* The role of liver resection at the time of secondary cytoreduction in patients with recurrent ovarian cancer. Int J Gynecol Cancer 2014; 24(1): 70-4.
[http://dx.doi.org/10.1097/IGC.0000000000000026] [PMID: 24356412]

[50]   Weber AM, Kennedy AW. The role of bowel resection in the primary surgical debulking of carcinoma of the ovary. J Am Coll Surg 1994; 179(4): 465-70.
[PMID: 7921399]

[51]   Scarabelli C, Gallo A, Franceschi S, *et al.* Primary cytoreductive surgery with rectosigmoid colon resection for patients with advanced epithelial ovarian carcinoma. Cancer 2000; 88(2): 389-97.
[http://dx.doi.org/10.1002/(SICI)1097-0142(20000115)88:2<389::AID-CNCR21>3.0.CO;2-W] [PMID: 10640973]

[52]   Tebes SJ, Cardosi R, Hoffman MS. Colorectal resection in patients with ovarian and primary peritoneal carcinoma. Am J Obstet Gynecol 2006; 195(2): 585-9.
[http://dx.doi.org/10.1016/j.ajog.2006.03.079] [PMID: 16730631]

[53]   Hacker NF, Berek JS, Lagasse LD, Nieberg RK, Elashoff RM. Primary cytoreductive surgery for epithelial ovarian cancer. Obstet Gynecol 1983; 61(4): 413-20.
[PMID: 6828269]

[54]   Chi DS, Eisenhauer EL, Zivanovic O, *et al.* Improved progression-free and overall survival in advanced ovarian cancer as a result of a change in surgical paradigm. Gynecol Oncol 2009; 114(1): 26-31.
[http://dx.doi.org/10.1016/j.ygyno.2009.03.018] [PMID: 19395008]

[55]   Potter ME, Partridge EE, Hatch KD, Soong SJ, Austin JM, Shingleton HM. Primary surgical therapy of ovarian cancer: how much and when. Gynecol Oncol 1991; 40(3): 195-200.
[http://dx.doi.org/10.1016/0090-8258(90)90277-R] [PMID: 2013440]

[56]   Magtibay PM, Adams PB, Silverman MB, Cha SS, Podratz KC. Splenectomy as part of cytoreductive surgery in ovarian cancer. Gynecol Oncol 2006; 102(2): 369-74.
[http://dx.doi.org/10.1016/j.ygyno.2006.03.028] [PMID: 16631919]

[57]   Eisenkop SM, Spirtos NM, Lin WC. Splenectomy in the context of primary cytoreductive operations for advanced epithelial ovarian cancer. Gynecol Oncol 2006; 100(2): 344-8.
[http://dx.doi.org/10.1016/j.ygyno.2005.08.036] [PMID: 16202446]

[58]   Berek JS, Hacker NF, Lagasse LD, Leuchter RS. Lower urinary tract resection as part of cytoreductive surgery for ovarian cancer. Gynecol Oncol 1982; 13(1): 87-92.
[http://dx.doi.org/10.1016/0090-8258(82)90012-9] [PMID: 7060996]

[59]   Fanfani F, Fagotti A, Gallotta V, *et al.* Upper abdominal surgery in advanced and recurrent ovarian cancer: role of diaphragmatic surgery. Gynecol Oncol 2010; 116(3): 497-501.
[http://dx.doi.org/10.1016/j.ygyno.2009.11.023] [PMID: 20004958]

[60]   Kapnick SJ, Griffiths CT, Finkler NJ. Occult pleural involvement in stage III ovarian carcinoma: role of diaphragm resection. Gynecol Oncol 1990; 39(2): 135-8.
[http://dx.doi.org/10.1016/0090-8258(90)90420-P] [PMID: 2227587]

[61]   Tsolakidis D, Amant F, Van Gorp T, Leunen K, Neven P, Vergote I. Diaphragmatic surgery during primary debulking in 89 patients with stage IIIB-IV epithelial ovarian cancer. Gynecol Oncol 2010; 116(3): 489-96.
[http://dx.doi.org/10.1016/j.ygyno.2009.07.014] [PMID: 19954825]

[62]   Bristow RE, Lagasse LD, Karlan BY. Secondary surgical cytoreduction for advanced epithelial ovarian cancer. Patient selection and review of the literature. Cancer 1996; 78(10): 2049-62.
[http://dx.doi.org/10.1002/(SICI)1097-0142(19961115)78:10<2049::AID-CNCR4>3.0.CO;2-J] [PMID: 8918397]

[63]   Chi DS, McCaughty K, Diaz JP, *et al.* Guidelines and selection criteria for secondary cytoreductive surgery in patients with recurrent, platinum-sensitive epithelial ovarian carcinoma. Cancer 2006; 106(9): 1933-9.
[http://dx.doi.org/10.1002/cncr.21845] [PMID: 16572412]

[64]   Tian WJ, Chi DS, Sehouli J, *et al.* A risk model for secondary cytoreductive surgery in recurrent ovarian cancer: an evidence-based proposal for patient selection. Ann Surg Oncol 2012; 19(2): 597-604.
[http://dx.doi.org/10.1245/s10434-011-1873-2] [PMID: 21732142]

[65]   Segna RA, Dottino PR, Mandeli JP, Konsker K, Cohen CJ. Secondary cytoreduction for ovarian cancer following cisplatin therapy. J Clin Oncol 1993; 11(3): 434-9.
[http://dx.doi.org/10.1200/JCO.1993.11.3.434] [PMID: 8445417]

[66]   Nezhat FR, Finger TN, Vetere P, *et al.* Comparison of perioperative outcomes and complication rates between conventional *versus* robotic-assisted laparoscopy in the evaluation and management of early, advanced, and recurrent stage ovarian, fallopian tube, and primary peritoneal cancer. Int J Gynecol Cancer 2014; 24(3): 600-7.
[http://dx.doi.org/10.1097/IGC.0000000000000096] [PMID: 24557439]

[67]   Lancaster JM, Powell CB, Chen LM, Richardson DL. SGO Clinical Practice Committee Society of Gynecologic Oncology statement on risk assessment for inherited gynecologic cancer predispositions.

Gynecol Oncol 2015; 136(1): 3-7.
[http://dx.doi.org/10.1016/j.ygyno.2014.09.009] [PMID: 25238946]

[68]   NIH Consensus Development Panel on Ovarian Cancer. NIH consensus conference. Ovarian cancer. Screening, treatment, and follow-up. JAMA 1995; 273(6): 491-7.
[http://dx.doi.org/10.1001/jama.1995.03520300065039] [PMID: 7837369]

[69]   Finch A, Beiner M, Lubinski J, *et al.* Hereditary Ovarian Cancer Clinical Study Group Salpingo-oophorectomy and the risk of ovarian, fallopian tube, and peritoneal cancers in women with a BRCA1 or BRCA2 Mutation. JAMA 2006; 296(2): 185-92.
[http://dx.doi.org/10.1001/jama.296.2.185] [PMID: 16835424]

[70]   Eisen A, Lubinski J, Klijn J, *et al.* Breast cancer risk following bilateral oophorectomy in BRCA1 and BRCA2 mutation carriers: an international case-control study. J Clin Oncol 2005; 23(30): 7491-6.
[http://dx.doi.org/10.1200/JCO.2004.00.7138] [PMID: 16234515]

[71]   Domchek SM, Friebel TM, Neuhausen SL, *et al.* Mortality after bilateral salpingo-oophorectomy in BRCA1 and BRCA2 mutation carriers: a prospective cohort study. Lancet Oncol 2006; 7(3): 223-9.
[http://dx.doi.org/10.1016/S1470-2045(06)70585-X] [PMID: 16510331]

[72]   Finch AP, Lubinski J, Møller P, *et al.* Impact of oophorectomy on cancer incidence and mortality in women with a BRCA1 or BRCA2 mutation. J Clin Oncol 2014; 32(15): 1547-53.
[http://dx.doi.org/10.1200/JCO.2013.53.2820] [PMID: 24567435]

[73]   Finch A, Wang M, Fine A, *et al.* Genetic testing for BRCA1 and BRCA2 in the Province of Ontario. Clin Genet 2016; 89(3): 304-11.
[http://dx.doi.org/10.1111/cge.12647] [PMID: 26219728]

[74]   LaDuca H, Stuenkel AJ, Dolinsky JS, *et al.* Utilization of multigene panels in hereditary cancer predisposition testing: analysis of more than 2,000 patients. Genet Med 2014; 16(11): 830-7.
[http://dx.doi.org/10.1038/gim.2014.40] [PMID: 24763289]

[75]   Tung N, Battelli C, Allen B, *et al.* Frequency of mutations in individuals with breast cancer referred for BRCA1 and BRCA2 testing using next-generation sequencing with a 25-gene panel. Cancer 2015; 121(1): 25-33.
[http://dx.doi.org/10.1002/cncr.29010] [PMID: 25186627]

[76]   Greene MH, Mai PL, Schwartz PE. Does bilateral salpingectomy with ovarian retention warrant consideration as a temporary bridge to risk-reducing bilateral oophorectomy in BRCA1/2 mutation carriers? Am J Obstet Gynecol 2011; 204(1): 19 e-1-6.

[77]   McAlpine JN, Hanley GE, Woo MM, *et al.* Opportunistic salpingectomy: uptake, risks, and complications of a regional initiative for ovarian cancer prevention. Am J Obstet Gynecol 2014; 210(5): 471 e1-11.
[http://dx.doi.org/10.1016/j.ajog.2014.01.003]

[78]   Committee on Gynecologic Practice. Committee opinion no. 620: Salpingectomy for ovarian cancer prevention. Obstet Gynecol 2015; 125(1): 279-81.
[http://dx.doi.org/10.1097/01.AOG.0000459871.88564.09] [PMID: 25560145]

[79]   Song T, Kim MK, Kim ML, *et al.* Impact of opportunistic salpingectomy on anti-Müllerian hormone in patients undergoing laparoscopic hysterectomy: a multicentre randomised controlled trial. BJOG 2017; 124(2): 314-20.
[http://dx.doi.org/10.1111/1471-0528.14182] [PMID: 27342222]

[80]   Morelli M, Venturella R, Mocciaro R, *et al.* Prophylactic salpingectomy in premenopausal low-risk women for ovarian cancer: primum non nocere. Gynecol Oncol 2013; 129(3): 448-51.
[http://dx.doi.org/10.1016/j.ygyno.2013.03.023] [PMID: 23558052]

[81]   McGowan L, Lesher LP, Norris HJ, Barnett M. Misstaging of ovarian cancer. Obstet Gynecol 1985; 65(4): 568-72.
[PMID: 3982731]

[82]   Nguyen HN, Averette HE, Hoskins W, Penalver M, Sevin BU, Steren A. National survey of ovarian carcinoma. Part V. The impact of physician's specialty on patients' survival. Cancer 1993; 72(12): 3663-70.
[http://dx.doi.org/10.1002/1097-0142(19931215)72:12<3663::AID-CNCR2820721218>3.0.CO;2-S]
[PMID: 8252483]

[83]   Mayer AR, Chambers SK, Graves E, *et al.* Ovarian cancer staging: does it require a gynecologic oncologist? Gynecol Oncol 1992; 47(2): 223-7.
[http://dx.doi.org/10.1016/0090-8258(92)90110-5] [PMID: 1468701]

[84]   Eisenkop SM, Spirtos NM, Montag TW, Nalick RH, Wang HJ. The impact of subspecialty training on the management of advanced ovarian cancer. Gynecol Oncol 1992; 47(2): 203-9.
[http://dx.doi.org/10.1016/0090-8258(92)90107-T] [PMID: 1468698]

[85]   Bristow RE, Chang J, Ziogas A, Randall LM, Anton-Culver H. High-volume ovarian cancer care: survival impact and disparities in access for advanced-stage disease. Gynecol Oncol 2014; 132(2): 403-10.
[http://dx.doi.org/10.1016/j.ygyno.2013.12.017] [PMID: 24361578]

[86]   Reich H, McGlynn F, Wilkie W. Laparoscopic management of stage I ovarian cancer. A case report J Rep Med 1990; 35(6): 601-4. discussion 4-5

[87]   Nezhat F, Yadav J, Rahaman J, Gretz H III, Gardner GJ, Cohen CJ. Laparoscopic lymphadenectomy for gynecologic malignancies using ultrasonically activated shears: analysis of first 100 cases. Gynecol Oncol 2005; 97(3): 813-9.
[http://dx.doi.org/10.1016/j.ygyno.2005.02.005] [PMID: 15943988]

[88]   Dottino PR, Tobias DH, Beddoe A, Golden AL, Cohen CJ. Laparoscopic lymphadenectomy for gynecologic malignancies. Gynecol Oncol 1999; 73(3): 383-8.
[http://dx.doi.org/10.1006/gyno.1999.5376] [PMID: 10366464]

[89]   Querleu D, LeBlanc E. Laparoscopic infrarenal paraaortic lymph node dissection for restaging of carcinoma of the ovary or fallopian tube. Cancer 1994; 73(5): 1467-71.
[http://dx.doi.org/10.1002/1097-0142(19940301)73:5<1467::AID-CNCR2820730524>3.0.CO;2-B]
[PMID: 8111714]

[90]   Childers JM, Lang J, Surwit EA, Hatch KD. Laparoscopic surgical staging of ovarian cancer. Gynecol Oncol 1995; 59(1): 25-33.
[http://dx.doi.org/10.1006/gyno.1995.1263] [PMID: 7557611]

[91]   Possover M, Krause N, Plaul K, Kühne-Heid R, Schneider A. Laparoscopic para-aortic and pelvic lymphadenectomy: experience with 150 patients and review of the literature. Gynecol Oncol 1998; 71(1): 19-28.
[http://dx.doi.org/10.1006/gyno.1998.5107] [PMID: 9784314]

[92]   Park HJ, Kim DW, Yim GW, *et al.* Staging laparoscopy for the management of early-stage ovarian cancer: a metaanalysis. Am J Obstet Gynecol 2013; 209(1): 58 -e1-8.
[http://dx.doi.org/10.1016/j.ajog.2013.04.013]

[93]   Park JY, Kim DY, Suh DS, *et al.* Comparison of laparoscopy and laparotomy in surgical staging of early-stage ovarian and fallopian tubal cancer. Ann Surg Oncol 2008; 15(7): 2012-9.
[http://dx.doi.org/10.1245/s10434-008-9893-2] [PMID: 18437497]

[94]   Chi DS, Abu-Rustum NR, Sonoda Y, *et al.* The safety and efficacy of laparoscopic surgical staging of apparent stage I ovarian and fallopian tube cancers. Am J Obstet Gynecol 2005; 192(5): 1614-9.
[http://dx.doi.org/10.1016/j.ajog.2004.11.018] [PMID: 15902166]

[95]   Nezhat FR, Ezzati M, Chuang L. Laparoscopic management of early ovarian and fallopian tube cancers: surgical and survival outcome. Am J Obstet Gynecol 2009; 200(1): 83-e1-6.
[http://dx.doi.org/10.1016/j.ajog.2008.08.013]

[96]   Ghezzi F, Cromi A, Uccella S, *et al.* Laparoscopy *versus* laparotomy for the surgical management of

apparent early stage ovarian cancer. Gynecol Oncol 2007; 105(2): 409-13.
[http://dx.doi.org/10.1016/j.ygyno.2006.12.025] [PMID: 17275077]

[97]   Melamed A, Keating NL, Clemmer JT, *et al.* Laparoscopic staging for apparent stage I epithelial ovarian cancer. Am J Obstet Gynecol 2017; 216(1): 50-e1- e12..
[http://dx.doi.org/10.1016/j.ajog.2016.08.030]

[98]   Rabinovich A. Robotic surgery for ovarian cancers: individualization of the surgical approach to select ovarian cancer patients. Int J Med Robot 2016; 12(3): 547-53.
[http://dx.doi.org/10.1002/rcs.1684] [PMID: 26173832]

[99]   Minig L, Padilla Iserte P, Zorrero C, Zanagnolo V. Robotic Surgery in Women With Ovarian Cancer: Surgical Technique and Evidence of Clinical Outcomes. J Minim Invasive Gynecol 2016; 23(3): 309-16.
[http://dx.doi.org/10.1016/j.jmig.2015.10.014] [PMID: 26538410]

[100] Fornalik H, Brooks H, Moore ES, Flanders NL, Callahan MJ, Sutton GP. Hand-Assisted Robotic Surgery for Staging of Ovarian Cancer and Uterine Cancers With High Risk of Peritoneal Spread: A Retrospective Cohort Study. Int J Gynecol Cancer 2015; 25(8): 1488-93.
[http://dx.doi.org/10.1097/IGC.0000000000000508] [PMID: 26270117]

[101] Finger TN, Nezhat FR. Robotic-assisted fertility-sparing surgery for early ovarian cancer. JSLS : J Soc of Laparoendoscopic Surgeons 2014; 18(2): 308-13.
[http://dx.doi.org/10.4293/108680813X13654754535557] [PMID: 24960498]

[102] Escobar PF, Levinson KL, Magrina J, *et al.* Feasibility and perioperative outcomes of robotic-assisted surgery in the management of recurrent ovarian cancer: a multi-institutional study. Gynecol Oncol 2014; 134(2): 253-6.
[http://dx.doi.org/10.1016/j.ygyno.2014.05.007] [PMID: 24844594]

[103] Melamed A, Nitecki R, Boruta DM II, *et al.* Laparoscopy Compared With Laparotomy for Debulking Ovarian Cancer After Neoadjuvant Chemotherapy. Obstet Gynecol 2017; 129(5): 861-9.
[http://dx.doi.org/10.1097/AOG.0000000000001851] [PMID: 28383367]

[104] Covens A, Carey M, Bryson P, Verma S, Fung Kee Fung M, Johnston M. Systematic review of first-line chemotherapy for newly diagnosed postoperative patients with stage II, III, or IV epithelial ovarian cancer. Gynecol Oncol 2002; 85(1): 71-80.
[http://dx.doi.org/10.1006/gyno.2001.6552] [PMID: 11925123]

[105] Morice P, Wicart-Poque F, Rey A, *et al.* Results of conservative treatment in epithelial ovarian carcinoma. Cancer 2001; 92(9): 2412-8.
[http://dx.doi.org/10.1002/1097-0142(20011101)92:9<2412::AID-CNCR1590>3.0.CO;2-7] [PMID: 11745298]

[106] Trimbos JB, Parmar M, Vergote I, *et al.* International Collaborative Ovarian Neoplasm 1 European Organisation for Research and Treatment of Cancer Collaborators-Adjuvant ChemoTherapy un Ovarian Neoplasm International Collaborative Ovarian Neoplasm trial 1 and Adjuvant ChemoTherapy In Ovarian Neoplasm trial: two parallel randomized phase III trials of adjuvant chemotherapy in patients with early-stage ovarian carcinoma. J Natl Cancer Inst 2003; 95(2): 105-12.
[http://dx.doi.org/10.1093/jnci/95.2.113] [PMID: 12529343]

[107] Colombo N, Pecorelli S. What have we learned from ICON1 and ACTION? Int J Gynecol Cancer 2003; 13 (Suppl. 2): 140-3.
[http://dx.doi.org/10.1136/ijgc-00009577-200311001-00002] [PMID: 14656270]

[108] Colombo N, Guthrie D, Chiari S, *et al.* International Collaborative Ovarian Neoplasm (ICON) collaborators International Collaborative Ovarian Neoplasm trial 1: a randomized trial of adjuvant chemotherapy in women with early-stage ovarian cancer. J Natl Cancer Inst 2003; 95(2): 125-32.
[http://dx.doi.org/10.1093/jnci/95.2.125] [PMID: 12529345]

[109] Bell J, Brady MF, Young RC, *et al.* Gynecologic Oncology Group Randomized phase III trial of three *versus* six cycles of adjuvant carboplatin and paclitaxel in early stage epithelial ovarian carcinoma: a

Gynecologic Oncology Group study. Gynecol Oncol 2006; 102(3): 432-9.
[http://dx.doi.org/10.1016/j.ygyno.2006.06.013] [PMID: 16860852]

[110]   Pignata S, Scambia G, Ferrandina G, *et al.* Carboplatin plus paclitaxel *versus* carboplatin plus pegylated liposomal doxorubicin as first-line treatment for patients with ovarian cancer: the MITO-2 randomized phase III trial. J Clin Oncol 2011; 29(27): 3628-35.
[http://dx.doi.org/10.1200/JCO.2010.33.8566] [PMID: 21844495]

[111]   Armstrong DK, Bundy B, Wenzel L, *et al.* Gynecologic Oncology Group Intraperitoneal cisplatin and paclitaxel in ovarian cancer. N Engl J Med 2006; 354(1): 34-43.
[http://dx.doi.org/10.1056/NEJMoa052985] [PMID: 16394300]

[112]   Alberts DS, Liu PY, Hannigan EV, *et al.* Intraperitoneal cisplatin plus intravenous cyclophosphamide *versus* intravenous cisplatin plus intravenous cyclophosphamide for stage III ovarian cancer. N Engl J Med 1996; 335(26): 1950-5.
[http://dx.doi.org/10.1056/NEJM199612263352603] [PMID: 8960474]

[113]   Markman M, Bundy BN, Alberts DS, *et al.* Phase III trial of standard-dose intravenous cisplatin plus paclitaxel *versus* moderately high-dose carboplatin followed by intravenous paclitaxel and intraperitoneal cisplatin in small-volume stage III ovarian carcinoma: an intergroup study of the Gynecologic Oncology Group, Southwestern Oncology Group, and Eastern Cooperative Oncology Group. J Clin Oncol 2001; 19(4): 1001-7.
[http://dx.doi.org/10.1200/JCO.2001.19.4.1001] [PMID: 11181662]

[114]   Walker JL, Armstrong DK, Huang HQ, *et al.* Intraperitoneal catheter outcomes in a phase III trial of intravenous *versus* intraperitoneal chemotherapy in optimal stage III ovarian and primary peritoneal cancer: a Gynecologic Oncology Group Study. Gynecol Oncol 2006; 100(1): 27-32.
[http://dx.doi.org/10.1016/j.ygyno.2005.11.013] [PMID: 16368440]

[115]   Katsumata N, Yasuda M, Takahashi F, *et al.* Japanese Gynecologic Oncology Group Dose-dense paclitaxel once a week in combination with carboplatin every 3 weeks for advanced ovarian cancer: a phase 3, open-label, randomised controlled trial. Lancet 2009; 374(9698): 1331-8.
[http://dx.doi.org/10.1016/S0140-6736(09)61157-0] [PMID: 19767092]

[116]   Katsumata N, Yasuda M, Isonishi S, *et al.* Japanese Gynecologic Oncology Group Long-term results of dose-dense paclitaxel and carboplatin *versus* conventional paclitaxel and carboplatin for treatment of advanced epithelial ovarian, fallopian tube, or primary peritoneal cancer (JGOG 3016): a randomised, controlled, open-label trial. Lancet Oncol 2013; 14(10): 1020-6.
[http://dx.doi.org/10.1016/S1470-2045(13)70363-2] [PMID: 23948349]

[117]   Walker JL BM, DiSilvestro PA, *et al.* A Phase III Clinical Trial of Bevacizumab with IV versus IP Chemotherapy in Ovarian, Fallopian Tube, and Primary Peritoneal Carcinoma (GOG 252) 2016.

[118]   Vergote I, Tropé CG, Amant F, *et al.* European Organization for Research and Treatment of Cancer-Gynaecological Cancer Group NCIC Clinical Trials Group Neoadjuvant chemotherapy or primary surgery in stage IIIC or IV ovarian cancer. N Engl J Med 2010; 363(10): 943-53.
[http://dx.doi.org/10.1056/NEJMoa0908806] [PMID: 20818904]

[119]   Kehoe S, Hook J, Nankivell M, *et al.* Primary chemotherapy *versus* primary surgery for newly diagnosed advanced ovarian cancer (CHORUS): an open-label, randomised, controlled, non-inferiority trial. Lancet 2015; 386(9990): 249-57.
[http://dx.doi.org/10.1016/S0140-6736(14)62223-6] [PMID: 26002111]

[120]   Blackledge G, Lawton F, Redman C, Kelly K. Response of patients in phase II studies of chemotherapy in ovarian cancer: implications for patient treatment and the design of phase II trials. Br J Cancer 1989; 59(4): 650-3.
[http://dx.doi.org/10.1038/bjc.1989.132] [PMID: 2713253]

[121]   Markman M, Hoskins W. Responses to salvage chemotherapy in ovarian cancer: a critical need for precise definitions of the treated population. J Clin Oncol 1992; 10(4): 513-4.
[http://dx.doi.org/10.1200/JCO.1992.10.4.513] [PMID: 1548513]

[122] Markman M, Rothman R, Hakes T, *et al.* Second-line platinum therapy in patients with ovarian cancer previously treated with cisplatin. J Clin Oncol 1991; 9(3): 389-93.
[http://dx.doi.org/10.1200/JCO.1991.9.3.389] [PMID: 1999708]

[123] Parmar MK, Ledermann JA, Colombo N, *et al.* ICON and AGO Collaborators Paclitaxel plus platinum-based chemotherapy *versus* conventional platinum-based chemotherapy in women with relapsed ovarian cancer: the ICON4/AGO-OVAR-2.2 trial. Lancet 2003; 361(9375): 2099-106.
[http://dx.doi.org/10.1016/S0140-6736(03)13718-X] [PMID: 12826431]

[124] Pfisterer J, Plante M, Vergote I, *et al.* AGO-OVAR NCIC CTG EORTC GCG Gemcitabine plus carboplatin compared with carboplatin in patients with platinum-sensitive recurrent ovarian cancer: an intergroup trial of the AGO-OVAR, the NCIC CTG, and the EORTC GCG. J Clin Oncol 2006; 24(29): 4699-707.
[http://dx.doi.org/10.1200/JCO.2006.06.0913] [PMID: 16966687]

[125] Pujade-Lauraine E, Wagner U, Aavall-Lundqvist E, *et al.* Pegylated liposomal Doxorubicin and Carboplatin compared with Paclitaxel and Carboplatin for patients with platinum-sensitive ovarian cancer in late relapse. J Clin Oncol 2010; 28(20): 3323-9.
[http://dx.doi.org/10.1200/JCO.2009.25.7519] [PMID: 20498395]

[126] Lawrie TA, Bryant A, Cameron A, Gray E, Morrison J. Pegylated liposomal doxorubicin for relapsed epithelial ovarian cancer. Cochrane Database Syst Rev 2013; (7): CD006910
[http://dx.doi.org/10.1002/14651858.CD006910.pub2] [PMID: 23835762]

[127] Gordon AN, Fleagle JT, Guthrie D, Parkin DE, Gore ME, Lacave AJ. Recurrent epithelial ovarian carcinoma: a randomized phase III study of pegylated liposomal doxorubicin *versus* topotecan. J Clin Oncol 2001; 19(14): 3312-22.
[http://dx.doi.org/10.1200/JCO.2001.19.14.3312] [PMID: 11454878]

[128] Rose PG, Smrekar M, Fusco N. A phase II trial of weekly paclitaxel and every 3 weeks of carboplatin in potentially platinum-sensitive ovarian and peritoneal carcinoma. Gynecol Oncol 2005; 96(2): 296-300.
[http://dx.doi.org/10.1016/j.ygyno.2004.03.046] [PMID: 15661211]

[129] Strauss HG, Henze A, Teichmann A, *et al.* Phase II trial of docetaxel and carboplatin in recurrent platinum-sensitive ovarian, peritoneal and tubal cancer. Gynecol Oncol 2007; 104(3): 612-6.
[http://dx.doi.org/10.1016/j.ygyno.2006.09.023] [PMID: 17069876]

[130] Ferrandina G, Ludovisi M, Lorusso D, *et al.* Phase III trial of gemcitabine compared with pegylated liposomal doxorubicin in progressive or recurrent ovarian cancer. J Clin Oncol 2008; 26(6): 890-6.
[http://dx.doi.org/10.1200/JCO.2007.13.6606] [PMID: 18281662]

[131] Morris R, Alvarez RD, Andrews S, *et al.* Topotecan weekly bolus chemotherapy for relapsed platinum-sensitive ovarian and peritoneal cancers. Gynecol Oncol 2008; 109(3): 346-52.
[http://dx.doi.org/10.1016/j.ygyno.2008.02.028] [PMID: 18410954]

[132] Rose PG, Blessing JA, Mayer AR, Homesley HD. Prolonged oral etoposide as second-line therapy for platinum-resistant and platinum-sensitive ovarian carcinoma: a Gynecologic Oncology Group study. J Clin Oncol 1998; 16(2): 405-10.
[http://dx.doi.org/10.1200/JCO.1998.16.2.405] [PMID: 9469322]

[133] Markman M, Blessing J, Rubin SC, Connor J, Hanjani P, Waggoner S. Gynecologic Oncology Group Phase II trial of weekly paclitaxel (80 mg/m2) in platinum and paclitaxel-resistant ovarian and primary peritoneal cancers: a Gynecologic Oncology Group study. Gynecol Oncol 2006; 101(3): 436-40.
[http://dx.doi.org/10.1016/j.ygyno.2005.10.036] [PMID: 16325893]

[134] Gore ME, Levy V, Rustin G, *et al.* Paclitaxel (Taxol) in relapsed and refractory ovarian cancer: the UK and Eire experience. Br J Cancer 1995; 72(4): 1016-9.
[http://dx.doi.org/10.1038/bjc.1995.453] [PMID: 7547214]

[135] Verschraegen CF, Sittisomwong T, Kudelka AP, *et al.* Docetaxel for patients with paclitaxel-resistant

Müllerian carcinoma. J Clin Oncol 2000; 18(14): 2733-9.
[http://dx.doi.org/10.1200/JCO.2000.18.14.2733] [PMID: 10894873]

[136]   Coleman RL, Brady WE, McMeekin DS, *et al.* A phase II evaluation of nanoparticle, albumin-bound
        (nab) paclitaxel in the treatment of recurrent or persistent platinum-resistant ovarian, fallopian tube, or
        primary peritoneal cancer: a Gynecologic Oncology Group study. Gynecol Oncol 2011; 122(1): 111-5.
        [http://dx.doi.org/10.1016/j.ygyno.2011.03.036] [PMID: 21497382]

[137]   Peng LH, Chen XY, Wu TX. Topotecan for ovarian cancer. Cochrane Database Syst Rev 2008; (2):
        CD005589
        [PMID: 18425923]

[138]   Gordon AN, Tonda M, Sun S, Rackoff W. Doxil Study 30-49 Investigators Long-term survival
        advantage for women treated with pegylated liposomal doxorubicin compared with topotecan in a
        phase 3 randomized study of recurrent and refractory epithelial ovarian cancer. Gynecol Oncol 2004;
        95(1): 1-8.
        [http://dx.doi.org/10.1016/j.ygyno.2004.07.011] [PMID: 15385103]

[139]   Sehouli J, Stengel D, Harter P, *et al.* Topotecan weekly versus conventional 5-day schedule in patients
        with platinum-resistant ovarian cancer: a randomized multicenter phase ii trial of the north-eastern
        german society of gynecological oncology ovarian cancer study group J cClin Oncol 2011; 29(2): 242-
        8.

[140]   Mutch DG, Orlando M, Goss T, *et al.* Randomized phase III trial of gemcitabine compared with
        pegylated liposomal doxorubicin in patients with platinum-resistant ovarian cancer. J Clin Oncol 2007;
        25(19): 2811-8.
        [http://dx.doi.org/10.1200/JCO.2006.09.6735] [PMID: 17602086]

[141]   Dorval T, Soussain C, Beuzeboc P, *et al.* Ifosfamide seven-day infusion for recurrent and cisplatin
        refractory ovarian cancer. J Infus Chemother 1996; 6(1): 47-9.
        [PMID: 8748008]

[142]   Willemse PH, vd Burg ME, vd Gaast A, *et al.* Ifosfamide given as a 24-h infusion with mesna in
        patients with recurrent ovarian cancer: preliminary results. Cancer Chemother Pharmacol 1990; 26
        (Suppl.): S51-4.
        [http://dx.doi.org/10.1007/BF00685420] [PMID: 2112053]

[143]   Burger RA, DiSaia PJ, Roberts JA, *et al.* Phase II trial of vinorelbine in recurrent and progressive
        epithelial ovarian cancer. Gynecol Oncol 1999; 72(2): 148-53.
        [http://dx.doi.org/10.1006/gyno.1998.5243] [PMID: 10021293]

[144]   Rothenberg ML, Liu PY, Wilczynski S, *et al.* Phase II trial of vinorelbine for relapsed ovarian cancer:
        a Southwest Oncology Group study. Gynecol Oncol 2004; 95(3): 506-12.
        [http://dx.doi.org/10.1016/j.ygyno.2004.09.004] [PMID: 15581954]

[145]   Miller DS, Blessing JA, Krasner CN, *et al.* Phase II evaluation of pemetrexed in the treatment of
        recurrent or persistent platinum-resistant ovarian or primary peritoneal carcinoma: a study of the
        Gynecologic Oncology Group. J Clin Oncol 2009; 27(16): 2686-91.
        [http://dx.doi.org/10.1200/JCO.2008.19.2963] [PMID: 19332726]

[146]   Teplinsky E, Herzog TJ. The efficacy of trabectedin in treating ovarian cancer. Expert Opin
        Pharmacother 2017; 18(3): 313-23.
        [http://dx.doi.org/10.1080/14656566.2017.1285282] [PMID: 28140689]

[147]   del Campo JM, Sessa C, Krasner CN, *et al.* Trabectedin as single agent in relapsed advanced ovarian
        cancer: results from a retrospective pooled analysis of three phase II trials. Med Oncol 2013; 30(1):
        435.
        [http://dx.doi.org/10.1007/s12032-012-0435-1] [PMID: 23397080]

[148]   Garcia AA, Hirte H, Fleming G, *et al.* Phase II clinical trial of bevacizumab and low-dose metronomic
        oral cyclophosphamide in recurrent ovarian cancer: a trial of the California, Chicago, and Princess
        Margaret Hospital phase II consortia. J Clin Oncol 2008; 26(1): 76-82.

[http://dx.doi.org/10.1200/JCO.2007.12.1939] [PMID: 18165643]

[149]   Burger RA, Brady MF, Bookman MA, *et al.* Gynecologic Oncology GroupIncorporation of beva-cizumab in the primary treatment of ovarian cancer. N Engl J Med 2011; 365(26): 2473-83.
[http://dx.doi.org/10.1056/NEJMoa1104390] [PMID: 22204724]

[150]   Ferriss JS, Java JJ, Bookman MA, *et al.* Ascites predicts treatment benefit of bevacizumab in front-line therapy of advanced epithelial ovarian, fallopian tube and peritoneal cancers: an NRG Oncology/GOG study. Gynecol Oncol 2015; 139(1): 17-22.
[http://dx.doi.org/10.1016/j.ygyno.2015.07.103] [PMID: 26216729]

[151]   Perren TJ, Swart AM, Pfisterer J, *et al.* ICON7 Investigators A phase 3 trial of bevacizumab in ovarian cancer. N Engl J Med 2011; 365(26): 2484-96.
[http://dx.doi.org/10.1056/NEJMoa1103799] [PMID: 22204725]

[152]   Oza AM, Cook AD, Pfisterer J, *et al.* ICON7 trial investigators Standard chemotherapy with or without bevacizumab for women with newly diagnosed ovarian cancer (ICON7): overall survival results of a phase 3 randomised trial. Lancet Oncol 2015; 16(8): 928-36.
[http://dx.doi.org/10.1016/S1470-2045(15)00086-8] [PMID: 26115797]

[153]   Aghajanian C, Goff B, Nycum LR, Wang YV, Husain A, Blank SV. Final overall survival and safety analysis of OCEANS, a phase 3 trial of chemotherapy with or without bevacizumab in patients with platinum-sensitive recurrent ovarian cancer. Gynecol Oncol 2015; 139(1): 10-6.
[http://dx.doi.org/10.1016/j.ygyno.2015.08.004] [PMID: 26271155]

[154]   Aghajanian C, Goff B, Nycum LR, Wang Y, Husain A, Blank S. Independent radiologic review: bevacizumab in combination with gemcitabine and carboplatin in recurrent ovarian cancer. Gynecol Oncol 2014; 133(1): 105-10.
[http://dx.doi.org/10.1016/j.ygyno.2014.02.003] [PMID: 24508841]

[155]   Aghajanian C, Blank SV, Goff BA, *et al.* OCEANS: a randomized, double-blind, placebo-controlled phase III trial of chemotherapy with or without bevacizumab in patients with platinum-sensitive recurrent epithelial ovarian, primary peritoneal, or fallopian tube cancer. J Clin Oncol 2012; 30(17): 2039-45.
[http://dx.doi.org/10.1200/JCO.2012.42.0505] [PMID: 22529265]

[156]   Coleman RL BM, Herzog TJ, *et al.* A phase III randomized controlled clinical trial of carboplatin and paclitaxel alone or in combination with bevacizumab followed by bevacizumab and secondary cytoreductive surgery in platinum-sensitive, recurrent ovarian, peritoneal primary and fallopian tube cancer (Gynecologic Oncology Group 0213) 2015.

[157]   Pujade-Lauraine E, Hilpert F, Weber B, *et al.* Bevacizumab combined with chemotherapy for platinum-resistant recurrent ovarian cancer: The AURELIA open-label randomized phase III trial. J Clin Oncol 2014; 32(13): 1302-8.
[http://dx.doi.org/10.1200/JCO.2013.51.4489] [PMID: 24637997]

[158]   Poveda AM, Selle F, Hilpert F, *et al.* Bevacizumab Combined With Weekly Paclitaxel, Pegylated Liposomal Doxorubicin, or Topotecan in Platinum-Resistant Recurrent Ovarian Cancer: Analysis by Chemotherapy Cohort of the Randomized Phase III AURELIA Trial. J Clin Oncol 2015; 33(32): 3836-8.
[http://dx.doi.org/10.1200/JCO.2015.63.1408] [PMID: 26282651]

[159]   Ledermann JA, Embleton AC, Raja F, *et al.* ICON6 collaborators Cediranib in patients with relapsed platinum-sensitive ovarian cancer (ICON6): a randomised, double-blind, placebo-controlled phase 3 trial. Lancet 2016; 387(10023): 1066-74.
[http://dx.doi.org/10.1016/S0140-6736(15)01167-8] [PMID: 27025186]

[160]   du Bois A, Floquet A, Kim JW, *et al.* Incorporation of pazopanib in maintenance therapy of ovarian cancer. J Clin Oncol 2014; 32(30): 3374-82.
[http://dx.doi.org/10.1200/JCO.2014.55.7348] [PMID: 25225436]

[161]   Williams CJ. Tamoxifen for relapse of ovarian cancer. Cochrane Database Syst Rev 2001; (1):

CD001034
[PMID: 11279703]

[162] Lindemann K, Gibbs E, Åvall-Lundqvist E, *et al.* Chemotherapy *vs.* tamoxifen in platinum-resistant ovarian cancer: a phase III, randomised, multicentre trial (Ovaresist). Br J Cancer 2017; 116(4): 455-63.
[http://dx.doi.org/10.1038/bjc.2016.435] [PMID: 28118323]

[163] Smyth JF, Gourley C, Walker G, *et al.* Antiestrogen therapy is active in selected ovarian cancer cases: the use of letrozole in estrogen receptor-positive patients. Clin Cancer Res 2007; 13(12): 3617-22.
[http://dx.doi.org/10.1158/1078-0432.CCR-06-2878] [PMID: 17575226]

[164] Kaufman B, Shapira-Frommer R, Schmutzler RK, *et al.* Olaparib monotherapy in patients with advanced cancer and a germline BRCA1/2 mutation. J Clin Oncol 2015; 33(3): 244-50.
[http://dx.doi.org/10.1200/JCO.2014.56.2728] [PMID: 25366685]

[165] Matulonis UA, Penson RT, Domchek SM, *et al.* Olaparib monotherapy in patients with advanced relapsed ovarian cancer and a germline BRCA1/2 mutation: a multistudy analysis of response rates and safety. Ann Oncol 2016; 27(6): 1013-9.
[http://dx.doi.org/10.1093/annonc/mdw133] [PMID: 26961146]

[166] Kristeleit RSS-FR, Oaknin A, Blamana J, *et al.* Clinical activity of the poly(ADP-ribose) polymerase (PARP) inhibitor rucaparib in patients (pts) with high-grade ovarian carcinoma (HGOC) and a BRCA mutation (BRCAmut): Analysis of pooled data from Study 10 (parts 1, 2a, and 3) and ARIEL2 (parts 1 and 2). ESMO 2016; 2016: 856O.
[http://dx.doi.org/10.1093/annonc/mdw374.03]

[167] Mirza MR, Monk BJ, Herrstedt J, *et al.* ENGOT-OV16/NOVA Investigators Niraparib Maintenance Therapy in Platinum-Sensitive, Recurrent Ovarian Cancer. N Engl J Med 2016; 375(22): 2154-64.
[http://dx.doi.org/10.1056/NEJMoa1611310] [PMID: 27717299]

[168] Ledermann J, Harter P, Gourley C, *et al.* Olaparib maintenance therapy in patients with platinum-sensitive relapsed serous ovarian cancer: a preplanned retrospective analysis of outcomes by BRCA status in a randomised phase 2 trial. Lancet Oncol 2014; 15(8): 852-61.
[http://dx.doi.org/10.1016/S1470-2045(14)70228-1] [PMID: 24882434]

[169] Pujade-Lauraine E, Ledermann JA, Selle F, *et al.* SOLO2/ENGOT-Ov21 investigators Olaparib tablets as maintenance therapy in patients with platinum-sensitive, relapsed ovarian cancer and a BRCA1/2 mutation (SOLO2/ENGOT-Ov21): a double-blind, randomised, placebo-controlled, phase 3 trial. Lancet Oncol 2017; 18(9): 1274-84.
[http://dx.doi.org/10.1016/S1470-2045(17)30469-2] [PMID: 28754483]

[170] Argenta PA, Sueblinvong T, Geller MA, *et al.* Hyperthermic intraperitoneal chemotherapy with carboplatin for optimally-cytoreduced, recurrent, platinum-sensitive ovarian carcinoma: a pilot study. Gynecol Oncol 2013; 129(1): 81-5.
[http://dx.doi.org/10.1016/j.ygyno.2013.01.010] [PMID: 23352917]

[171] Andikyan VTP, Farag S, Fields J, *et al.* Hyperthermic intraperitoneal chemotherapy for treatment of ovarian and primary peritoneal cancer: single institutional experience. Int J Gynecol Obstet Res 2015; 3: 53-9.
[http://dx.doi.org/10.1016/j.ygyno.2015.01.434]

[172] Bakrin N, Cotte E, Golfier F, *et al.* Cytoreductive surgery and hyperthermic intraperitoneal chemotherapy (HIPEC) for persistent and recurrent advanced ovarian carcinoma: a multicenter, prospective study of 246 patients. Ann Surg Oncol 2012; 19(13): 4052-8.
[http://dx.doi.org/10.1245/s10434-012-2510-4] [PMID: 22825772]

[173] van Driel WJ, Koole SN, Sikorska K, *et al.* Hyperthermic Intraperitoneal Chemotherapy in Ovarian Cancer. N Engl J Med 2018; 378(3): 230-40.
[http://dx.doi.org/10.1056/NEJMoa1708618] [PMID: 29342393]

[174] Hamanishi J, Mandai M, Ikeda T, *et al.* Safety and Antitumor Activity of Anti-PD-1 Antibody,

Nivolumab, in Patients With Platinum-Resistant Ovarian Cancer. J Clin Oncol 2015; 33(34): 4015-22.
[http://dx.doi.org/10.1200/JCO.2015.62.3397] [PMID: 26351349]

[175] Dobrzanski MJ, Rewers-Felkins KA, Quinlin IS, *et al.* Autologous MUC1-specific Th1 effector cell
immunotherapy induces differential levels of systemic TReg cell subpopulations that result in
increased ovarian cancer patient survival. Clin Immunol 2009; 133(3): 333-52.
[http://dx.doi.org/10.1016/j.clim.2009.08.007] [PMID: 19762283]

[176] Sakakura K, Chikamatsu K, Furuya N, Appella E, Whiteside TL, Deleo AB. Toward the development
of multi-epitope p53 cancer vaccines: an *in vitro* assessment of CD8(+) T cell responses to HLA class
I-restricted wild-type sequence p53 peptides. Clin Immunol 2007; 125(1): 43-51.
[http://dx.doi.org/10.1016/j.clim.2007.05.015] [PMID: 17631051]

[177] Correa I, Plunkett T. Update on HER-2 as a target for cancer therapy: HER2/neu peptides as tumour
vaccines for T cell recognition. Breast Cancer Res 2001; 3(6): 399-403.
[http://dx.doi.org/10.1186/bcr330] [PMID: 11737893]

[178] Odunsi K, Matsuzaki J, Karbach J, *et al.* Efficacy of vaccination with recombinant vaccinia and
fowlpox vectors expressing NY-ESO-1 antigen in ovarian cancer and melanoma patients. Proc Natl
Acad Sci USA 2012; 109(15): 5797-802.
[http://dx.doi.org/10.1073/pnas.1117208109] [PMID: 22454499]

[179] Odunsi K, Matsuzaki J, James SR, *et al.* Epigenetic potentiation of NY-ESO-1 vaccine therapy in
human ovarian cancer. Cancer Immunol Res 2014; 2(1): 37-49.
[http://dx.doi.org/10.1158/2326-6066.CIR-13-0126] [PMID: 24535937]

[180] Moore KN, Martin LP, O'Malley DM, *et al.* Safety and Activity of Mirvetuximab Soravtansine
(IMGN853), a Folate Receptor Alpha-Targeting Antibody-Drug Conjugate, in Platinum-Resistant
Ovarian, Fallopian Tube, or Primary Peritoneal Cancer: A Phase I Expansion Study. J Clin Oncol
2017; 35(10): 1112-8.
[http://dx.doi.org/10.1200/JCO.2016.69.9538] [PMID: 28029313]

[181] Weekes CD, Lamberts LE, Borad MJ, *et al.* Phase I Study of DMOT4039A, an Antibody-Drug
Conjugate Targeting Mesothelin, in Patients with Unresectable Pancreatic or Platinum-Resistant
Ovarian Cancer. Mol Cancer Ther 2016; 15(3): 439-47.
[http://dx.doi.org/10.1158/1535-7163.MCT-15-0693] [PMID: 26823490]

[182] Matei D, Fang F, Shen C, *et al.* Epigenetic resensitization to platinum in ovarian cancer. Cancer Res
2012; 72(9): 2197-205.
[http://dx.doi.org/10.1158/0008-5472.CAN-11-3909] [PMID: 22549947]

[183] Herzog T, Armstrong D. First-line chemotherapy for advanced (stage III or IV) epithelial ovarian,
fallopian tubal, and peritoneal cancer . November 2018. Available from:. www.uptodate.com/contents/
first-line-chemotherapy-for-advanced-stage-iii-or-iv-epithelial-ovarian-fallopian-tubal--
nd-peritoneal-cancer

[184] Coleman RL, Sabbatini P. Medical treatment for relapsed epithelial ovarian, fallopian tubal, or
peritoneal cancer: Platinum-sensitive disease November 2018. Available from:. www.uptodate.com/
contents/medical-treatment-for-relapsed-epithelial-ovarian-fallopian-tubal-or-periton-
al-cancer-platinum-sensitive-disease

[185] Birrer M, Fujiwara K. Medical treatment for relapsed epithelial ovarian, fallopian tubal, or peritoneal
cancer: Platinum-resistant disease November 2018. Available from:. https://www.uptodate.com/
contents/medical-treatment-for-relapsed-epithelial-ovarian-fallopian-tubal-or-periton-
al-cancer-platinum-resistant-disease

CHAPTER 2

Pathology of Ovarian Cancer

Jessica Beyda[1,*] and **Sedef Everest**[2]

1 St. Francis Hospital Roslyn, N.Y., USA

2 The Mount Sinai Health System, N.Y., USA

Abstract: Ovarian cancer is the fifth leading cause of cancer death in American women. The term 'ovarian cancer' is loosely used by laymen to refer to ovarian malignancies from all classes of ovarian tumors (sex-cord stromal, germ cell and epithelial). In this chapter, we will discuss specifically the ovarian carcinomas, derived from epithelium, historically thought to be derived from the germinal epithelium but now shown to include fallopian tube epithelium. Ovarian carcinomas constitute a diverse group of neoplasms for which this chapter will discuss: clinical features including symptoms, gross findings, tumor histology with illustrations, immunohistochemical features used in working up the pathologic diagnosis, molecular features, and prognosis.

Keywords: BRCA, Borderline, Clear cell, ERBB2, Endometrioid, Hereditary, HNPCC, KRAS, Low-grade, Mucinous, P53, PIK3CA, Pathogenesis, Prognosis, RRSO, Serous, STIC, PTEN, STIL.

INTRODUCTION

Ovarian cancer is a deadly disease, ranking fifth in cancer deaths among women in the United States. According to the American Cancer Society, in 2016, there are 22,000 new cases of ovarian cancer reported; however, it is disproportionally lethal, accounting for 14,000 deaths [1]. In fact, ovarian cancer is responsible for more deaths in the United States than any other gynecologic malignancy. The disproportionate high mortality rate can be attributed to a combined result of nonspecific symptoms, late stage, and a lack of an effective, sensitive screening test. Vaginal ultrasound and serum CA125 are ovarian cancer screening techniques that lack sensitivity and specificity to detect these lesions at a curable stage due to the microscopic size at the origin, even when disseminated. Therefore, patients ultimately present at an advanced stage (stage III) and little chance of achieving a cure as most cannot be eradicated at surgery.

* **Corresponding author Jessica Beyda:** St. Francis Hospital Roslyn, N.Y., USA; Tel: (516) 562-6525; E-mail: Jessica.beyda@chsli.org

Typically, ovarian carcinoma occurs in the postmenopausal setting, in women over the age of 60. In the United States, the median age at diagnosis is 63 years and at death is 71 years [2]. White women have a higher incidence of ovarian cancer than blacks and Asians. Several risk factors for developing ovarian cancer have been identified. These include advanced age, nulliparity, high socioeconomic status, personal history of ovarian cancer and family history of ovarian, breast or colorectal carcinoma. Several iatrogenic risk factors have also been pinpointed such as increased use of birth control pills, gynecologic surgery (including tubal ligation) are associated with a decreased risk, while fertility drugs (Clomid) and hormone replacement therapy have been associated with an increased risk. Interestingly, environment is implicated as a risk factor as migration studies have shown ovarian cancer rates are similar to the place of immigration rather than emigration [3].

There has been increasing interest in family cancer syndromes, such as BRCA1 and BRCA2 mutations; 40% and 18%, respectively, of these women will develop ovarian cancer by age 70 without intervention, *i.e.* risk-reducing salpingo-oophorectomy (RRSO) [4]. It is important to note that RRSO is not a complete reduction of cancer risk and the risk of primary peritoneal serous carcinoma is significant at a rate of 0.2-0.35% per year after salpingo-oophorectomy, with BRCA1 mutations showing a slightly higher risk [5]. At least 10% of ovarian cancers are due to genetic predisposition and of these, 90% are due to BRCA germline mutations [6]. Recently, hereditary ovarian cancer was classified as site-specific ovarian cancer, hereditary breast/ovarian cancer (BRCA1 and BRCA2), and hereditary non-polyposis colorectal cancer (HNPCC, Lynch syndrome II). Site-specific ovarian cancer, considered "ovarian-specific" variant of hereditary breast/ovarian cancer, refers to families with two or more first- or first- and second-degree relatives with ovarian cancer and a life time risk three times higher than the general population. HNPCC is an autosomal dominant syndrome with increased risk of colon and endometrial cancer, and less commonly, accounts for 2% of ovarian cancers [6, 7]. Compared to sporadic ovarian cancer, familial ovarian cancer occurs at a younger age, is of higher grade and stage yet the prognosis is better for BRCA associated familial cases of ovarian cancer [8].

Established prognostic factors for ovarian cancer patients are FIGO (Federation of International Gynecologic Oncology) stage and volume of residual disease after surgical staging with or without debulking in stage IIIC and IV patients [9]. Age is also a prognostic factor however, is likely not independent [10]. Although cell type, histopathologic grade, and tumor rupture are important factors for prognosis, they remain embedded in controversy [11].

Of note, ovarian carcinomas are only a subset of ovarian tumors. In fact, of primary ovarian tumors, 25% are malignant. Ovarian tumors are quite heterogeneous, reflecting the range of types of cells present in the ovary, such as epithelial surface cells, mesenchymal stromal cells with steroid producing cells, and germs cells. Ovarian tumors are broadly classified into three main groups based on cell of origin and morphology, as illustrated in Table **1** below: (i) epithelial, (ii) sex-cord stromal, and (iii) germ cell. Epithelial neoplasms are the most common of the groups, comprising 50% of ovarian tumors and up to 90% of ovarian malignancies [12]. As the largest of the groups, and in pathologic terms, ovarian carcinoma of epithelial origin is the most often diagnosis referred to in the colloquial diagnosis of "ovarian cancer."

Additionally, even though carcinomas are usually clinically regarded as a single group, each distinct subtype has a unique pathogenesis, behavior, and prognosis. The histopathologic classification is crucial as ovarian neoplasms often have a similar vague clinical presentation; such as abdominal pain or distension, occurring in women in their 40s-50s with solid and cystic masses on imaging studies. Accurate pathologic classification is essential as newer adjuvant therapies increasingly target specific tumor subtypes. Also, determining the carcinoma subtype may direct genetic testing, for example, BRCA testing in high grade serous carcinoma or Lynch testing in endometrioid or clear cell carcinomas.

The most common subtypes of ovarian carcinoma include: high grade serous carcinoma, low grade serous carcinoma, mucinous carcinoma, endometrioid carcinoma, and clear cell carcinoma. As a side note, each of the epithelial carcinomas has borderline counterparts with intermediate clinical and histological features between benign cystadenomas and carcinomas. This category was first introduced in the early 1970s to describe a subset of ovarian epithelial tumors without invasion yet occasionally exhibiting malignant features [12]. Other terminology for borderline tumors includes atypical proliferative tumors and ovarian tumors of low malignant potential. It used to be widely accepted that benign, borderline, and malignant ovarian tumors are progressions of malignant transformation; however, newer studies have proved that this not often the case for some serous carcinomas. Furthermore, serous carcinomas are also subdivided into high grade and low-grade carcinomas, which are thought to develop separately.

Table **1** shows that there are many subtypes of ovarian cancers. The majority of ovarian "cancers" are the high-grade serous carcinomas. These tumors have distinct histologic features which distinguish them from the other ovarian carcinomas, as will be discussed subsequently.

Table 1. Main categories of primary ovarian malignancy.

Epithelial Tumors	Sex-Cord Stromal Tumors	Germ Cell Tumors
Serous carcinoma, high grade Serous carcinoma, low grade Mucinous carcinomas Endometrioid carcinomas Clear cell carcinomas Others	Granulosa cell tumors Others	Malignant transformation in Mature teratoma ('dermoid') Yolk sack tumor Dysgerminoma Others

Tumor Subtypes: Low-grade Serous (Type I), High-grade Serous (Type II)

Serous carcinoma is separated into two categories: type I (low grade serous carcinoma) and type II (high grade serous carcinoma). These carcinomas arise from different and independent molecular events. Low grade serous carcinomas often have KRAS and BRAF mutations and occur in younger patients, associated with slow-growing borderline tumors which appear to arise from cystadenomas. In contrast, high grade serous carcinomas have p53 mutations with a high rate of genetic instability and rapid tumor growth which is often detected and diagnosed in late stages. This high rate of genetic instability found in most ovarian carcinomas, Type II, proves to be extraordinarily difficult when targeting molecular defects for screening and therapy purposes. Additionally, due to a low proliferative index, low grade serous carcinomas are often more chemoresistant than high grade serous carcinomas.

Histogenesis: Ovarian Surface Epithelium *versus* Fallopian Tube (STIC)

There are different models hypothesizing the origin of high grade serous carcinomas. Historically, it was widely accepted that serous carcinomas originate from the ovary, shedding from the ovarian surface and spreading into the peritoneal cavity. According to the classic model of ovarian carcinoma, tumor cells arise from ovarian surface mesothelium undergoing tubal-type metaplastic change and malignant transformation, presumably after repeated ovulation induced trauma. A significant portion of ovarian tumors, specifically type 1, do appear to arise from cortical inclusion cysts thus suggesting a gradual progression from precursor to cancer. However, with increased awareness of BRCA mutations and prophylactic salpingo-oopherectomies, the classic model of the origin of high grade serous carcinoma has evolved. As more cases of early, small, non-invasive serous carcinomas (serous tubal intraepithelial carcinoma or STIC, pictured in Fig. (1)) have been identified, particularly involving the fimbriated end of fallopian tubes in prophylactic cases, a newer hypothesis of tubal origin of high grade serous carcinoma has been supported. Prophylactic specimens from women with BRCA mutations have shown tubal epithelium atypia, carcinoma *in situ*, and high-grade serous tubal carcinoma [13]. Molecular studies have provided additional support for tubal origin of some high-grade serous carcinomas. These studies not only demonstrated that STIC lesions also harbor p53 mutations, a recent study found STIC and concurrent ovarian high-grade serous carcinoma share identical p53 mutations [14]. Further evidence in support of tubal origin in serous carcinogenesis, several studies have shown an association with chronic salpingitis and ovarian and tubal serous carcinoma suggesting that inflammatory changes are possibly involved in carcinogenesis and may lead to fimbrial epithelium deposition in the ovarian surface and cortex [15 - 18]. According to data from the World Health Organization (WHO) in 2015, it has been reported that up to 60% of extrauterine high grade serous carcinomas have concurrent STIC. Of note, while ovarian and fallopian tube serous carcinomas are staged and treated similarly, there is no clinical standard regarding management of STIC.

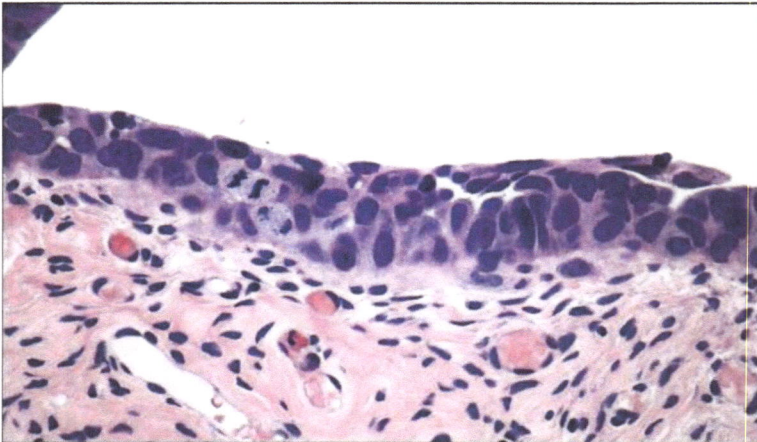

Fig. (1). STIC (400x) Tubal epithelium showing expansion, loss of polarity, tufting, and mitoses. Cytologically, increased nuclear-to-cytoplasmic ratios, nuclear pleomorphism, hyperchomasia, and conspicuous nucleoli.

As aforementioned, many studies have shown that a significant portion of pelvic serous carcinomas arise in the fimbria as STIC, as well as a high percentage of early carcinomas found in BRCA positive women arise in the fimbria. The diagnosis of STIC, in addition to atypical and malignant tubal epithelium, requires p53 mutations, confirmed by strong and diffuse p53 immunohistochemistry (IHC), and a proliferative index greater than 10%. To increase the likelihood of detecting early tubal cancer, the Sectioning and Extensively Examining the Fimbriated end (SEE-FIM) protocol was developed to expose maximum surface area of the fimbria [19]. With the advent of the SEE-FIM protocol facilitating meticulous histopathologic and immunohistochemical evaluation of the tube, more and more studies continue to elucidate the serous carcinogenesis model. A putative, latent precursor to pelvic serous carcinoma, the p53 signature, has been described and shares the following with serous carcinoma: fimbrial location, cell of origin (secretory cell), DNA damage, and p53 mutations; however, the mucosa is otherwise benign [14]. Subsequently described is an intermediary between p53 signatures and STIC, termed serous tubal intraepithelial lesion (STIL), which in addition to DNA damage and p53 mutation, has epithelial expansion and proliferation. p53 signature and STIL are not established diagnoses and their clinical relevance is unknown thus only applicable in the research setting. A recent study sheds additional light on the fimbria's role in carcinogenesis by describing the tubal peritoneal junction (TPJ), where peritoneum and fimbrial epithelium meet. As junctions between different epithelia and transitional metaplasias, also found at the TPJ, are known for malignant potential, this phenomenon suggests the TPJ of the fimbria is indeed the site of serous carcinogenesis [12].

Another hypothesis relating to the origin of high grade serous carcinoma is that there is a field effect where native or metaplastic tubal-type epithelium are under the same influences, leading to multifocal lesions, rather than there being a direct precursor from either the ovary or the fallopian tube. Either way, the site of origin of the tumor is often difficult to discern due to massive, bulky disease and currently there is little clinical relevance.

The second most common ovarian cancer is endometrioid carcinoma comprising up to 25% of primary cancers [20]. These Type I lesions are the subset of ovarian cancers arising from cysts and show mutations in K-ras, pTEN, and CTNNB1 (β-catenin encoding gene) [3]. Due to the slow growth of these tumors from benign cysts that grow quite large before transforming to cancer, most patients are diagnosed with a large pelvic mass on pelvic examination facilitating treatment at an earlier and more curable stage, also reflecting the associated favorable prognosis. There is associated endometriosis in up to 15% of endometrioid carcinomas with many tumors seen directly arising from endometriotic cysts; occasionally the full morphologic spectrum of endometriosis with hyperplasia to atypical hyperplasia to carcinoma is appreciable [21]. Less common than endometrioid carcinoma, clear cell carcinoma has the highest association of all with endometriosis and with atypical changes in the vicinity. Endometriosis can be found in up to 10% of reproductive-age women, however malignant transformation is low, 0.3% develop cancer [22]. The mean age of endometrioid cancer associated with endometriosis is younger, 50 years, than unassociated endometrioid cancer, 55-58 years [23]. Since Type I slow growing tumors arise in endometriosis, the likelihood of identifying the precursor lesion is greater thus endometriosis is the best documented and most readily appreciated precursor of ovarian cancer. The proposed origin of type I tumors is retrograde menstruation leading to endometriosis of the ovary followed by atypical proliferative tumors which may develop into endometrioid or clear cell carcinomas. Endometriosis of the ovary is significantly more likely to give rise to cancer than extraovarian endometriosis [24]. Additional support for the premalignant potential of endometriosis is shown by molecular alterations, such as loss of heterozygosity in the PTEN gene and microsatellite instability, indicating neoplastic changes [25].

SEROUS TUMORS

Serous Cystadenoma

(Adenofibroma, cystadenofibroma, surface papillomas): Cyst lined by fallopian-tube type cells. Comprise two-thirds of benign OSE tumors, however most are cystically dilated inclusions and recently shown to be polyclonal and thus not neoplastic [26, 27].

Clinical: Age 40-60. Asymptomatic, or nonspecific pelvic pain/discomfort, 12-23% bilateral [3].

Gross findings: At least 1 cm and up to 30 cm, with average size of 5-8 cm. Thin walled cysts filled with serous (watery) or seromucinous (slightly viscous) fluid. Variable papillary excrescences on the surface and lining. Adenofibromas present as rubbery nodules.

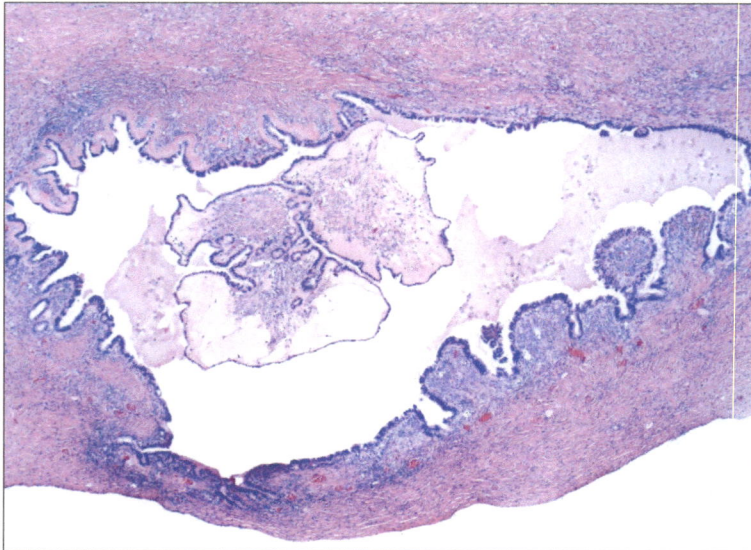

Fig. (2). Serous cystadenofibroma (40x) Thick fibrous papillae lined by a single layer of Mullerian epithelium project into the cyst lumen.

Histology (Figs. **2**, **3**): Psuedostratified columnar cells (secretory and ciliated cells). Also, may be a single layer of flat to cuboidal cells. Usually lack proliferation, atypia, and mitoses, however these findings must compromise less than 10% of tumor when present. Psammoma bodies are present in 15% of cases [3].

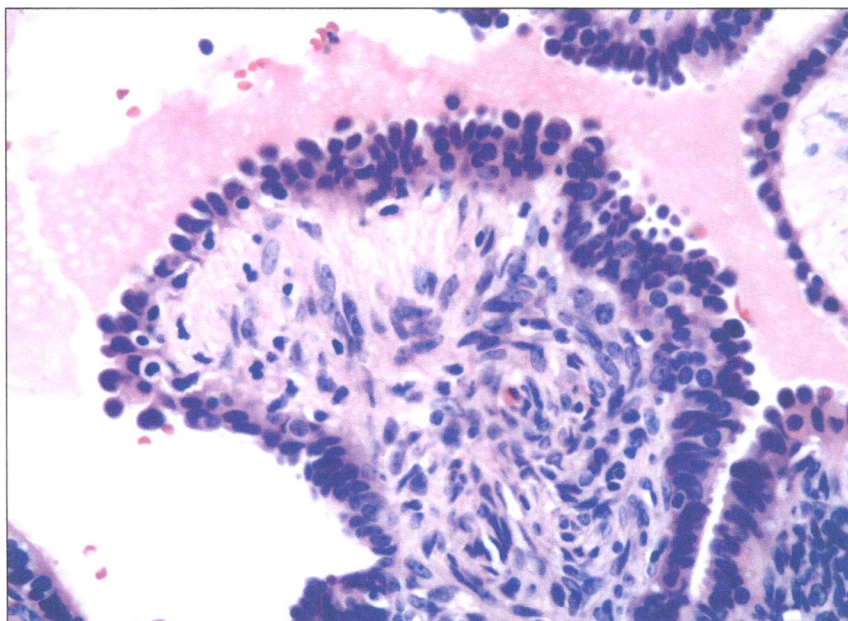

Fig. (3). Serous cystadenofibroma (400x) Thick fibrous papilla lined by a single layer of monomorphic Mullerian epithelium.

Prognosis: Benign, may recur.

Atypical Proliferative Serous Tumor (APST) or Serous Borderline Tumor (SBT)

Most common borderline variant (50%) [28]. Intermediary of cystadenomas and serous carcinoma displaying fallopian-tube type cells with proliferation and atypia. Peritoneal lesions associated with borderline tumors are classified as implants (noninvasive epithelial or desmoplastic-type) or metastatic low-grade serous carcinoma (invasive or noninvasive with micropapillae).

Clinical: Average age is 42. Approximately 55% are bilateral and 56% of bilateral tumors show extraovarian involvement [29]. Associated with infertility. BRCA mutations less likely.

Gross findings: Average size is 5 cm (8 cm for noninvasive MPSC) [30]. The mass is cystic with abundant delicate and friable papillary excrescences of the lining. Up to 70% showing involvement of the surface of the ovary, also more likely to be seen with peritoneal implants [29]. To exclude invasion, extensive sampling is required and recently 2 sections per cm are recommended rather than 1 section [3].

Histology (Figs. **4-9**): At least 10% of the tumor must show extensive epithelial stratification, tufting or budding, and detached cells or clusters, otherwise these lesions exhibit a wide spectrum of morphology. The lower, or benign, end of the spectrum shows cuboidal to columnar cells with a complex hierarchical branching pattern (where papillae become smaller as they separate from the main mass). Behaving like low-grade serous carcinoma at the upper end of the spectrum is noninvasive micropapillary serous carcinoma (MPSC), pictured in Figs. (**10-20**), showing long, delicate micropapillae with minimal fibrovascular stroma radiating directly from a thick, centrally located fibrovascular core; these features must be present in at least 5 mm of confluence or 10% of the tumor to qualify as this entity. Noninvasive MPSC is often referred to as "medusa head" in appearance. There is a strong association of noninvasive MPSC with metastatic low-grade serous carcinoma (invasive implants) [31]. Several proposed theories for this phenomenon include sampling error (missed occult invasion), the complex micropapillary growth is a form of invasion or a "carcinoma *in situ*" which exfoliates malignant cells onto peritoneal surfaces that seed and grow [31]. Further supporting noninvasive MPSC's malignant potential is the increased association with lymph node metastasis [32].

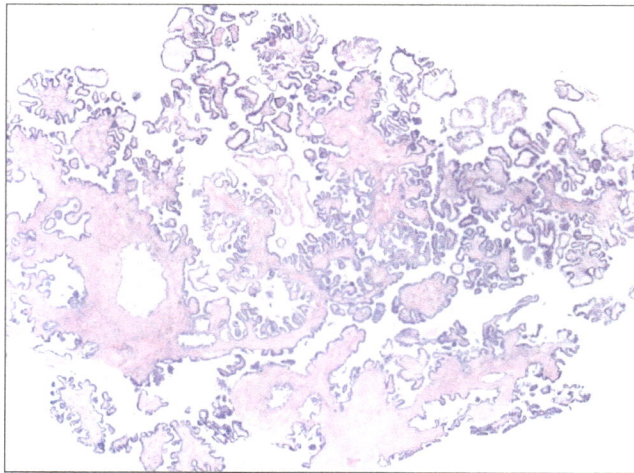

Fig. (4). APST (SBT) (20x) Characteristically seen is this complex hierarchical branching pattern where successive branching gives rise to smaller and smaller papillae.

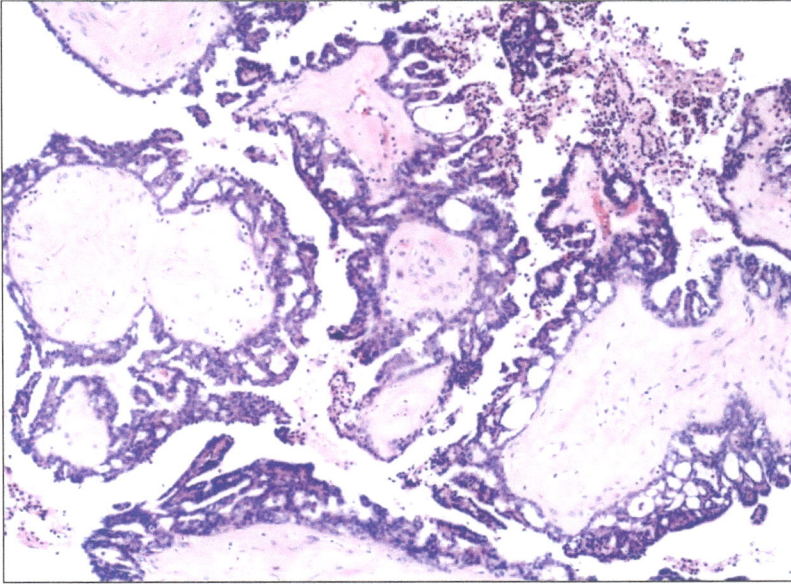

Fig. (5). APST (SBT) (100x) Characteristically seen is this complex hierarchical branching pattern where successive branching gives rise to smaller and smaller papillae and eventually detached cell clusters. Fusion of papillae imparts the appearance of Roman bridges and cribriforming.

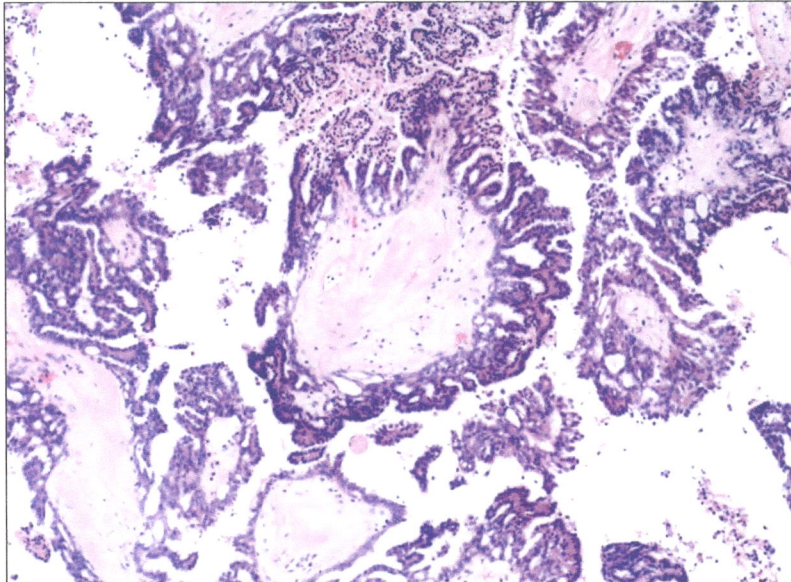

Fig. (6). APST (SBT) (100x) Characteristically seen is this complex hierarchical branching pattern where successive branching gives rise to smaller papillae and eventually detached cell clusters. Fusion of papillae imparts the appearance of Roman bridges and cribriforming.

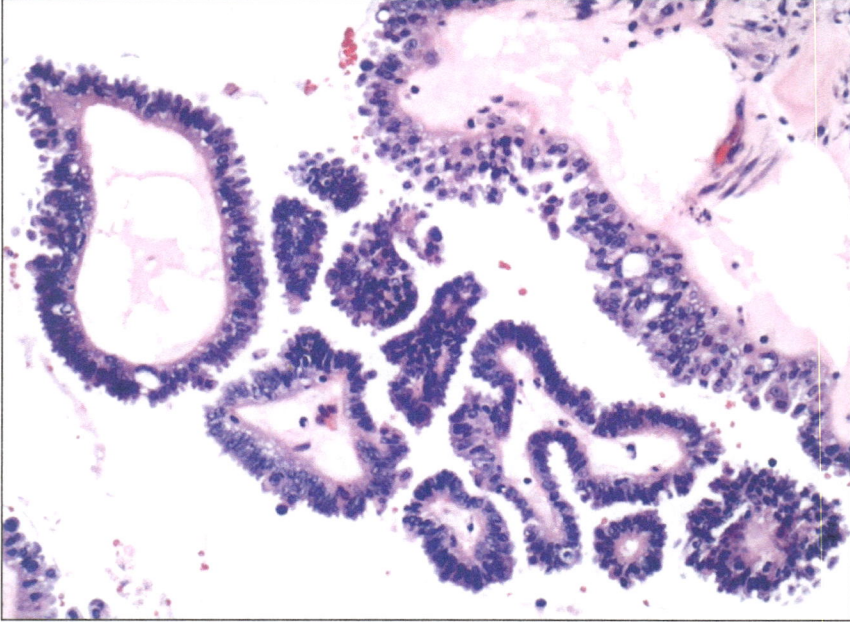

Fig. (7). APST (SBT) (200x) Small papillae and cell clusters detached from a larger papilla. Epithelium shows budding and tufting.

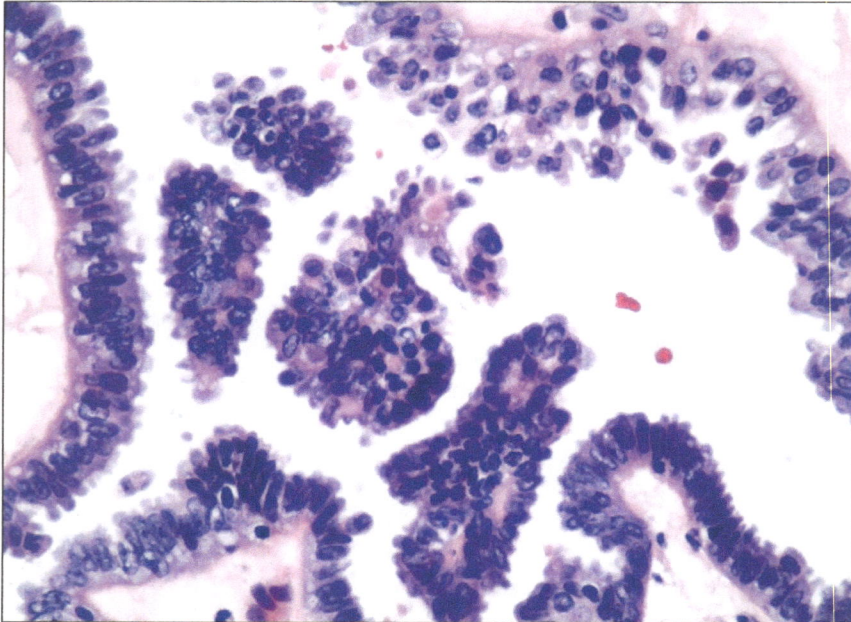

Fig. (8). APST (SBT) (400x) Mostly pseudostratified columnar, including some cuboidal, cells with mild to moderate nuclear atypia and small prominent nucleoli.

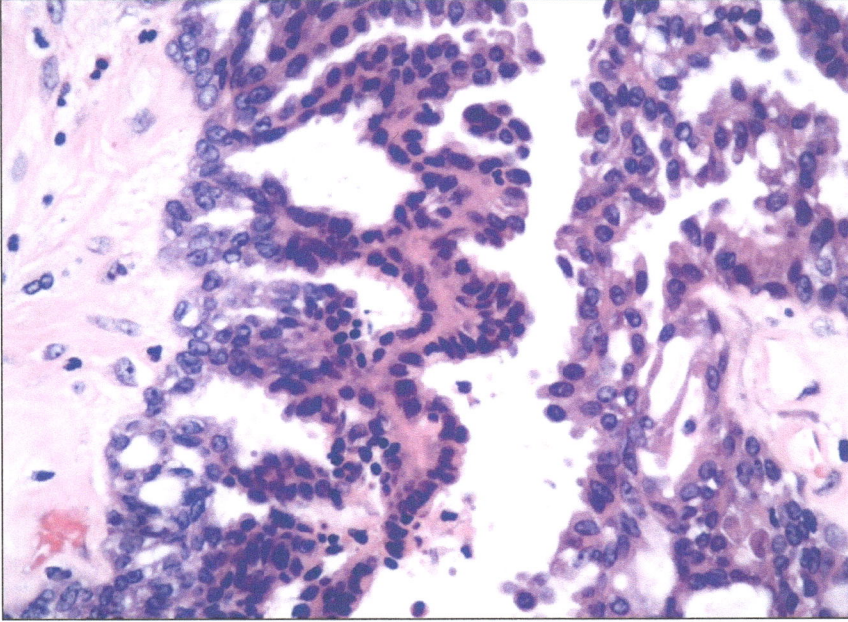

Fig. (9). APST (SBT) (400x) Fusion of papillae seen here as Roman bridging and cribriforming. Cytologic atypia is mild to moderate and small prominent nucleoli.

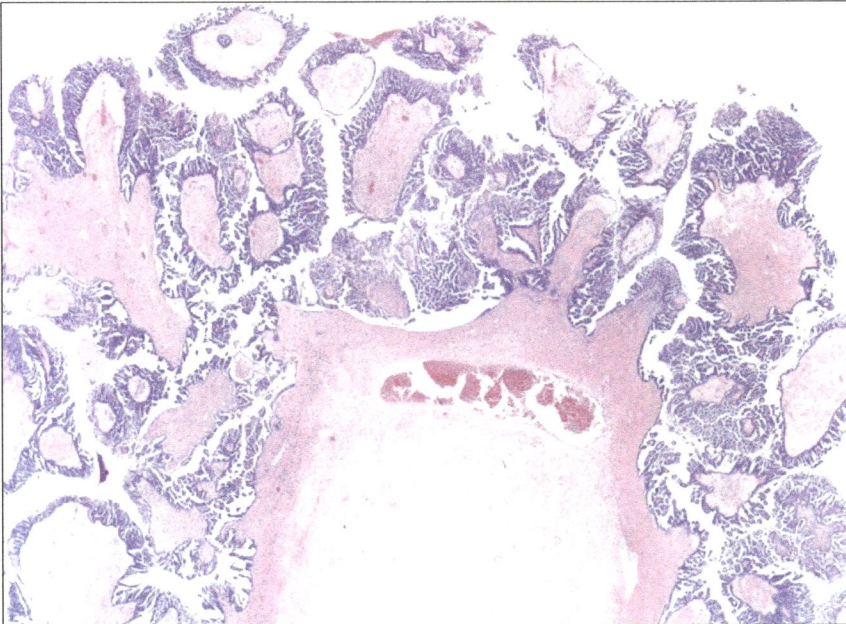

Fig. (10). Noninvasive micropapillary serous carcinoma (20x) Large, fibrotic papillae abruptly give rise to numerous long and thin micropapillae, the so-called Medusa head appearance.

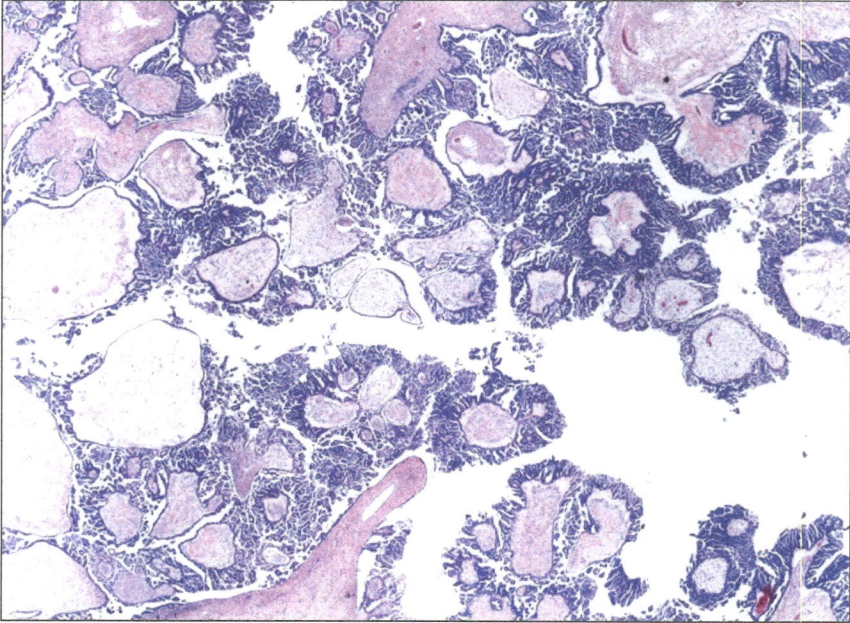

Fig. (11). Noninvasive micropapillary serous carcinoma (20x) Large, fibrotic papillae abruptly give rise to numerous long and thin micropapillae, the so-called Medusa head appearance.

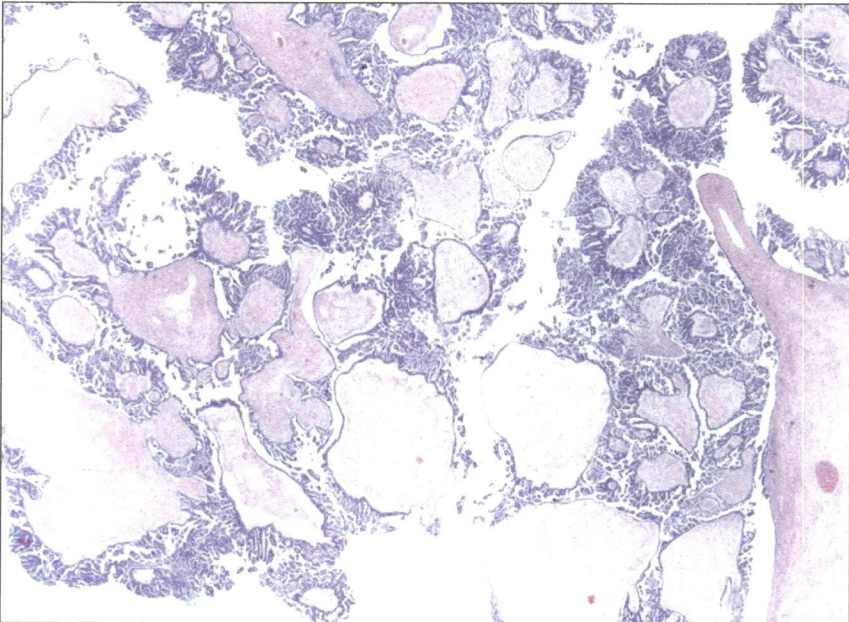

Fig. (12). Noninvasive micropapillary serous carcinoma (20x) Large, fibrotic papillae abruptly give rise to numerous long and thin micropapillae, the so-called Medusa head appearance.

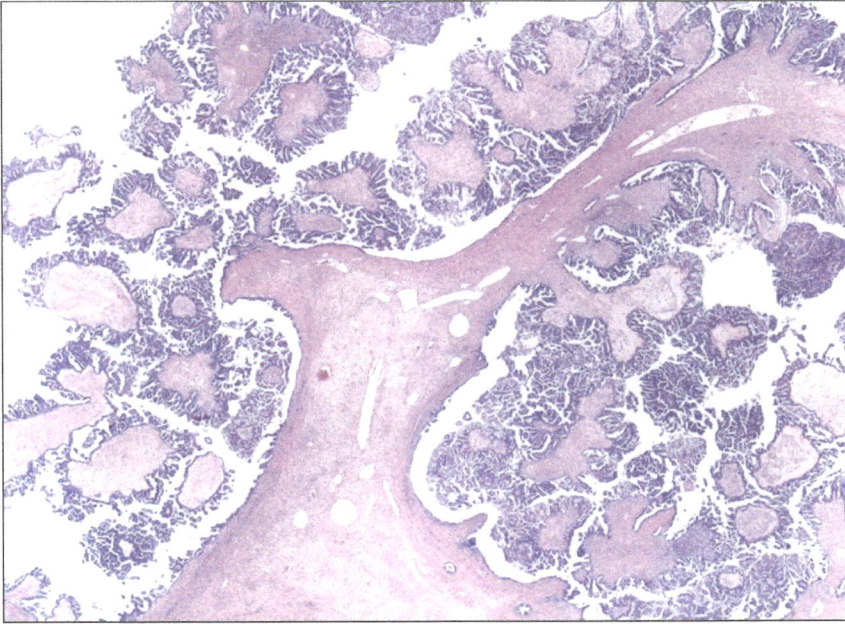

Fig. (13). Noninvasive micropapillary serous carcinoma (20x) Large, fibrotic papillae abruptly give rise to numerous long and thin micropapillae, the so-called Medusa head appearance.

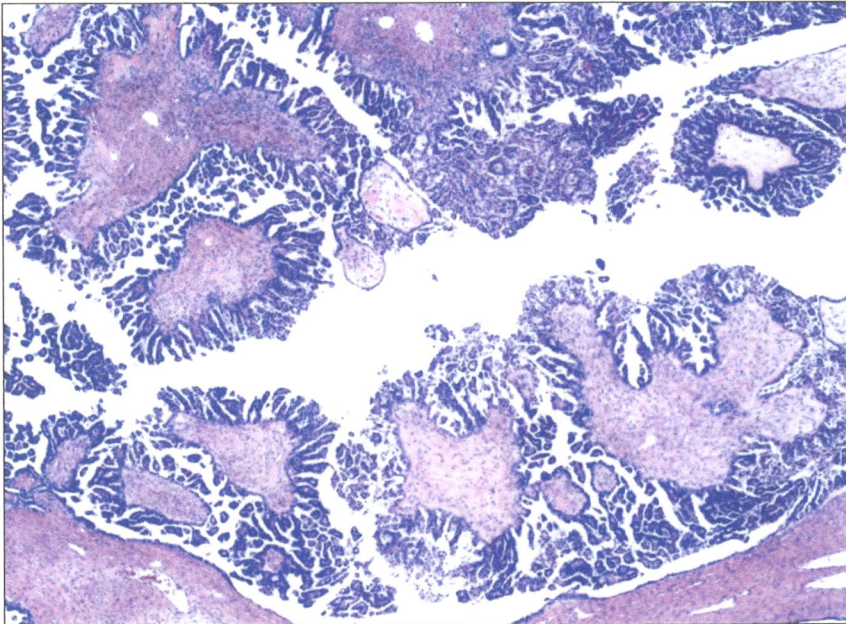

Fig. (14). Noninvasive micropapillary serous carcinoma (40x) Large, fibrotic papillae abruptly give rise to numerous long and thin micropapillae, the so-called Medusa head appearance.

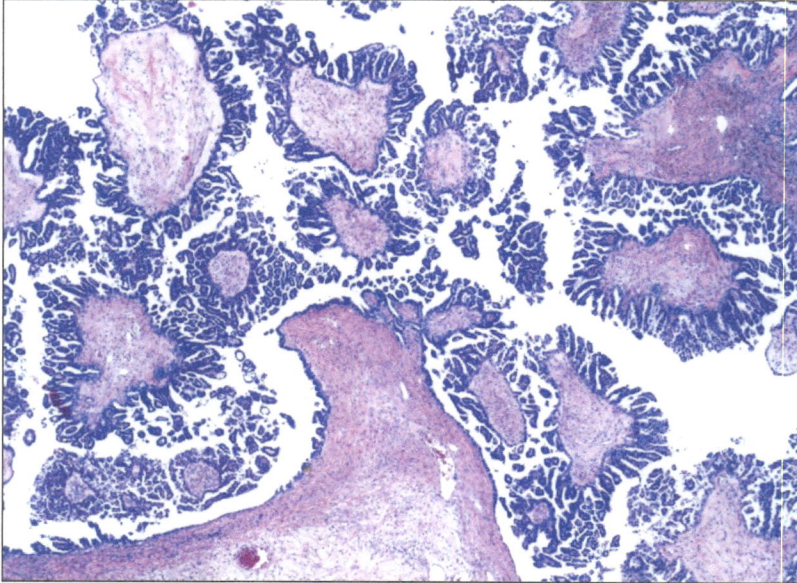

Fig. (15). Noninvasive micropapillary serous carcinoma (40x) Large, fibrotic papillae abruptly give rise to numerous long and thin micropapillae, the so-called Medusa head appearance.

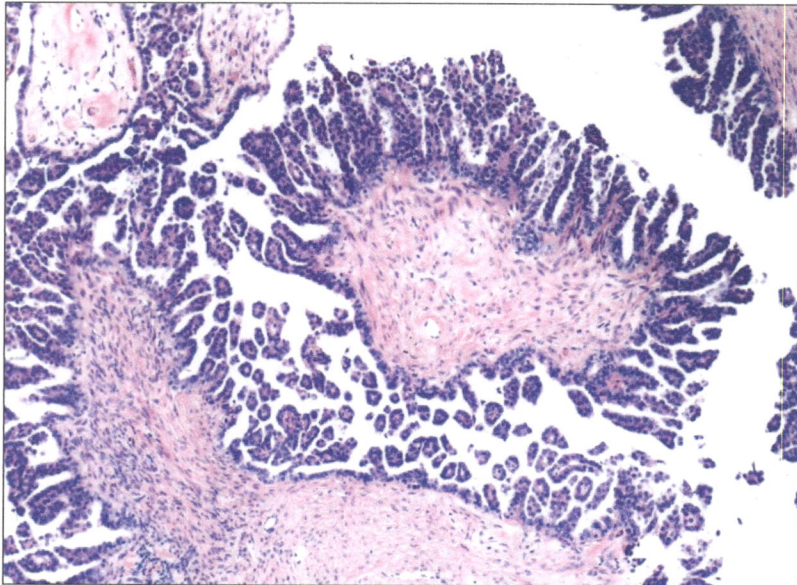

Fig. (16). Noninvasive micropapillary serous carcinoma (100x) Large, fibrotic papillae abruptly give rise to numerous long and thin micropapillae, the so-called Medusa head appearance. The delicate micropapillae lack significant fibrovascular cores.

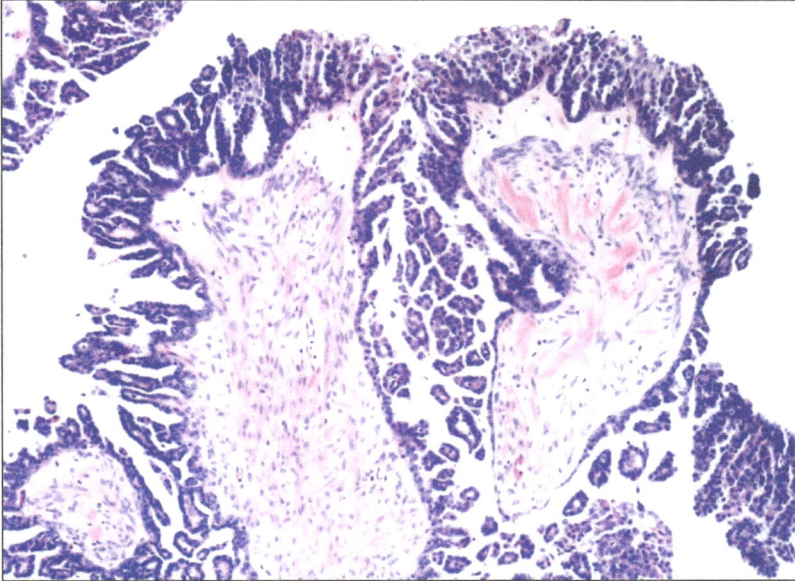

Fig. (17). Noninvasive micropapillary serous carcinoma (100x) Large, fibrotic papillae abruptly give rise to numerous long and thin micropapillae, the so-called Medusa head appearance. The delicate micropapillae lack significant fibrovascular cores.

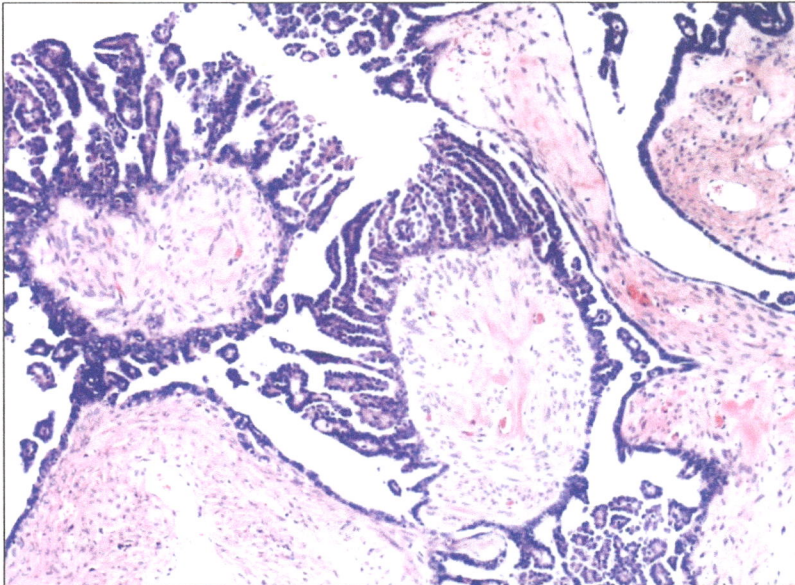

Fig. (18). Noninvasive micropapillary serous carcinoma (100x) Large, fibrotic papillae abruptly give rise to numerous long and thin micropapillae, the so-called Medusa head appearance. The delicate micropapillae lack significant fibrovascular cores.

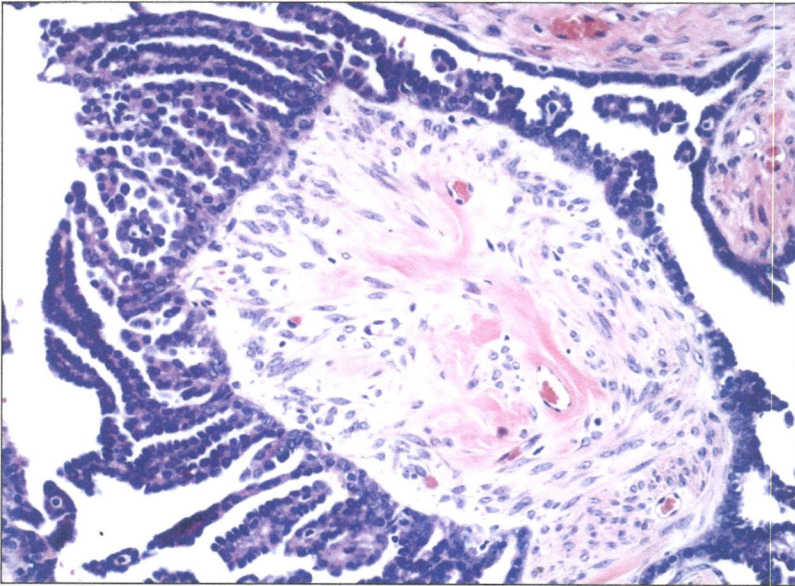

Fig. (19). Noninvasive micropapillary serous carcinoma (200x) Large, fibrotic papillae abruptly give rise to numerous long and thin micropapillae, the so-called Medusa head appearance. The delicate micropapillae lack significant fibrovascular cores and the epithelial lining shows hobnail cells.

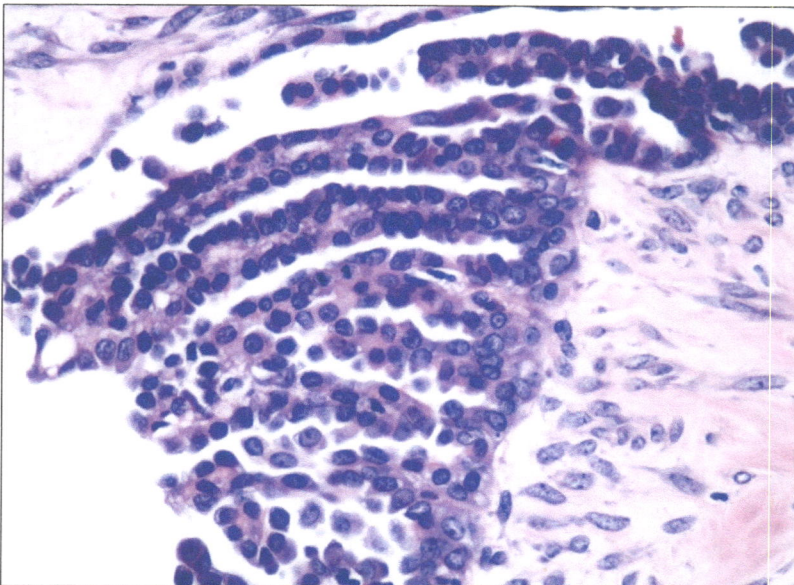

Fig. (20). Noninvasive micropapillary serous carcinoma (400x) The delicate papillae lack significant fibrovascular cores and show cuboidal cells with mild to moderate cytologic atypia, small prominent nucleoli, and a low mitotic rate.

Microinvasion is defined as <5 mm area of cells infiltrating the ovarian stroma. Stromal invaginations of the papillae on tangential sections are frequent and require distinction from invasion. Roman bridges or cribriforming may be seen when papillae fuse. Cells show epithelial, including ciliated cells like the fallopian tube, or mesothelial differentiation. Hobnail cells may be seen, where cell nuclei protrude from papillae into surrounding spaces. Cytologic atypia is mild, nuclei are ovoid or rounded with fine chromatin and inconspicuous nucleoli, and polarity is maintained. Mitoses are uncommon and are typically below four per ten high-power fields [33]. Psammoma bodies are common. Autoimplants, microscopically identical to noninvasive desmoplastic implants, may be present on the ovarian surface and in one third of cases show infarcted papillae [34].

Molecular: KRAS, BRAF, ERBB2 mutations (HER2/neu, only present with absent KRAS or BRAF mutations) [35].

Prognosis: Stage dependent. If confined to ovary (Stage I), no different than general population (100% survival), but may recur 20 years later [36]. Advanced stage noninvasive MPSC has a 5- and 10-year survival rate of 75-85% and 40-60%, respectively [37]. Microinvasion does not change the prognosis. Non-invasive implants have a high chance of recurrence. Most important factor is extra-ovarian invasive implants (low-grade serous carcinoma), shown to have a recurrence rate of 65% and a survival rate like low-grade serous carcinoma [38].

Low-grade Serous Carcinoma (Psammocarcinoma, MPSC)

Uncommon, 4% of ovarian carcinomas. Invasive lesion with low-grade cytologic atypia.

Clinical: Average age of 45 years, and 54 years for psammocarcinoma (psammomatous variant) [39]. Usually asymptomatic but advanced stage presents as abdominal pain, fullness, or distention; 80-90% are bilateral and 94% are advanced stage [37, 40].

Gross: Average size is 11 cm, 54% with ovarian surface lesions [37]. Cystic and papillary growth with a variable amount of friable tissue. Psammocarcinoma is associated with uterine serosal adhesions and invasion [39].

Histology (Figs. **21-24**): LGSC displays many architectural patterns, often complex papillary growth, with stromal invasion. The invasion is seen as disorganized infiltration by single cells, solid nests, micropapillae, and less commonly macropapillae; usually a clear space, or cleft, encompasses the invasive components [37]. The cause of these clefts is unknown, however recently some have been identified as lymphatic spaces. One third of MPSCs have intratumoral lymphatic invasion [41]. Aside from the invasion, noninvasive and

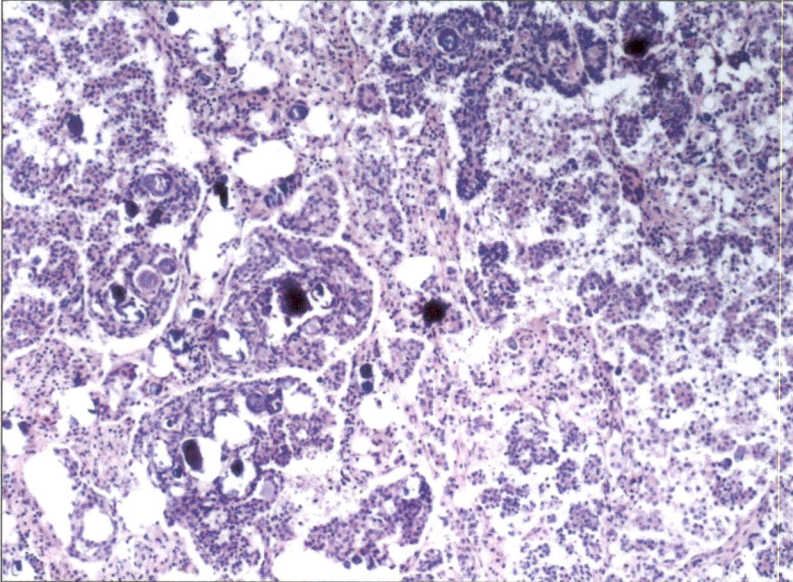

Fig. (21). Low grade serous carcinoma (100x) Confluent glandular and cribriform patterns on the *left* and micropapillary pattern on the *right*.

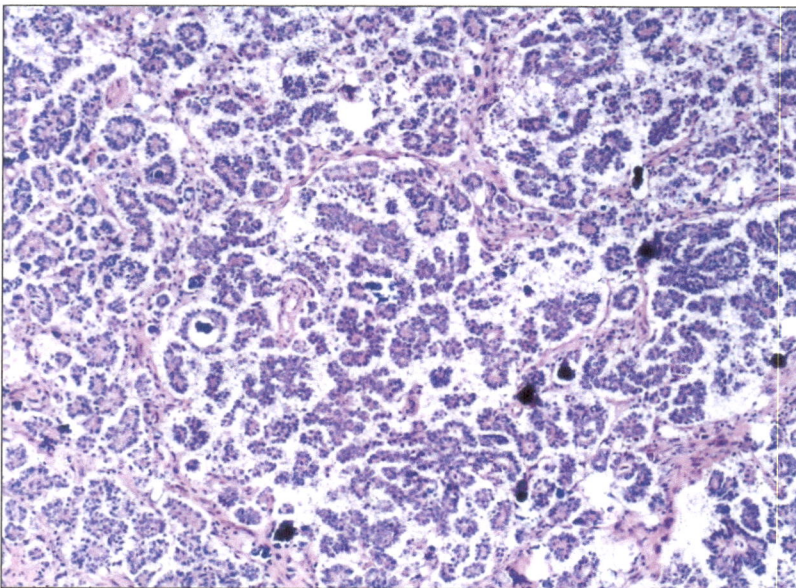

Fig. (22). Low grade serous carcinoma (100x) Confluent micropapillary pattern of growth seen as seemingly freely floating micropapillae and associated psammoma bodies.

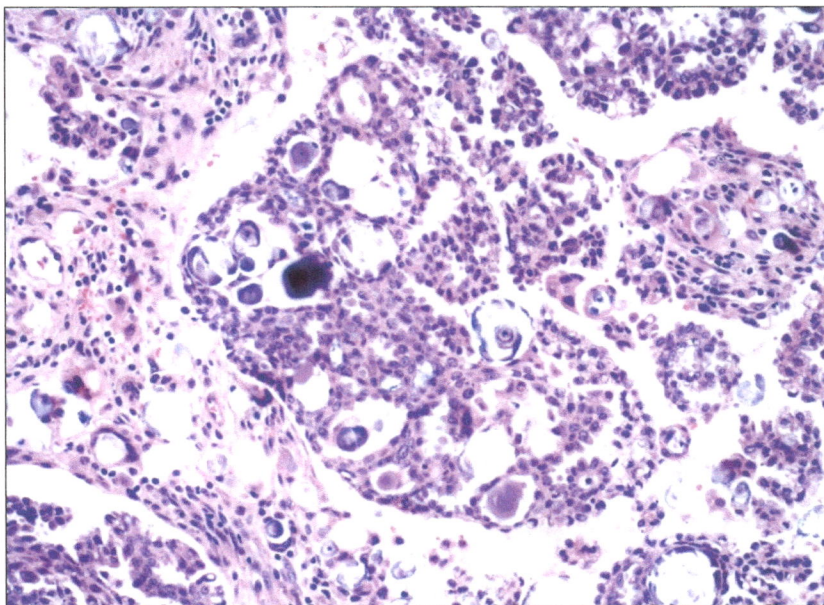

Fig. (23). Low grade serous carcinoma (200x) Cribriform pattern with psammoma bodies showing mild to moderate cytologic atypia.

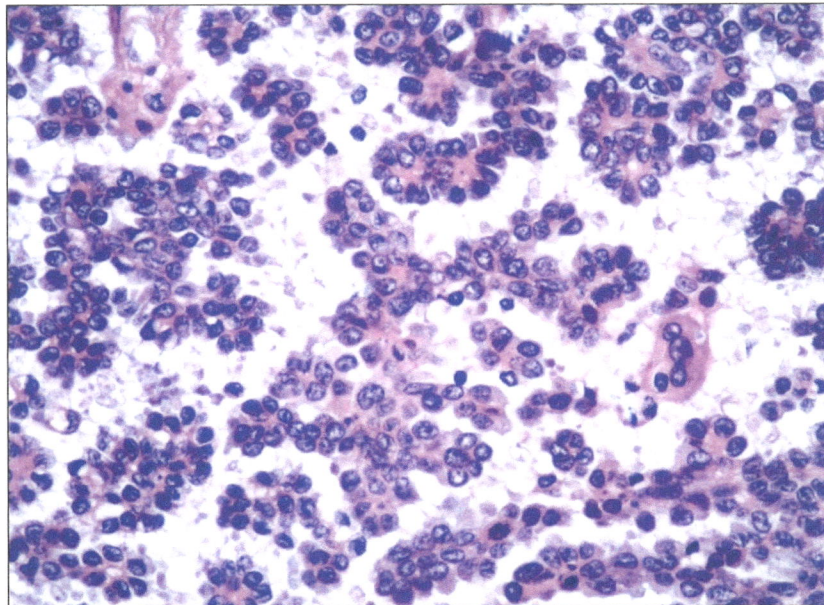

Fig. (24). Low grade serous carcinoma (400x) Micropapillary pattern showing moderate cytologic atypia. Chromatin pattern ranges from hyperchromatic to vesicular with clumpy chromatin, occasional small prominent nucleoli, and rare mitosis.

invasive MPSC are morphologically identical. When metastases (invasive implants) were identified, thorough histologic examination revealed invasion of the primary ovarian tumor [42]. Many cases have an associated serous borderline tumor component whereas high-grade serous carcinoma rarely does [37], again underscoring the different pathogenesis of low-grade and high-grade serous carcinomas. The cells are rounded with minimal cytoplasm, mild to moderate nuclear atypia with a small nucleolus, and limited nuclear pleomorphism [43]. If severe nuclear atypia is present without invasion, the diagnosis should be high-grade serous carcinoma. Frequent psammoma bodies are seen. More than 75% of psammocarcinoma papillae are replaced by psammoma bodies [39]. Necrosis is very rare and there is low mitotic activity (<3 per high power field) [37].

Immunohistochemistry: p53 is focal. WT1, ER/PR (50%), EMA, and CK7 are positive [3]. Ki-67 proliferation index is low.

Molecular: KRAS, BRAF, ERBB2 mutations (HER2/neu, only present with absent KRAS or BRAF mutations). Loss of 1p36 and CDKN2A/B [44].

Prognosis: Rarely Stage I (confined to the ovaries) which has an excellent prognosis and advanced stage can have mortality of 50%. Advanced stage low-grade serous carcinoma portends a better prognosis and smaller volume disease than stage matched high-grade serous carcinoma [36]; rarely transforms to high-grade serous carcinoma [45]. Progression free survival is 2 years and the median survival is 6-7 years [46]. Five-year survival rate is 75% for FIGO stage III [3]. Generally, these are slow growing tumors resistant to chemotherapy (platinum-taxane), however primary and secondary cytoreduction are efficacious [46, 47].

High-grade Serous Carcinoma (HGSC)

Most common and lethal ovarian carcinoma. Severe cytologic atypia is pathognomonic.

Clinical: Average age is 57 to 63 years [3]. The non-specific symptoms (abdominal pain, fullness, or distention) lead to a delayed diagnosis and presentation at advanced stage with extensive abdominopelvic disease either by direct extension or metastasis. Abdominal pain and distention are the most common presenting symptoms due to ascites or bulky tumor. Gastrointestinal and genitourinary symptoms, such as dysuria, urinary frequency, and vaginal bleeding, are also common. Asymptomatic, stage I presentation is exceedingly rare. Three fourths of women with a history of breast cancer presenting with peritoneal carcinomatosis have a primary ovarian or peritoneal serous carcinoma [48].

Gross: Range from microscopic to 20 cm multilocular, complex (solid and cystic) masses with delicate, friable papillary excrescences filling the cysts, and sometimes are entirely solid. Two thirds are bilateral [3]. External surface is smooth and may show papillary projections. Hemorrhage and necrosis are common. Omental cakes form by fusion of firm metastatic nodules. Microscopic tumor is detected in 22% of grossly normal omentectomy specimens [3].

Histology (Figs. **25-37**): Complex papillary, glandular, cribriform, or solid growth of severely cytologically atypical cells, the hallmark of high-grade serous carcinoma. Extensive bridging and fusing of papillae causes characteristic slit-like spaces. A villoglandular papillary pattern resembling endometrioid carcinoma may also be seen, however the high-grade cytology will exclude this entity. Foci of small, uniform cells does not exclude high-grade serous carcinoma, nor does cytoplasmic clearing akin to clear cell carcinoma (as diagnostic features for this lesion are absent). Cytologically, nuclei are large, bizarre, and pleomorphic with irregular chromatin distribution, often vesicular, with large, eosinophilic nucleoli. Large, angulated, and hyperchromatic nuclei with a smudgy quality, referred to as "smudge cells," are commonly seen. Multinucleated tumor giant cells or syncytial-like aggregates are common as well, especially in the solid growth pattern. Mitotic activity is brisk exceeding 12 mitotic figures per 10 HPF and includes atypical mitoses. Necrosis is common. Psammoma bodies are seen in 25% of these carcinomas [3].

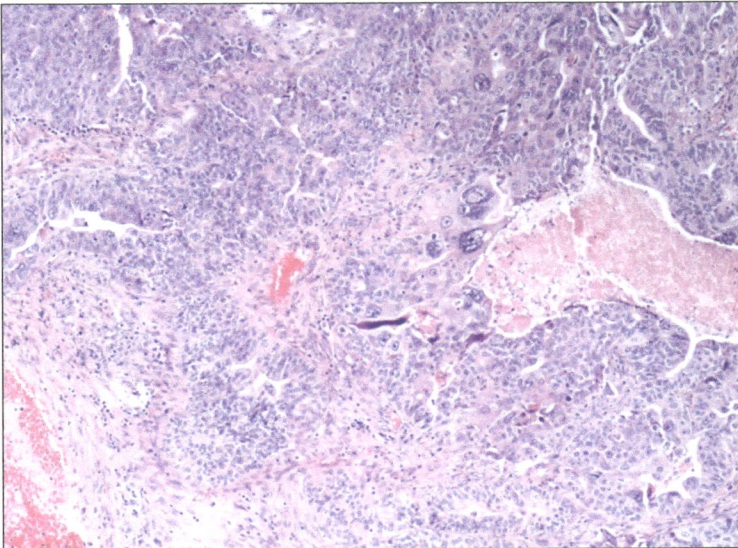

Fig. (25). HGSC (100x) Solid and glandular growth pattern with characteristic slit-like spaces, irregular luminal contours, necrosis, and severe cytologic atypia (*center right*).

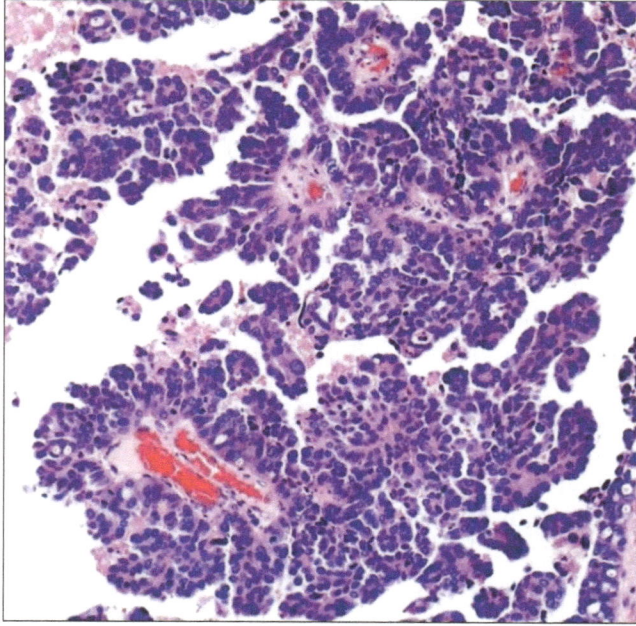

Fig. (26). HGSC 100x Papillary growth pattern with slit-like spaces due to papillary coalescence.

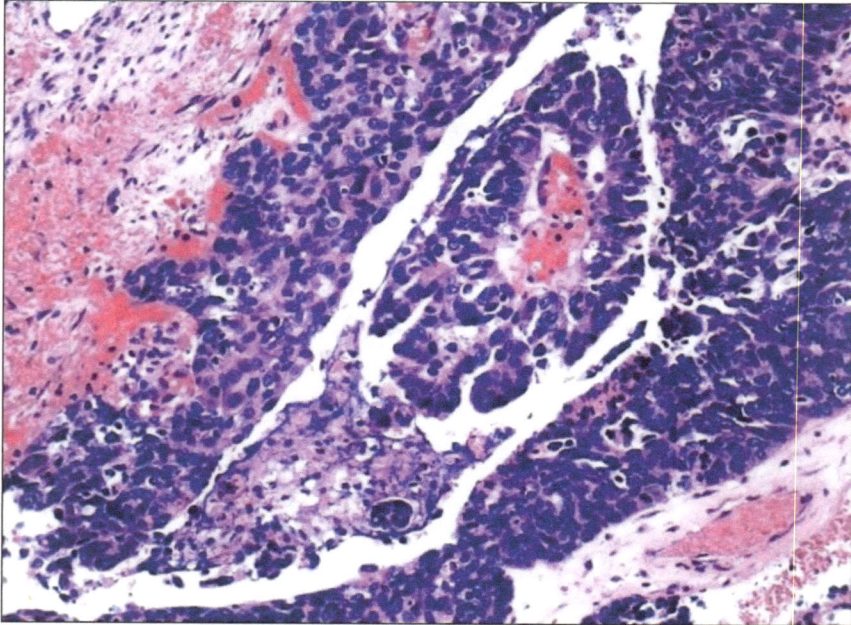

Fig. (27). HGSC 100x A papillae in the center flanked by solid growth with slit-like spaces.

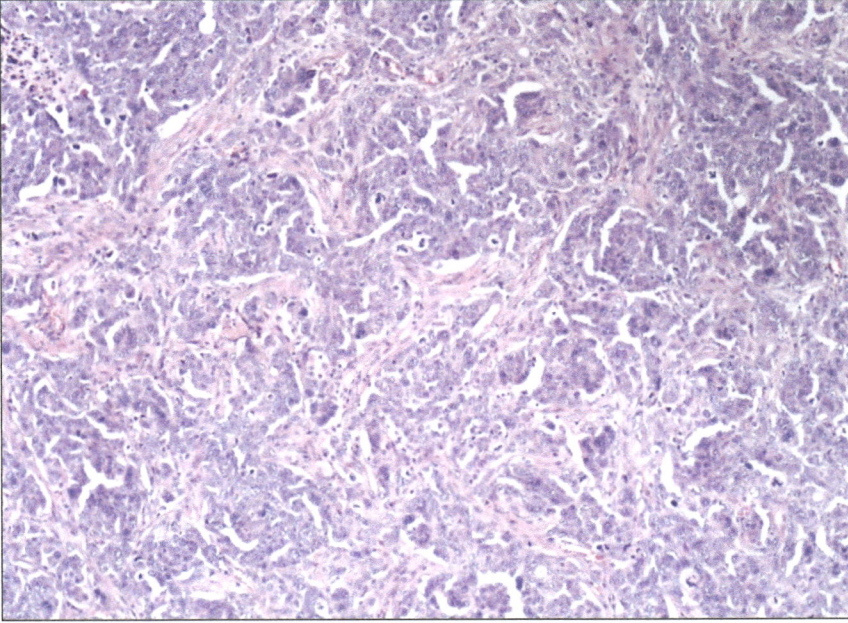

Fig. (28). HGSC (100x) Solid and glandular growth pattern with characteristic slit-like spaces.

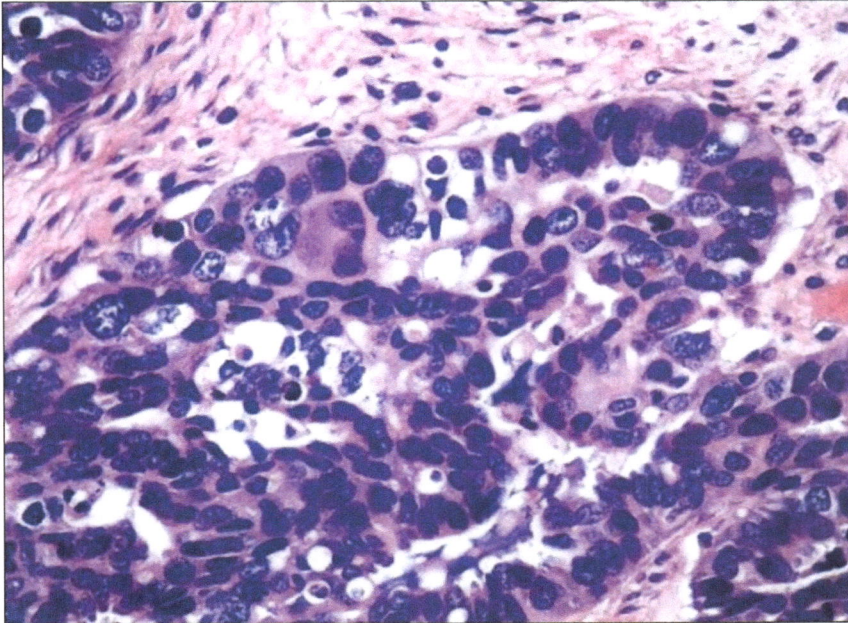

Fig. (29). HGSC 200x High grade cytology seen as prominent nuclear pleomorphism, hyperchromasia, and irregular chromatin patterns.

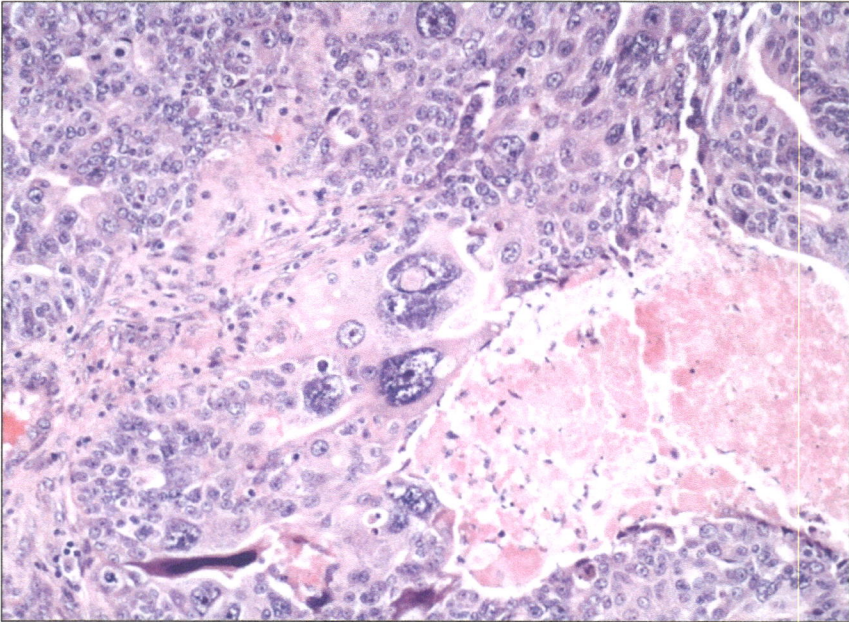

Fig. (30). HGSC (200x) Solid and glandular growth pattern with characteristic slit-like spaces, irregular luminal contours, necrosis, and severe cytologic atypia.

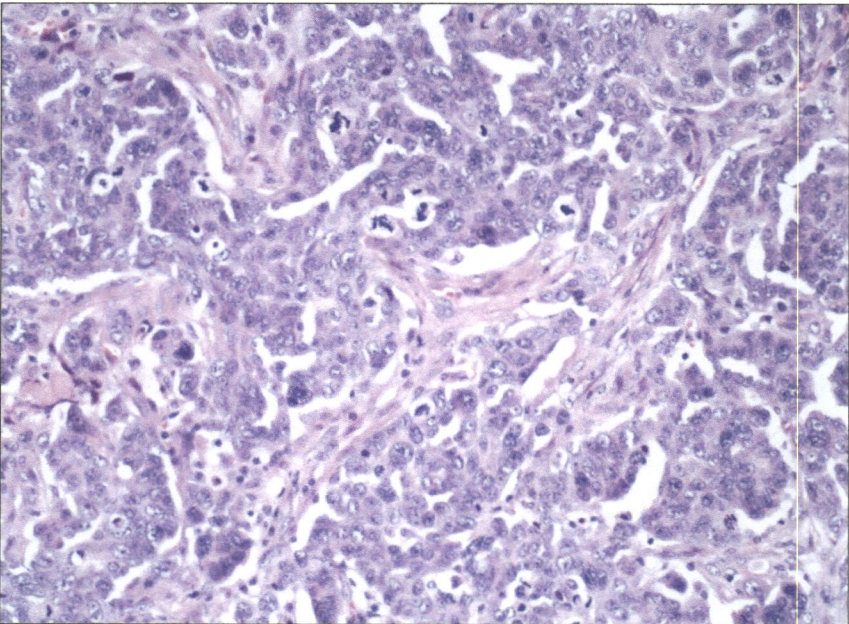

Fig. (31). HGSC (200x) Solid and glandular growth pattern with characteristic slit-like spaces, high grade cytology, and brisk mitoses.

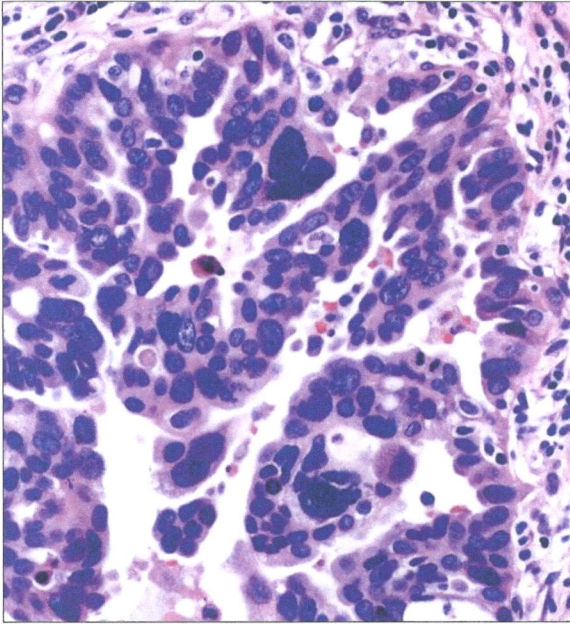

Fig. (32). HGSC 400x High grade cytology seen as prominent nuclear pleomorphism with large bizarre nuclei (*top*) and multinucleated tumor giant cells (*bottom*).

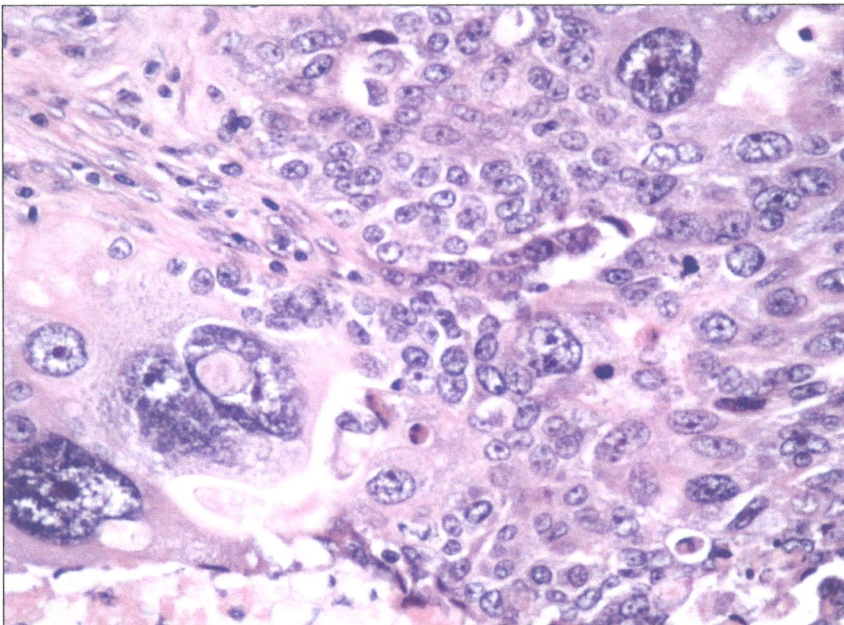

Fig. (33). HGSC (400x) Severe cytologic atypia seen as marked nuclear pleomorphism, giant and bizarre nuclei, and prominent macronucleoli.

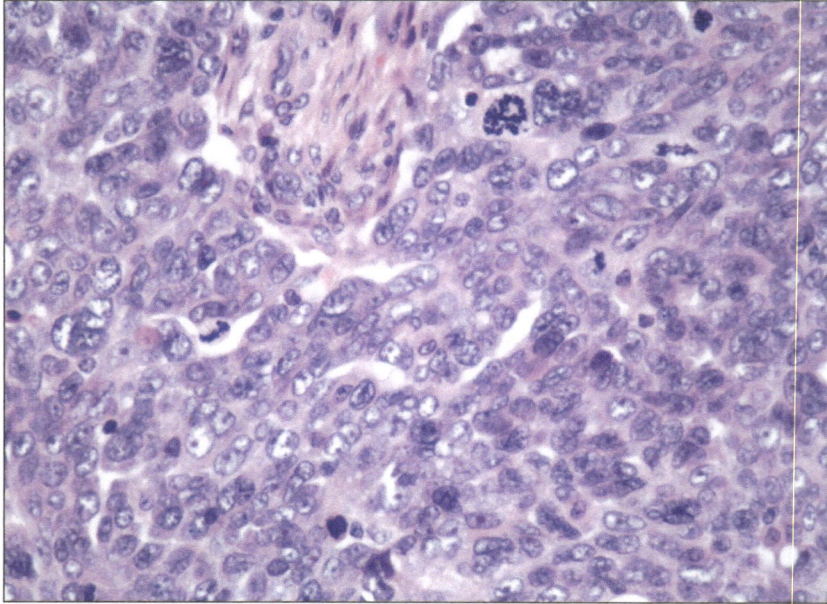

Fig. (34). HGSC (400x) Characteristic slit-like spaces with severe atypia seen as prominent nuclear pleomorphism, irregular and clumpy chromatin, and macronucleoli. Also present are multinucleated tumor cells and atypical mitoses.

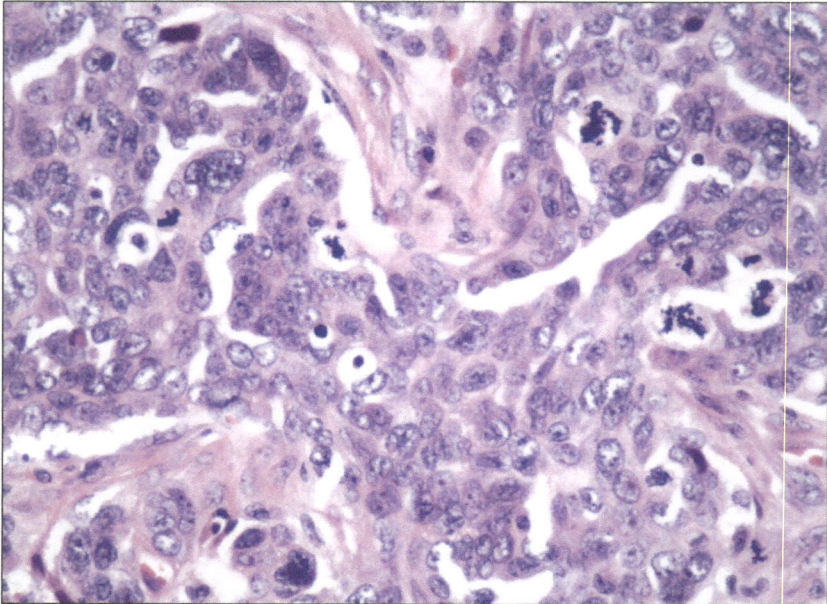

Fig. (35). HGSC (400x) Characteristic slit-like spaces with severe atypia seen as prominent nuclear pleomorphism, irregular and clumpy chromatin, and macronucleoli. Also present are multinucleated tumor cells and atypical mitoses.

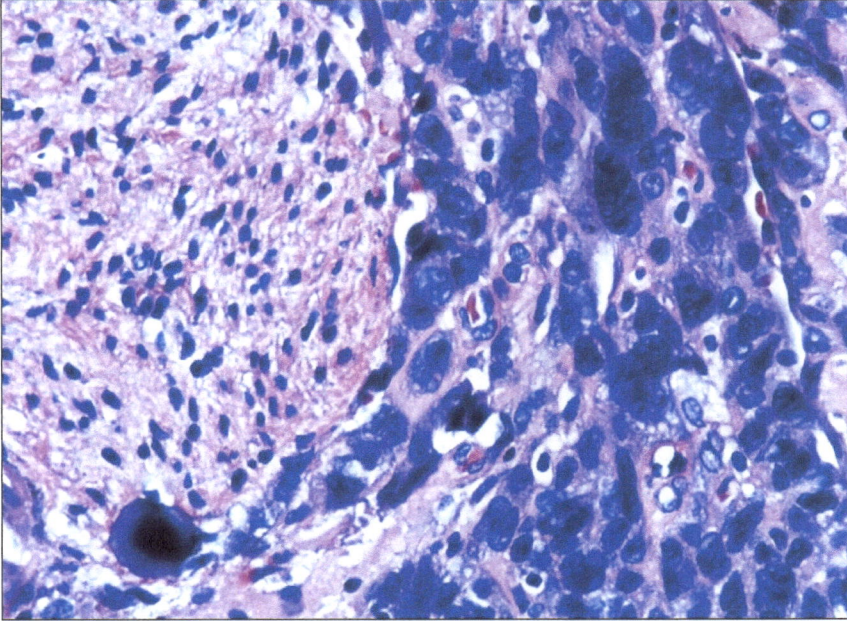

Fig. (36). HGSC (400x) Status-post neoadjuvant chemotherapy effect seen as nuclear and cytoplasmic vacuolation and a psammoma body (lamellated). Severe cytologic atypia and tumor giant cells.

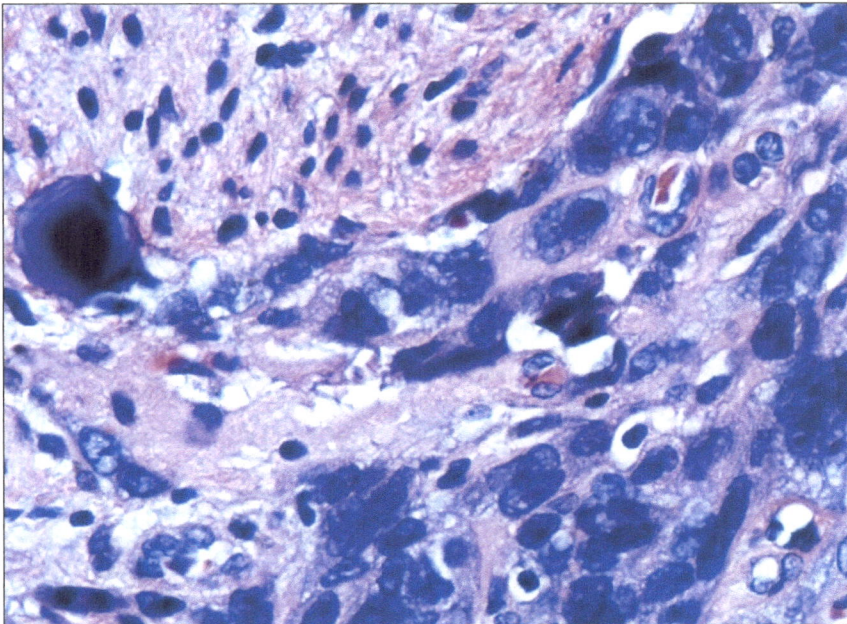

Fig. (37). HGSC (600x) Status-post neoadjuvant chemotherapy effect seen as nuclear and cytoplasmic vacuolation and psammoma body (lamellated). Severe cytologic atypia and tumor giant cells.

Many specimens are histopathologically evaluated after neoadjuvant chemotherapy as interval debulking and show extensive psammoma bodies, fibrosis, and foreign body giant cells admixed with microscopic residual carcinoma. These residual tumor cells display abundant clear, vacuolated, or eosinophilic cytoplasm and large macronucleoli (Fig. **37**). Other associated findings include lymphocytes, foamy macrophages, hemosiderin, and cholesterol clefts. Omental cakes are often reduced in size and show fat necrosis and fibrosis [49].

Immunohistochemistry: Positivity is seen with p53 (hallmark - strong diffuse nuclear staining or complete absence, null-type), p16 (strong diffuse nuclear), WT1 (90%), BRCA1, EMA, CAM5.2, CK7, BER-EP4 (95%), ER (88-95%), vimentin (45%), and CD99. Negative stains include PR, CK20 (majority), inhibin, p63, h-caldesmon, thrombomodulin, CA19-9, CD 15, and D2-40 [3].

Molecular: p53 mutations (~80%) [49], BRCA1/2, PTEN, PIK3CA [50], and high chromosomal instability.

Prognosis: Stage dependent with patients that have macroscopic disease completely resected having a better prognosis. Again, stage I is very rare and has a 5-year survival rate greater than 90%. Most are advanced stage (*i.e.* stage III and IV) with poor overall survival. The five-year survival rate is 35% for FIGO stage III [3]. As these tumors are very sensitive to platinum based chemotherapy, neoadjuvant chemotherapy is followed by interval debulking. Optimal debulking (less than 1 cm residual disease) increases the 5-year survival rate to 50%, and infrequently there are 10-year survivors [3]. Serum CA125 levels are followed to detect recurrence.

MUCINOUS TUMORS

Mucinous cystadenoma, borderline tumor, and carcinoma comprise the spectrum of events in the ovarian mucinous carcinogenesis sequence. Most importantly, distinguishing primary ovarian mucinous cancer from a metastatic mucinous cancer is a significant diagnostic challenge, and a critical distinction. Often a metastatic ovarian mucinous lesion is the initial presentation for an extraovarian primary, further complicating the dilemma. Also, ancillary diagnostic techniques such as immunohistochemistry are not helpful for this distinction. The most common mucinous tumors of the ovary with extraovarian primaries are from the gastrointestinal tract or of appendiceal origin, the latter often presenting as pseudomyxoma peritonei (PMP). In the early 2000s diagnostic criteria for ovarian mucinous neoplasms was refined to distinguish primary from metastatic. Prior to this many metastases were likely misclassified as primary ovarian mucinous neoplasms thus interpretation of older data is dubious. The refined diagnostic criteria demonstrated that primary ovarian mucinous carcinomas are far less common than previously believed [51].

Mucinous Cystadenoma

13% of benign ovarian epithelial neoplasms. Intestinal (80%) and endocervical types [3].

Clinical: Average age is 50 years.

Gross findings: Overwhelmingly unilateral masses that can reach more than 30 cm, with an average size of 10 cm. More often multilocular than unilocular cysts with thick, sticky contents. Capsule is thick, white, and with a smooth exterior.

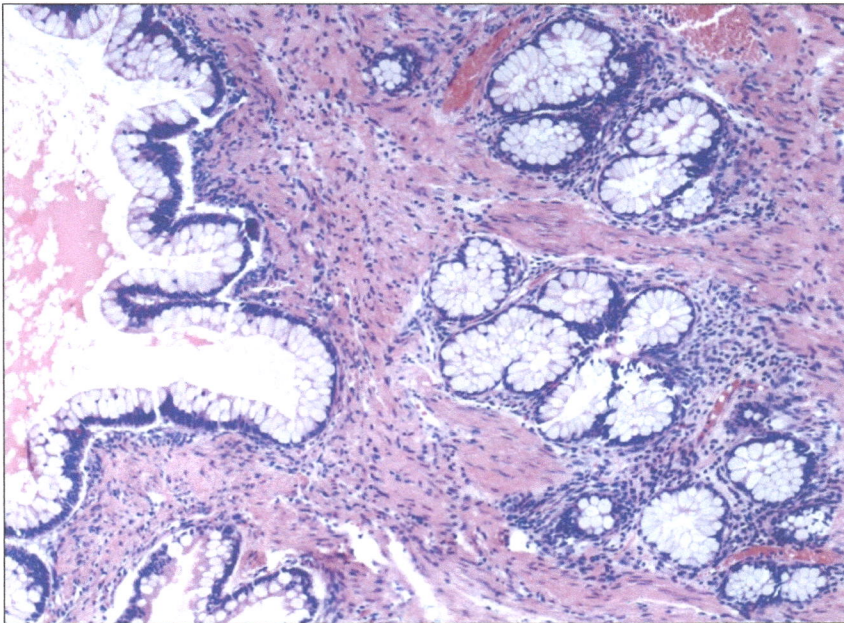

Fig. (38). Mucinous Cystadenoma (100x) Glands lined by a single layer of non-stratified intestinal-type epithelium.

Histology (Figs. **38**, **39**): Cysts and glands lined by a single layer of mucin producing columnar cells that resemble gastric foveolar-type, intestinal-type with goblet cells, or endocervical-type epithelium. Some crypts may show reactive nuclei and mitoses with focal mild or no atypia. Often, epithelium is undulating in appearance but generally lacks proliferation and budding. However up to 10% of the tumor may show proliferation or atypia rendering the diagnosis mucinous cystadenoma with focal proliferation or atypia [52]. Spiculated calcifications are common, as are muciphages, pseudoxanthoma cells, and luteinized stromal cells. Less common are multinucleated giant cells and pseudomyxoma ovarii, acellular mucin in the stroma [53]. Up to 18% of cases may be associated with a Brenner tumor, or transitional cell nests [53]. The endocervical-type mucinous, also referred to as müllerian-type or seromucinous, cystadenoma, show papillary structures with endocervical-like epithelium.

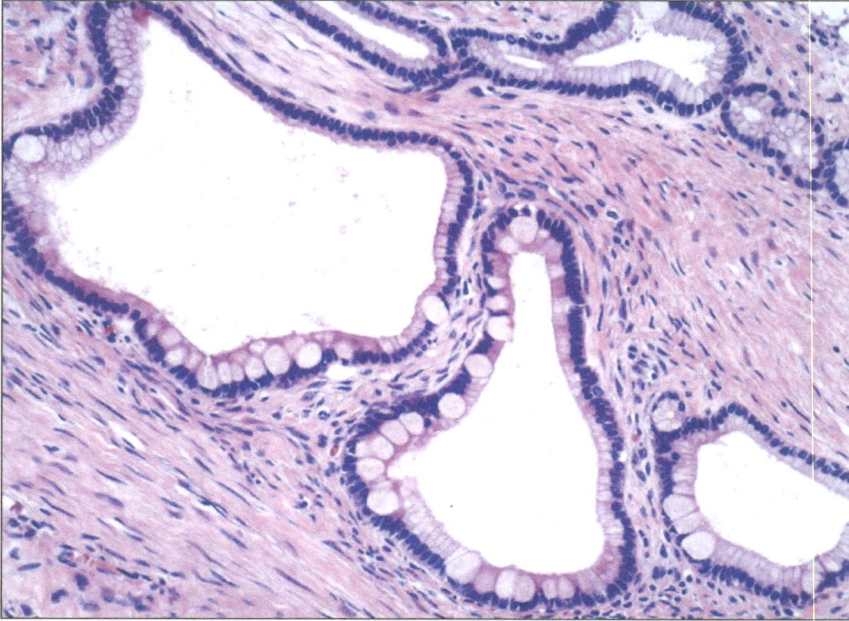

Fig. (39). Mucinous Cystadenoma (100x) Glands lined by a single layer of non-stratified intestinal-type epithelium with goblet cells.

Prognosis: Benign. Recurrence is associated with incomplete excision and not tumor rupture.

Atypical Proliferative Mucinous Tumor (APMT) or Mucinous Borderline Tumor

Gastrointestinal- or endocervical-type (much less common). Mucinous type cells with proliferation and atypia intermediary to cystadenoma and carcinoma.

Clinical: Average age is 40-49 years

Gross findings: Gastrointestinal-type: Average size of 20-22 cm, usually unilateral (95%), multiloculated mass with minimal solid areas and smooth capsule [54, 55]. Cyst lining is smooth and filled with gelatinous contents.

Endocervical-type: Smaller size and often bilateral.

Histology (Figs. **40-46**): Cysts with stratified gastrointestinal-type (most common) mucinous lining with increased proliferation showing tufting and villoglandular or papillary growth without stromal invasion. Nuclear atypia is mild to moderate. These features must be present in more than 10% of the tumor to qualify as APMT otherwise the diagnosis is mucinous cystadenoma. Microinvasion is defined by 5 mm of stromal invasion. APMT with microinvasion shows stromal invasion either by small foci of mucinous single cells, glands, or nests, or small foci of confluent or cribriform glandular growth; foci measure 2 to 5 mm [56]. The designation APMT with intraepithelial carcinoma should be given to those APMTs with marked nuclear atypia.

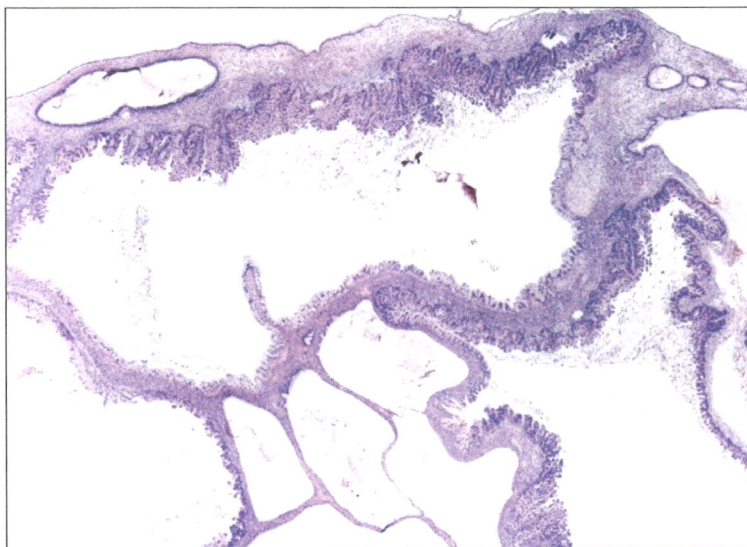

Fig. (40). Atypical Proliferative Mucinous Tumor or Mucinous Borderline Tumor (20x) Multiloculated cyst with some cysts showing epithelial proliferation while others do not.

Endocervical-type is associated with endometriosis and morphologically resembles APST. The epithelium is a combination of endocervical-type mucinous cells and serous-type cells that are ciliated, as well as other cell types may be seen (endometrioid, squamous, eosinophilic), with stromal acute inflammation; these features have also designated this type seromucinous-type APMT [57].

Immunohistochemistry: CK7, ER, and PR positive. CK 20 negative [58].

Prognosis: Virtually all are stage I tumors with excellent prognosis, 100% survival, and only rarely advancing to carcinoma.

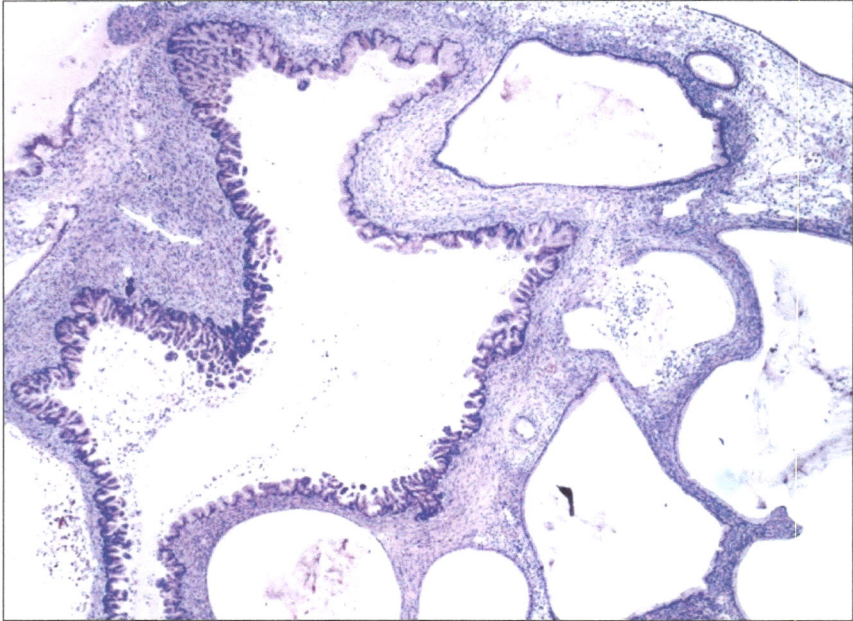

Fig. (41). Atypical Proliferative Mucinous Tumor or Mucinous Borderline Tumor (40x) Multiloculated cyst with some cysts showing epithelial proliferation while others do not.

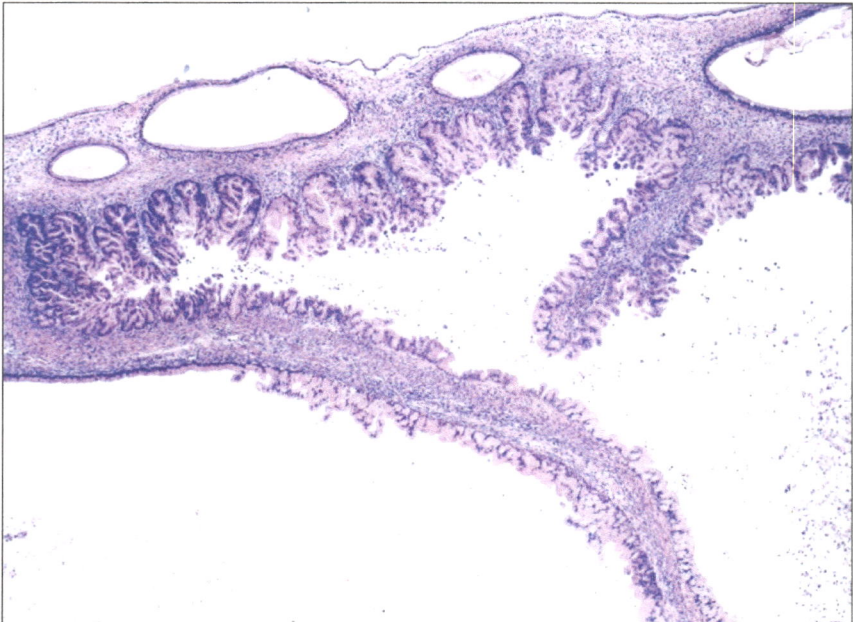

Fig. (42). Atypical Proliferative Mucinous Tumor or Mucinous Borderline Tumor (40x) Abundant epithelial proliferation with stratification, tufting, and foci of detached cells and clusters.

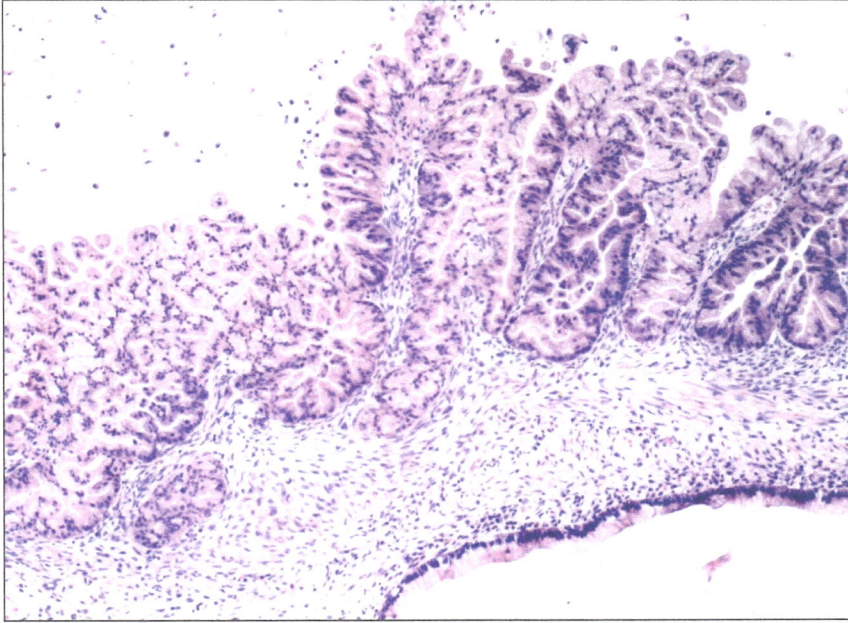

Fig. (43). Atypical Proliferative Mucinous Tumor or Mucinous Borderline Tumor (100x) Papillary fusion and epithelial proliferation with stratification, tufting, and detached cells and clusters.

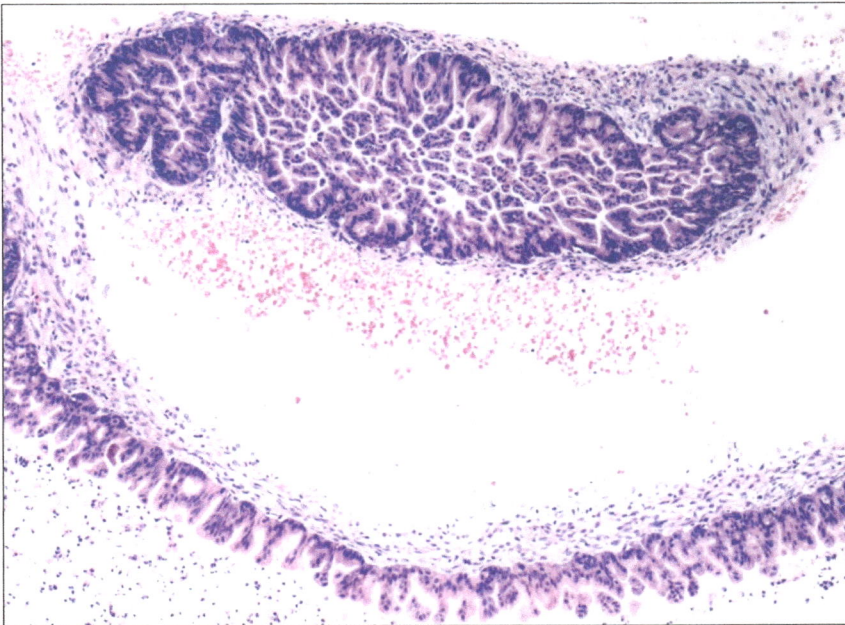

Fig. (44). Atypical Proliferative Mucinous Tumor or Mucinous Borderline Tumor (100x) Epithelial proliferation with stratification, tufting, and foci of detached cells and clusters.

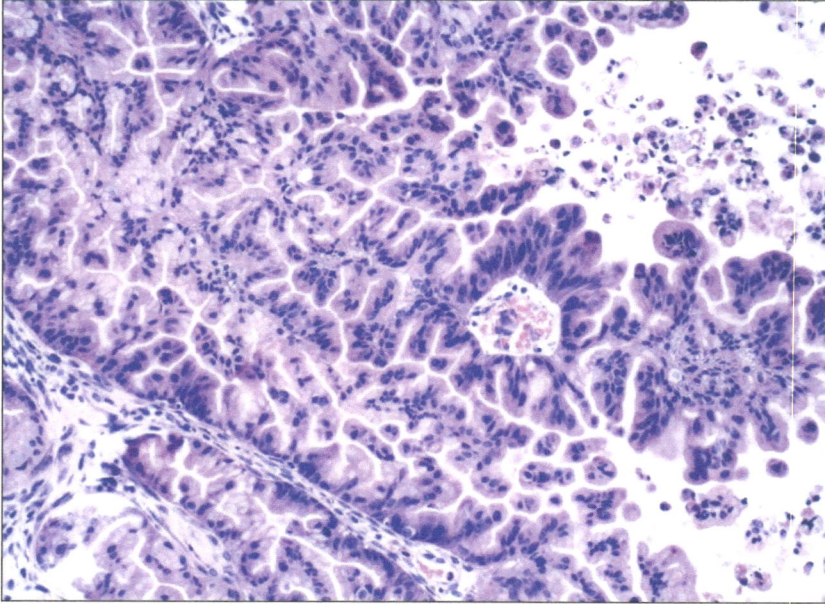

Fig. (45). Atypical Proliferative Mucinous Tumor or Mucinous Borderline Tumor (200x) Epithelial proliferation with stratification, tufting, and foci of detached cells and clusters. The mucinous epithelium is gastrointestinal-type with mild cytologic atypia and inconspicuous nucleoli.

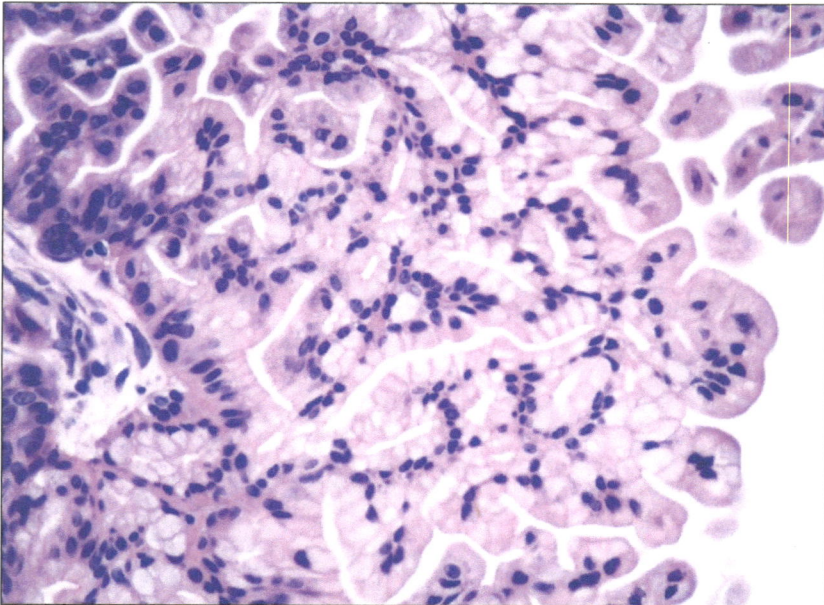

Fig. (46). Atypical Proliferative Mucinous Tumor or Mucinous Borderline Tumor (400x) The gastrointestinal-type mucinous epithelium shows goblet cells and mild cytologic atypia.

Mucinous Carcinoma

Rare, 2-3% of ovarian carcinomas [59]. Malignant mucinous cells invading ovarian stroma. Features favoring a metastatic mucinous carcinoma are bilateral involvement, size less than 13 cm, tumor on the ovarian surface, nodular growth, and a destructive pattern of stromal invasion [54].

Clinical: Average age is 44.

Gross: Average size is 18-22 cm. Large, unilateral, multicystic and mucinous mass with smooth white capsules [60]. Solid, necrotic, and hemorrhagic foci may be seen.

Histology (Figs. **47-50**): Well differentiated, complex glandular or papillary architecture with malignant mucinous epithelium showing invasion into stroma in either a destructive, infiltrative pattern or a confluent glandular or expansile pattern; often seen arising from an APMT. The expansile invasion is commonly seen in primary ovarian mucinous carcinomas and is associated with a better prognosis than destructive invasion [61]. An APMT with greater than 5 mm of confluent glandular growth qualifies for carcinoma. An associated teratoma and Brenner tumor may also be seen. Preferred nuclear grading is classified as low- or high-grade, and the latter is significantly more likely to be seen with the destructive pattern of invasion [62].

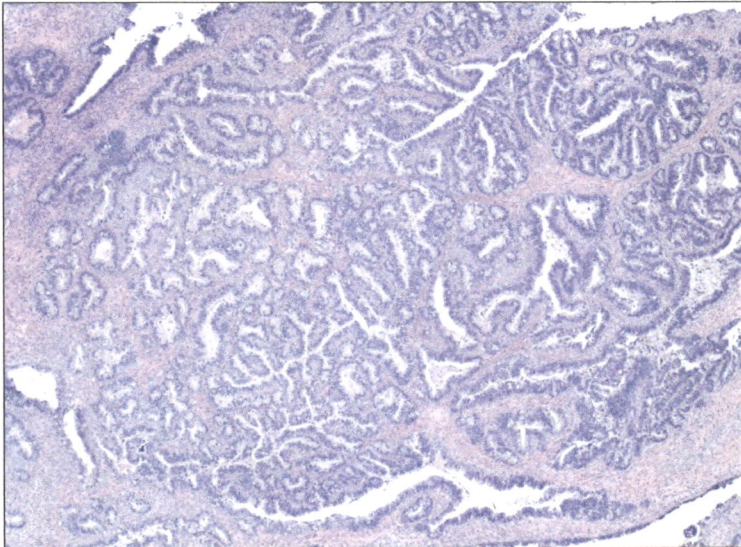

Fig. (47). Mucinous Carcinoma (40x) Complex and confluent glandular growth pattern.

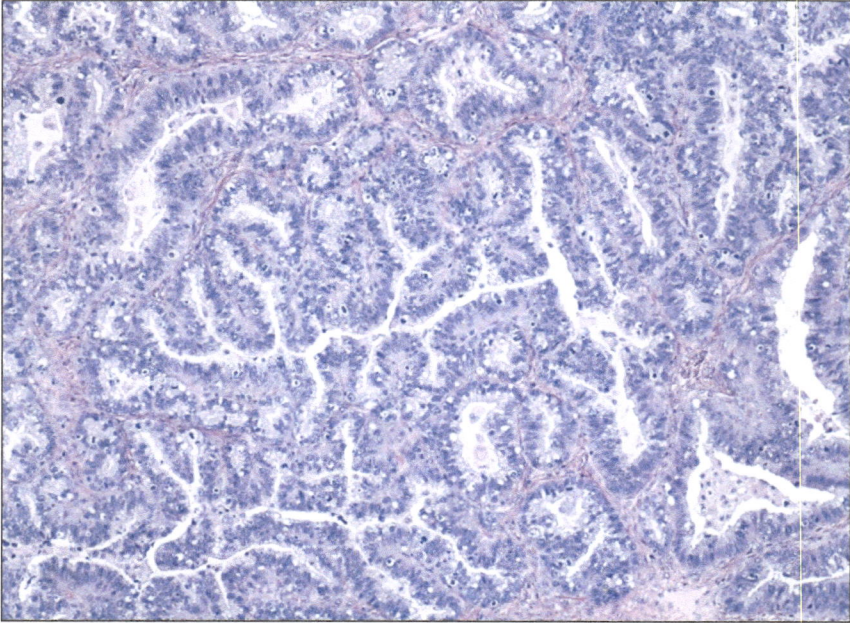

Fig. (48). Mucinous Carcinoma (100x) Complex and confluent glandular growth pattern.

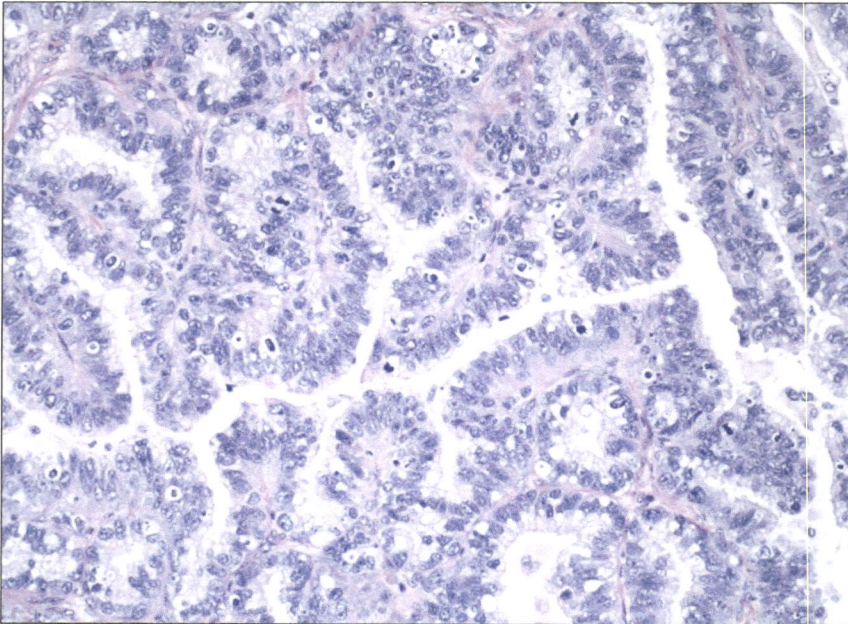

Fig. (49). Mucinous Carcinoma (200x) Complex and confluent glandular growth pattern with moderate cytologic atypia, goblet cells, and mitoses.

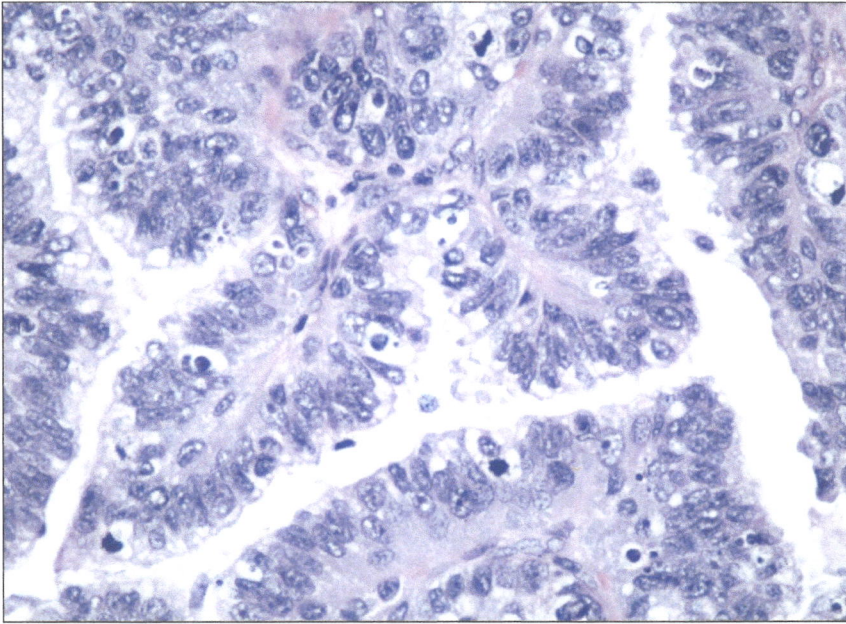

Fig. (50). Mucinous Carcinoma (400x) Complex and confluent glandular growth pattern with moderate cytologic atypia, goblet cells, and mitoses.

Immunohistochemistry: CK7 is diffusely positive. CK20 shows variable positivity, however when it is positive, it is not as diffuse as CK7 [63]. CDX2 may be positive and p16 is patchy positive. ER, PR, and CA125 are negative. If morphologically the tumor resembles lower gastrointestinal tumors and has pseudomyxoma ovarii, a CK7 negative and CK20 positive immunoprofile should raise concern for metastatic disease [64].

Molecular: KRAS mutations seen in at least 75% and the same KRAS mutations were found in adjacent mucinous cystadenomas, APMT, and carcinoma [65]. MUC2, MUC3, MUC17, CDX1, CDX2, and LGALS4 genes showed expression [66].

Prognosis: Very favorable, particularly if confined to the ovary. Stage 1 with expansile invasion has a 90% survival. Adverse prognosis is associated with destructive invasion [61]. Platinum-paclitaxel is effective.

ENDOMETRIOID TUMORS

Benign ovarian endometrioid neoplasms, cystadenofibromas and borderline tumors, are far less common than endometrioid carcinoma. As previously mentioned, endometrioid tumors are often seen arising from endometriosis, the majority of which are monoclonal and harbor chromosomal alterations signifying a neoplastic process [67].

Endometrioid Cystadenofibroma

Very rare, 1% of ovarian epithelial tumors [3].

Clinical: Average age is 57 years.

Gross: Average size is 10 cm. The ovarian capsule is smooth. The mass is fibrous with cystic areas containing serous fluid, imparting a honey comb appearance.

Histology (Fig. **51**): Adenofibroma or cystadenofibroma architecture showing glands or cysts with cellular or fibrotic stroma. The epithelium resembles proliferative endometrium, that is tall columnar cells with elongated nuclei, or less often, will resemble atrophic or inactive endometrium with flat or cuboidal cells. Ciliated cells are common resembling tubal epithelium. Secretory and squamous changes may also be seen. Mitoses are rare. Frequently, associated endometriosis is seen [3].

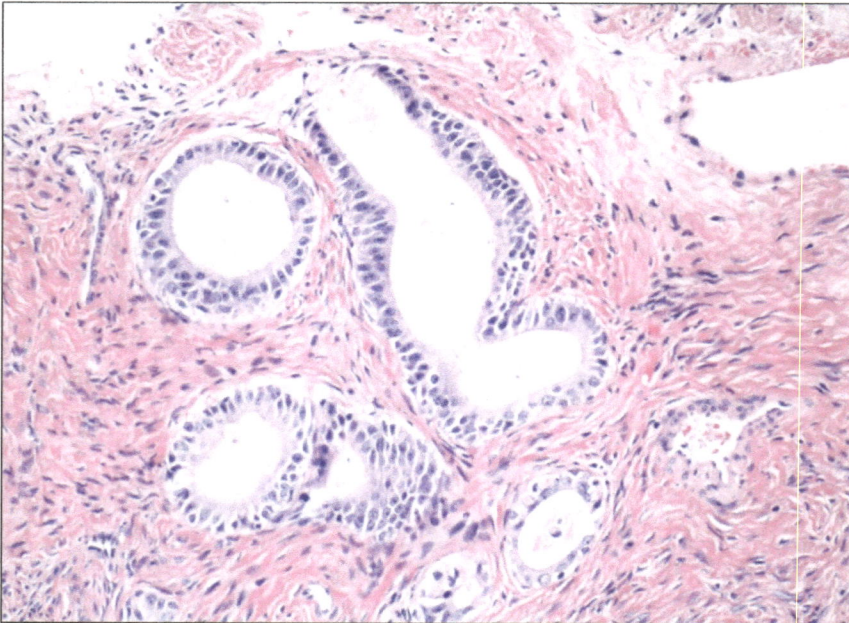

Fig. (51). Endometrioid Adenofibroma (200x) Benign Mullerian glands in a fibrotic stroma.

Molecular: PTEN mutations and loss of heterozygosity on 10q23.3 [68].

Prognosis: Benign, rarely recur.

Atypical Proliferative Endometrioid Tumor (APET)

Atypical Proliferative Endometrioid Tumor (APET) or Endometrioid Borderline Tumor: Also known as atypical endometrioid adenofibroma, proliferative endometrioid tumor, endometrioid tumor of low malignant potential. A spectrum of tumors ranging from glandular crowding with mild cytologic atypia to confluent glandular growth (5 mm) with cytologic atypia and even microinvasion (5 mm).

Clinical: Average age 51 [69]. Very rare, only 0.2% of ovarian epithelial tumors, with 63% having associated endometriosis [69].

Gross: Average size is 9 cm. Usually a unilateral, cystic mass, a minority have solid foci, with bloody, brown or green fluid [69].

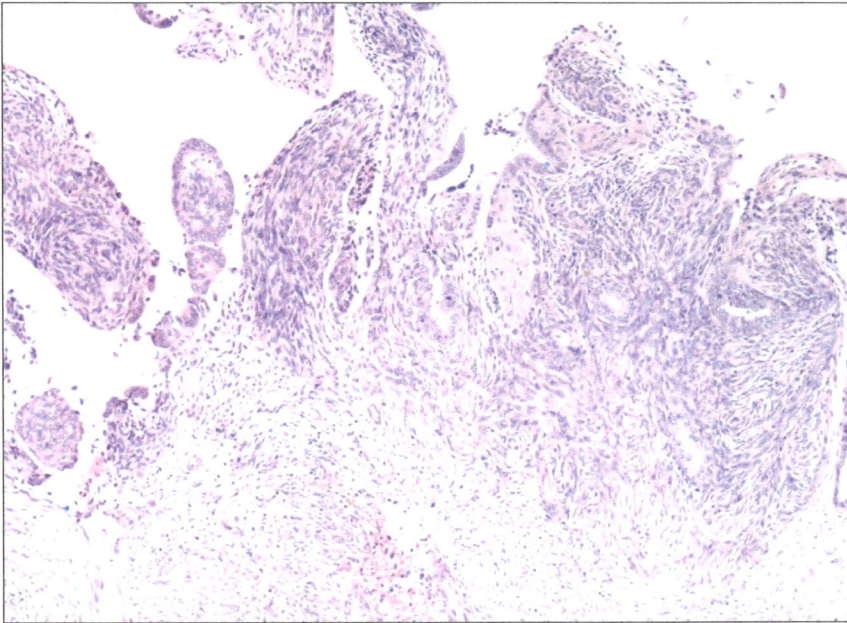

Fig. (52). Atypical Proliferative Endometrioid Tumors (APET) or Endometrioid Borderline Tumor (100x) Endometrioid glands with squamous metaplasia in a fibrotic stroma.

Histology (Figs. **52-54**): The classic morphology is adenofibromatous and glandular-papillary architecture, with an associated adenofibroma in half of cases [69]. The stratified epithelium exhibits a range of complexity and crowding, with confluent growth 5 mm qualifying for microinvasion; confluent growth or invasion (destructive or confluent) above 5 mm warrants diagnosis of carcinoma. Cytologic atypia is mild to moderate. Severe atypia is considered intraepithelial carcinoma, which is rare [70]. Additionally, epithelial tufting, bridging, cribriforming, and squamous metaplasia may be seen [69]. The stroma may be fibrotic or cellular, with increased cellularity surrounding the glands, *i.e.* periglandular cuffing [70]. Intraluminal or intracystic necrosis is common.

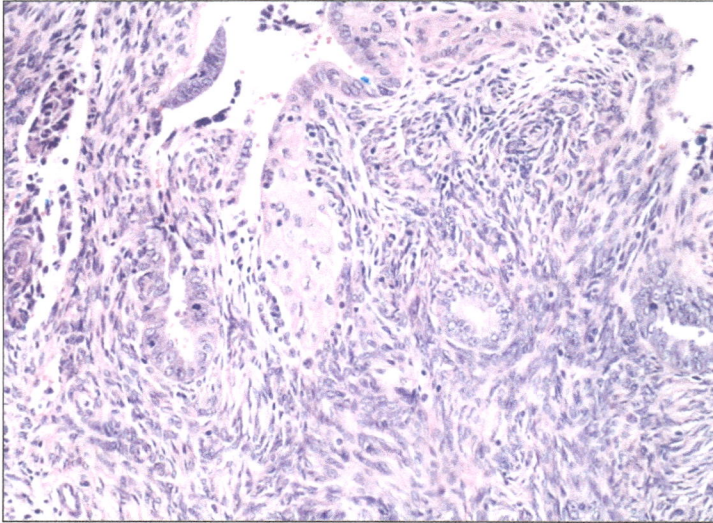

Fig. (53). Atypical Proliferative Endometrioid Tumors (APET) or Endometrioid Borderline Tumor (200x) Endometrioid glands with mild cytologic atypia and squamous metaplasia in a fibrotic stroma.

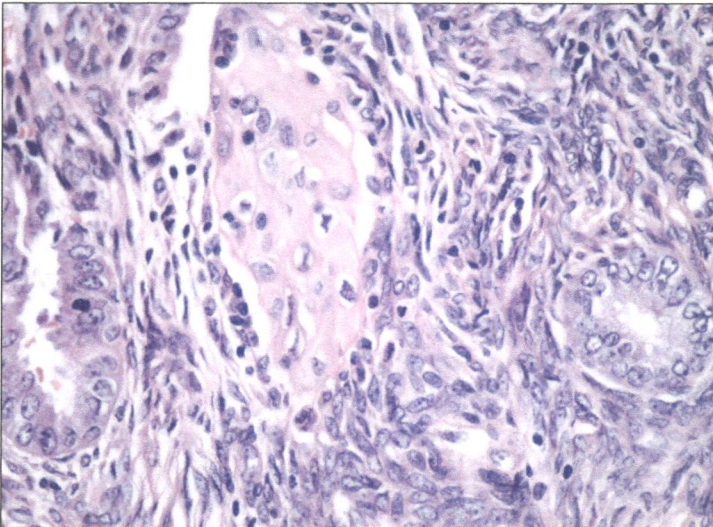

Fig. (54). Atypical Proliferative Endometrioid Tumors (APET) or Endometrioid Borderline Tumor (400x) Endometrioid glands with mild cytologic atypia, squamous metaplasia, and occasional mitoses in a fibrotic stroma.

Immunohistochemistry: Positive markers include EMA, cytokeratins, and p16 focally (50% of cases) [71].

Molecular: PTEN mutations and loss of heterozygosity on 10q23.3 [72].

Prognosis: Excellent; usually stage I, 5-year survival is 100%, including with microinvasion, however data regarding microinvasion and intraepithelial carcinoma is limited [69, 70].

Endometrioid Carcinoma

The second most common type of ovarian epithelial malignancy is characterized by invasive, endometrioid –type glands. An average of 15-20% and up to 42% of endometrioid carcinomas are associated with endometriosis [70]. Interestingly, 14% of ovarian endometrioid carcinomas are associated with synchronous endometrial carcinoma, also presenting a diagnostic challenge for pathologists to accurately classify the ovarian tumor as a synchronous primary or metastatic from the uterus [3].

Clinical: Average age is 55-58 years, significantly lower than serous carcinoma [73]. Commonly, presentation is abdominal distention and pain, vaginal bleeding, and adnexal mass on examination.

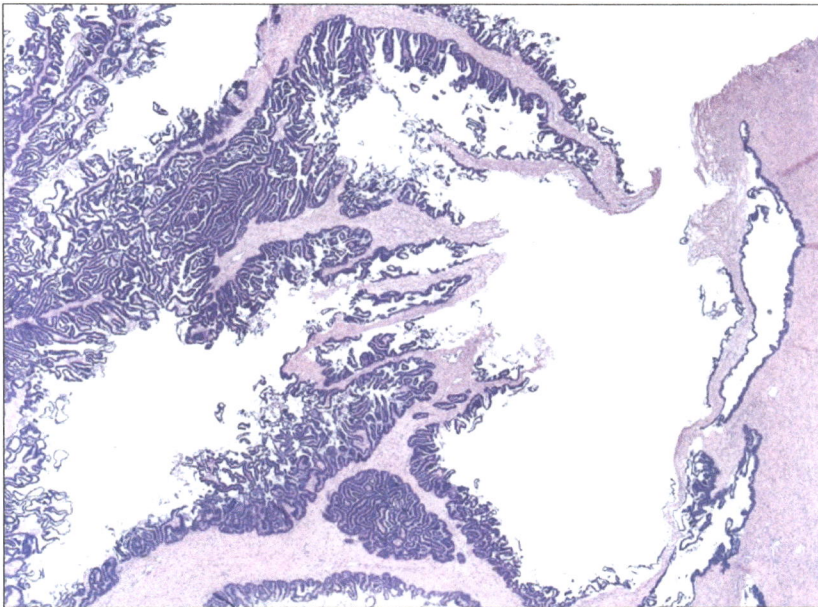

Fig. (55). **Endometrioid Carcinoma, Well-Differentiated (20x)** Confluent villoglandular growth pattern.

Gross: Average size is a 15-cm complex mass with smooth outer surfaces. The cysts contain friable tumor and bloody fluid. Less commonly, there is mucoid or greenish fluid or solid growth with hemorrhage and necrosis. Also, may be seen arising in an endometrioma with chocolate-like fluid and nodules or papillations of the lining.

Histology (Figs. **55-66**): The most common pattern of growth or invasion seen is the confluent or expansile pattern which must be greater than 5 mm [74]. Destructive infiltrative invasion is also seen as irregularly shaped glands, nests, solid sheets, or single cells surrounded by edema and inflammation [74]. More than half are associated with endometriosis, endometrioid adenofibroma, or APET, which also comprises a large portion of the tumor [60].

The most common histologic grade is well-differentiated endometrioid adenocarcinoma and is cribriform, confluent, or villoglandular growth lined by stratified tall, columnar epithelium with well-defined lumens. Foci of high-grade cytology are seen, and mitoses are frequent [36]. Occasionally, focal secretory-type epithelium is seen. Squamous differentiation occurs in up to 50% of cases [70].

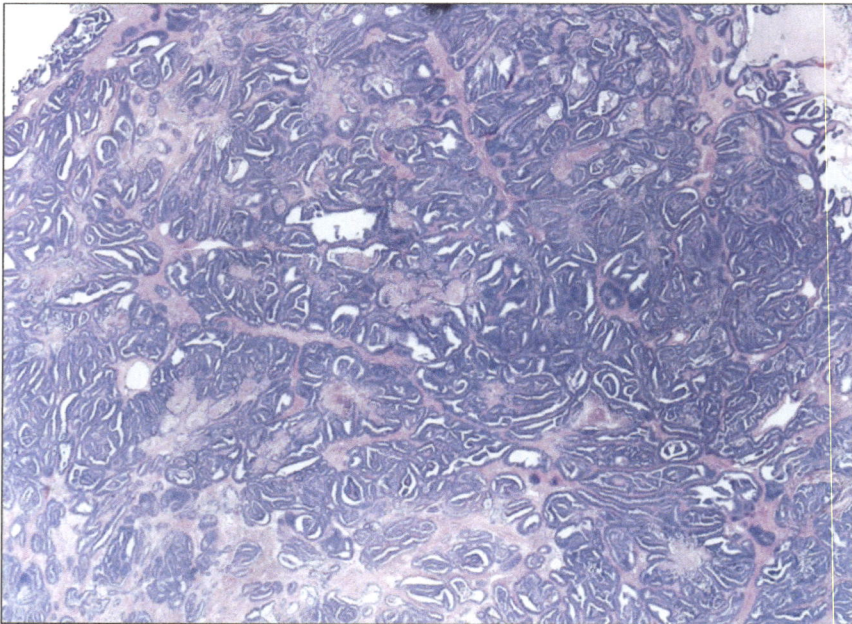

Fig. (56). Endometrioid Carcinoma, Well-Differentiated (20x) Confluent glandular growth pattern and back-to-back glands.

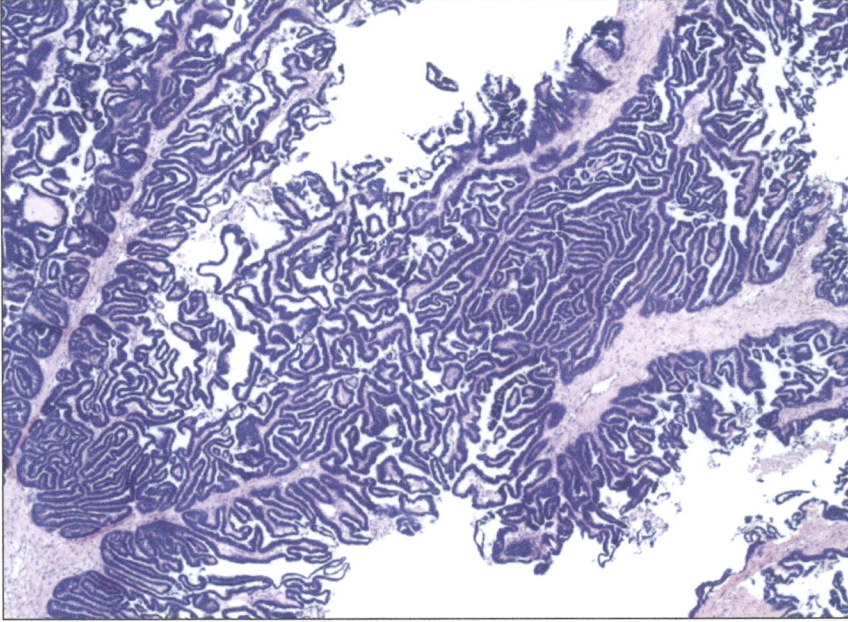

Fig. (57). Endometrioid Carcinoma, Well-Differentiated (40x) Confluent villoglandular growth pattern.

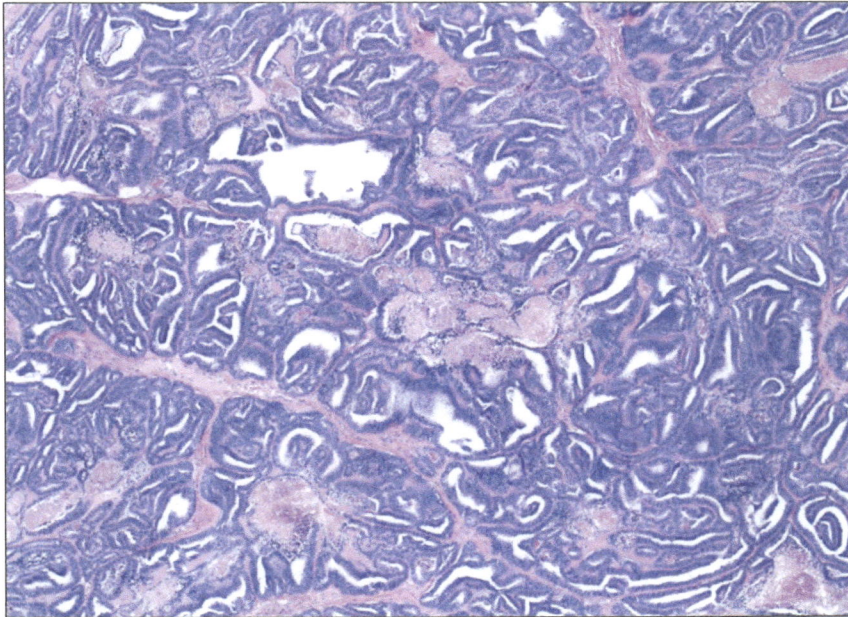

Fig. (58). Endometrioid Carcinoma, Well-Differentiated (40x) Confluent glandular growth pattern, back-to-back glands, and intraluminal necrosis.

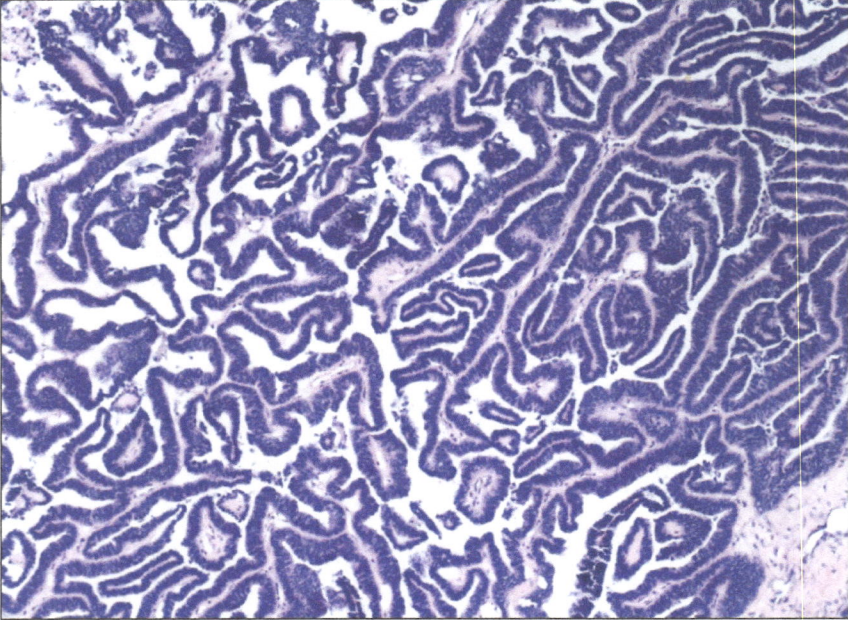

Fig. (59). Endometrioid Carcinoma, Well-Differentiated (100x) Confluent endometrioid villoglandular growth pattern.

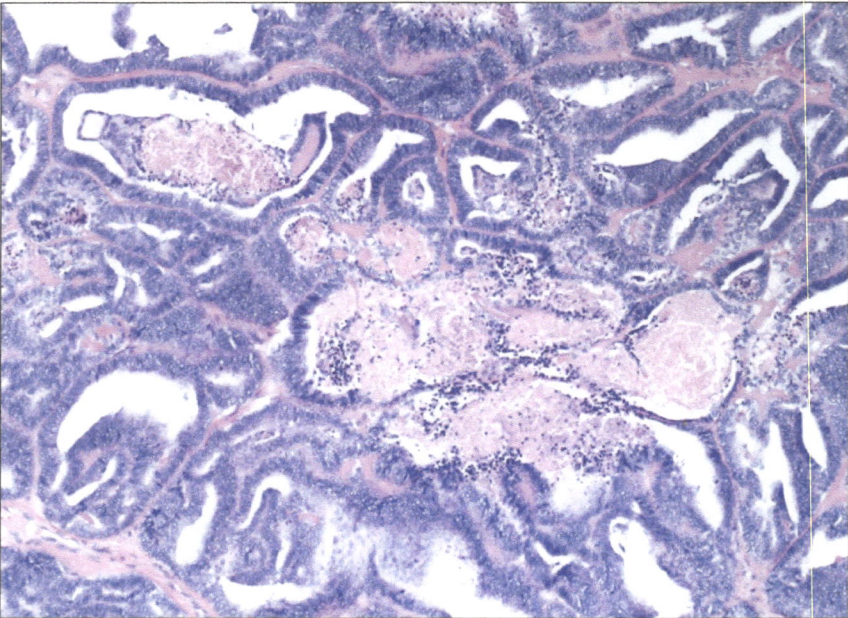

Fig. (60). Endometrioid Carcinoma, Well-Differentiated (100x) Endometrioid epithelium showing a confluent glandular growth pattern, back-to-back glands, and intraluminal necrosis.

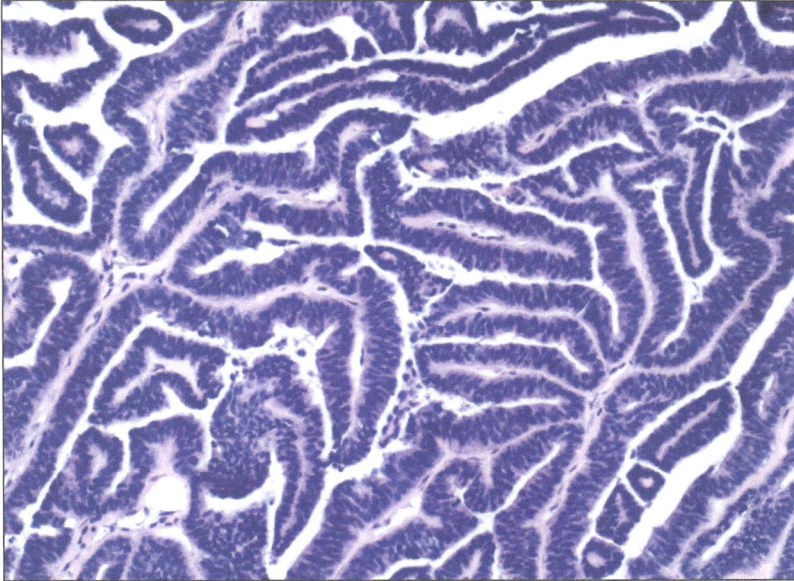

Fig. (61). Endometrioid Carcinoma, Well-Differentiated (200x) Confluent endometrioid villoglandular growth pattern. The epithelium mirrors proliferative-type endometrium with pseudostratified columnar cells.

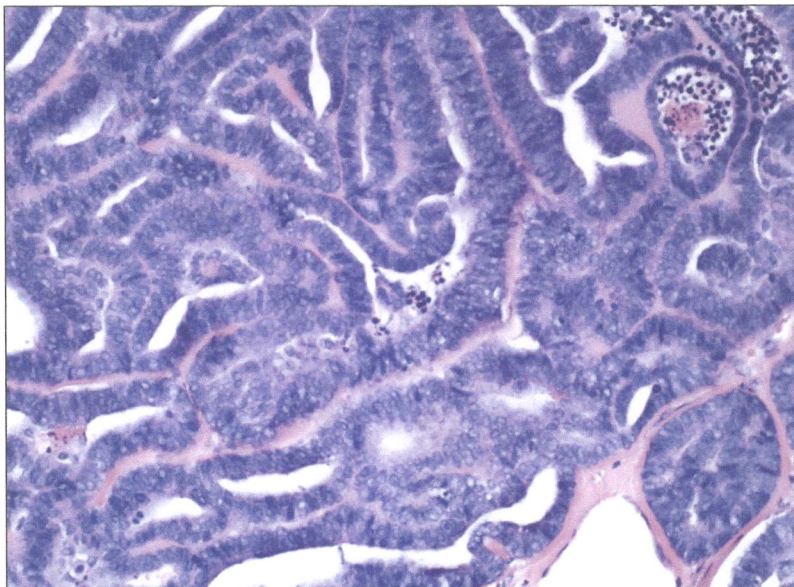

Fig. (62). Endometrioid Carcinoma, Well-Differentiated (200x) Endometrioid epithelium showing a confluent glandular growth pattern, back-to-back glands, and intraluminal necrosis (top right). The epithelium mirrors proliferative-type endometrium with pseudostratified columnar cells.

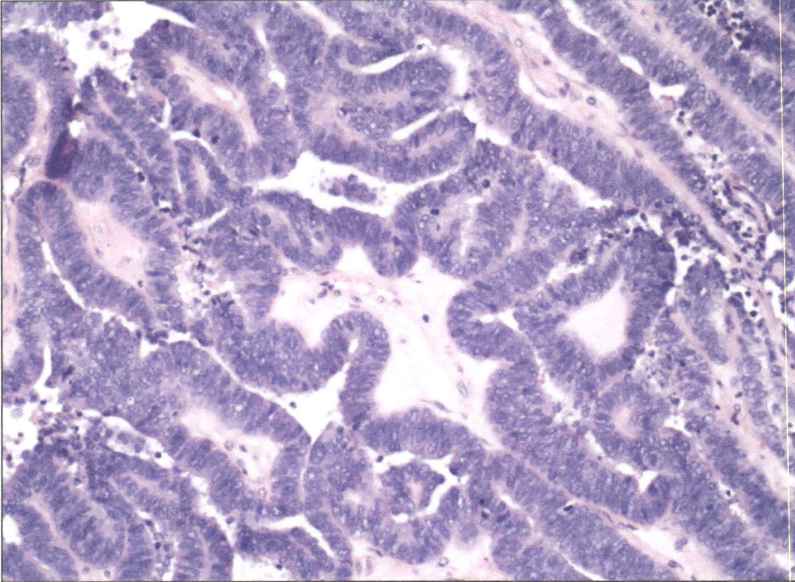

Fig. (63). Endometrioid Carcinoma, Well-Differentiated (200x) Endometrioid epithelium showing a confluent glandular growth pattern and back-to-back glands. The epithelium mirrors proliferative-type endometrium with pseudostratified columnar cells and mitoses.

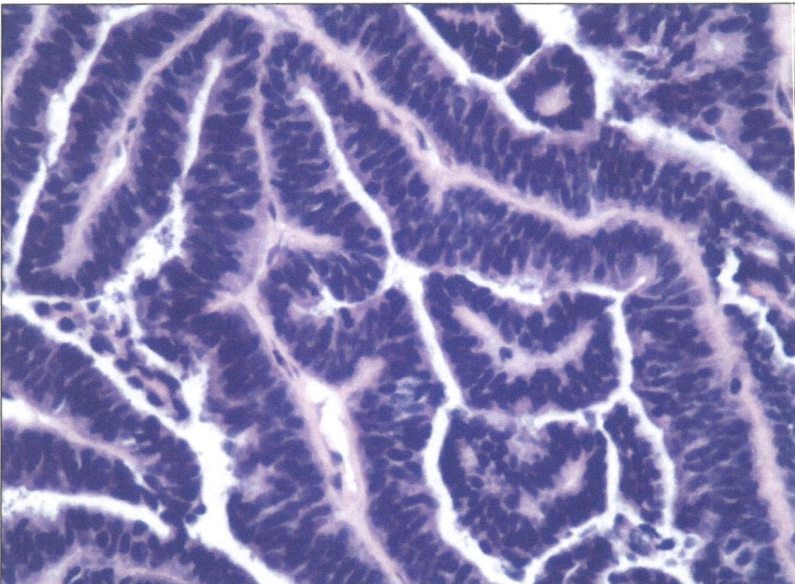

Fig. (64). Endometrioid Carcinoma, Well-Differentiated (400x) Confluent endometrioid villoglandular growth pattern. The epithelium mirrors proliferative-type endometrium with pseudostratified and cytologically bland columnar cells and occasional mitoses.

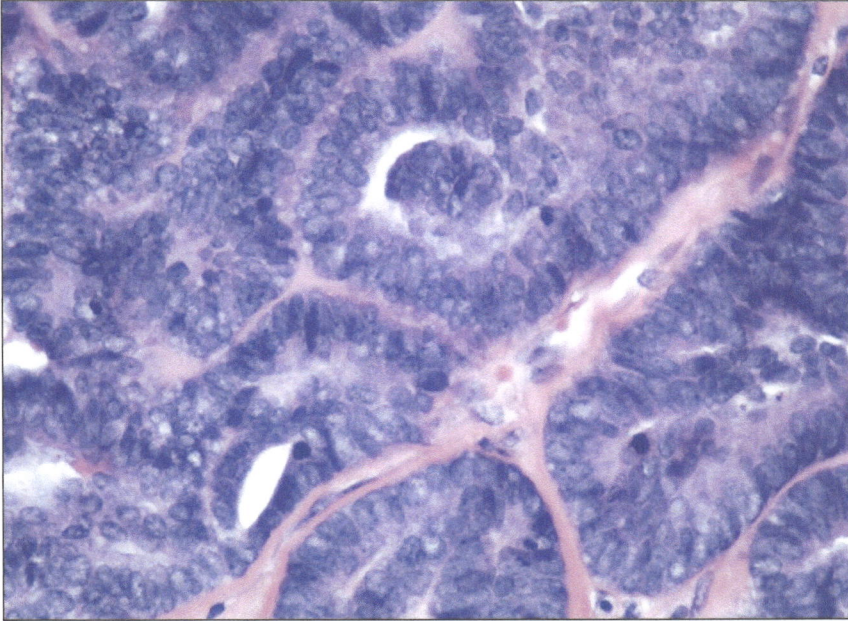

Fig. (65). Endometrioid Carcinoma, Well-Differentiated (400x) Proliferative-type endometrioid epithelium with pseudostratified columnar cells, mild cytologic atypia, and mitoses.

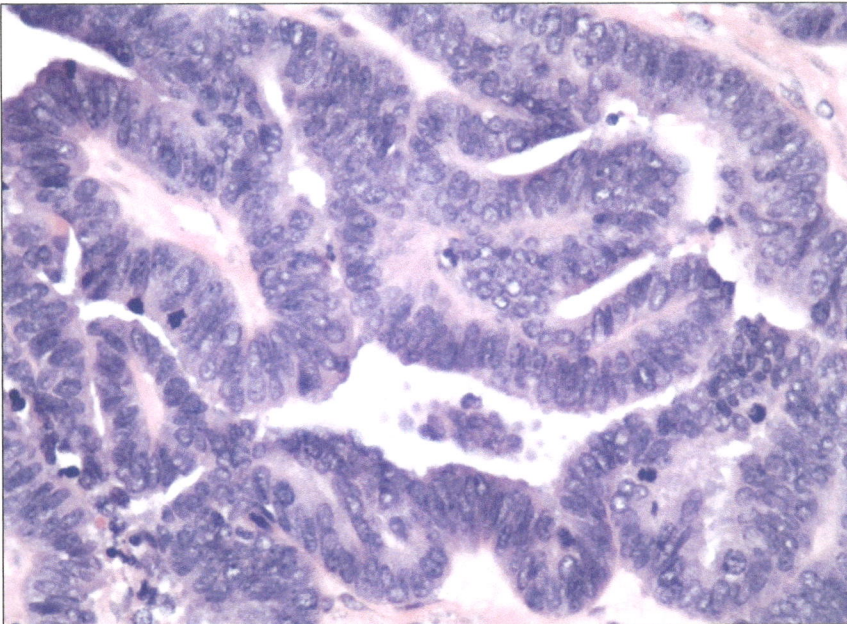

Fig. (66). Endometrioid Carcinoma, Well-Differentiated (400x) Proliferative-type endometrioid epithelium with pseudostratified columnar cells, mild cytologic atypia, and mitoses.

Moderately and poorly differentiated endometrioid carcinomas showing more solid growth, high-grade nuclei, and brisk mitoses may also be seen, however most of the poorly differentiated variety should be classified as high-grade serous [75]. Morphologically, ovarian endometrioid cancer should mirror endometrial endometrioid adenocarcinoma. Mixed serous-endometrioid carcinoma is a possibility, however these comprise 1.5% of ovarian carcinomas [3]. Importantly, a standardized grading system for ovarian endometrioid carcinoma has not been established, nor has the WHO 3-grade system or the binary system been validated for this entity [3]. Several rare variants of endometrioid carcinomas occur: secretory, ciliated, sertoliform, undifferentiated neuroendocrine, adenoid cystic-like, basaloid, and oxyphilic [3]. Post chemotherapy, endometrioid carcinomas show keratin granulomas secondary to necrosis of squamous metaplasia [3].

Immunohistochemistry: Positive markers include CK7, EMA, ER, PR, BRCA1, CD99, and p16 focally (50% of cases) [76]. WT1, inhibin, calretinin, and TTF1 are usually negative [3].

Molecular: CTNNB1 (well differentiated), pTEN, PIK3CA (well differentiated), K-ras, BRAF, and p53 (poorly differentiated) mutations [77]. Microsatellite instability can be seen in up to 20% cases (MLH1 and MSH2 loss of staining) [78].

Prognosis: Stage dependent with up to 78% survival in stage I tumors; more than half are stage I or II on diagnosis [79]. Higher grade tumors with more solid growth have a worse prognosis.

CLEAR CELL TUMORS

Although ovarian clear cell neoplasms were once believed to be derived from the mesonephric duct, their association with endometriosis, endometrioid adenocarcinomas, and DES-exposed vaginal adenosis substantiates a Müllerian origin. The occurrence of primary uterine clear cell carcinoma further supports the Müllerian origin of clear cell tumors.

Clear Cell Adenofibromas

Benign clear cell tumors are extremely rare and thus data are very limited.

Clinical: Average age is 45 years.

Gross: The average size is 12 cm and unilateral. The external surface is smooth and the multicystic lesion has a honey-comb appearance with clear fluid. The fibromatous stroma has a firm and rubbery consistency.

Histology: Tubules are lined by polyhedral, hobnail or flattened cells with either minimal cytoplasm or abundant clear, granular or eosinophilic cytoplasm. Cytoplasmic glycogen is usually present. Minimal cytologic atypia and mitoses are present if at all. The stroma is fibromatous and compact. Mucin may also be seen.

Prognosis: Benign.

Atypical Proliferative Clear Cell Tumors (APCCT), Clear Cell Borderline Tumors (CCBT)

Atypical Proliferative Clear Cell Tumors (APCCT), Clear Cell Borderline Tumors (CCBT), Clear Cell Tumor of Low Malignant Potential: This lesion resembles a clear cell adenofibroma and additionally shows moderate cytologic atypia and/or epithelial proliferation without invasion. These tumors are very rare, 0.2% of ovarian epithelial tumors [3]. This is a challenging diagnosis and the distinction between APCCT and carcinoma is believed to be amongst the most difficult distinctions in gynecologic pathology [80].

Clinical: Average age is 60-70 years.

Gross: Average size is 15 cm and resembles an adenofibroma with soft foci.

Histology: Morphologically, again resembles a clear cell adenofibroma however, there is a significant glandular crowding and epithelial proliferation with stratification and budding. There is also significant cytologic atypia with coarse chromatin, macronucleoli, and up to 3 mitoses per 10 HPF. The upper limit of glandular crowding in APCCT is not well defined, thus some are likely diagnosed as carcinoma. Atypical endometriosis is designated when the lining of the endometrioma shows clear cells with atypia [81]. Very rarely in this setting there is malignant cytology without invasion which is designated an APCCT with intraepithelial carcinoma.

Prognosis: Excellent survival in limited data available.

Clear Cell Carcinoma

Clear Cell Carcinoma (Figs. 67 - 69): Invasive, malignant clear and eosinophilic (pink) cells most often seen in association with its precursor, endometriosis with atypia. Clear cell carcinoma's association with endometriosis is the highest among all types of ovarian carcinomas.

Clinical: Average age is 50-53 years. Nonspecific symptoms associated with an abdominal or pelvic mass. Interestingly, clear cell carcinoma is the ovarian epithelial tumor most commonly associated with vascular thrombotic events and paraneoplastic hypercalcemia [82, 83].

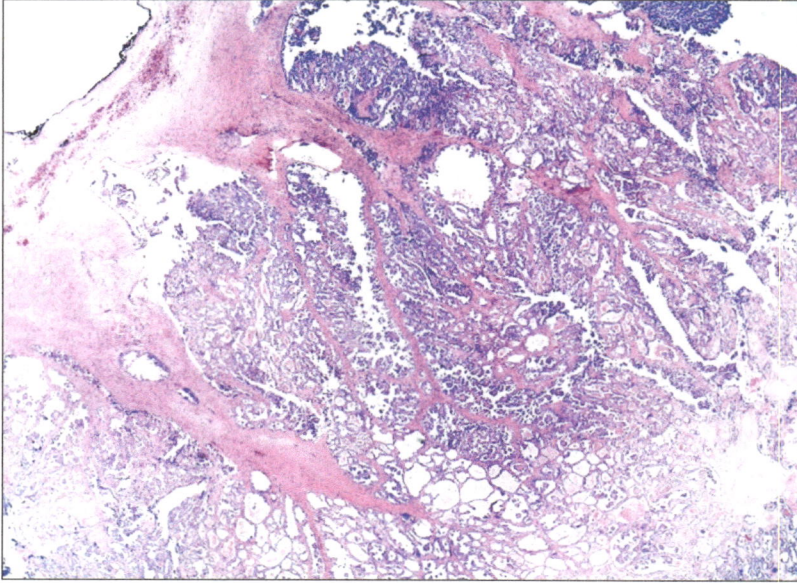

Fig. (67). Clear Cell Carcinoma (20x) Characteristic papillary and tubulocystic architecture and hyalinized stroma.

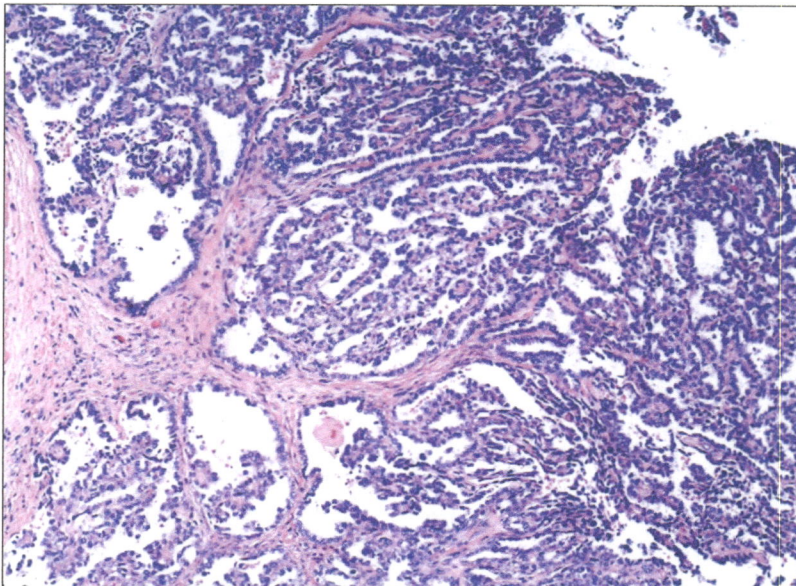

Fig. (68). Clear Cell Carcinoma (100x) Characteristic papillary and tubulocystic architecture and hyalinized stroma (pink). Clear cytoplasm and hobnail cells are seen.

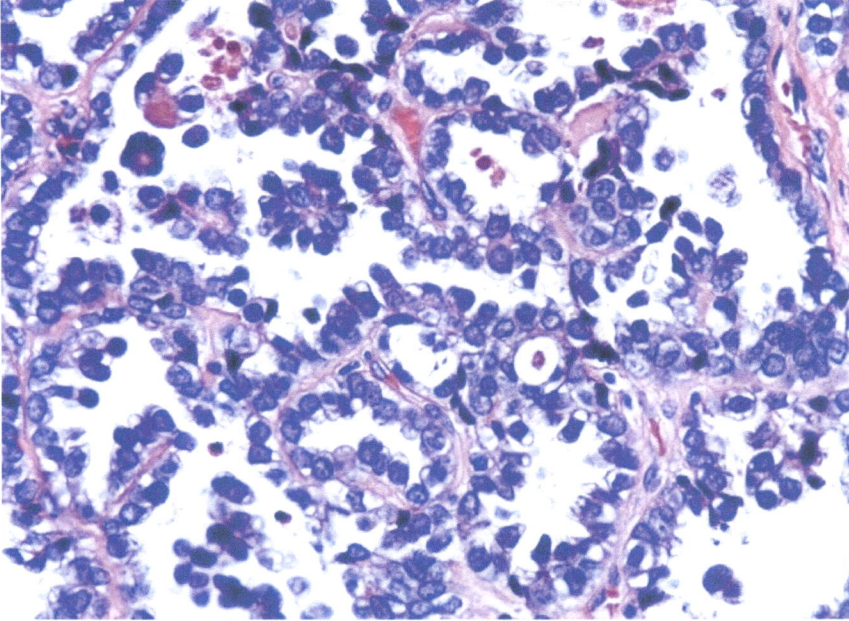

Fig. (69). Clear Cell Carcinoma (400x) Clear and hobnail cells with mild to moderate cytologic atypia and a hyalinized stroma.

Gross: Average size is 13-15 cm, ranges up to 30 cm and typically unilateral. Often associated with an endometriotic cyst filled with chocolate-like fluid and nodules or polypoid areas of the lining or a larger solid focus. Less commonly may present as a unilocular thick walled cyst with nodules of the lining or multilocular cystic mass with serous or mucinous fluid. Even less commonly seen is the gross appearance of a clear cell adenofibroma or APCCT described above [3].

Histology: Malignant cells with clear and slightly granular eosinophilic cytoplasm in multiple patterns, usually all present in combination in the same tumor: tubulocystic, papillary, and/or solid. The solid pattern shows sheets of polygonal clear cells separated by thin fibrovascular or dense fibrotic stroma. An adenofibromatous background may be present and is more often seen with the tubulocystic growth pattern, which has variable sized tubules and cysts [84]. Usually associated with endometriosis, the cystic tumors display papillary growth and characteristically, the papillae have hyalinized cores. Oxyphilic clear cell carcinoma refers to those tumors where cells predominately have abundant eosinophilic cytoplasm. The clear cytoplasm is due to glycogen and may also display intracytoplasmic mucinous inclusions. PAS positive hyaline globules are characteristic of clear cell carcinomas. Also, characteristically present in the papillary and tubulocystic patterns are hobnail cells, the seemingly naked nuclei protrude into the tubular lumen or cystic spaces. Nuclear features range from small and rounded to large and pleomorphic with macronucleoli. In fact, most tumors show a spectrum of mild to severe atypia, thus clear cell carcinomas are always high grade. Usually, mitoses are inconspicuous and necrosis, hemorrhage, psammoma bodies, and stromal inflammatory cells may be seen [84]. One third of clear cell carcinomas are cystic lesions arising directly from endometriosis as either gradual or abrupt transition from benign to malignant epithelium [84]. In comparison to the adenofibromatous type, the cystic type is significantly more likely to show endometriosis and atypical endometriosis [84]. Recent studies have shown that more than 50% of clear cell carcinomas are associated with endometriosis, ovarian or elsewhere in the peritoneal cavity [84].

Immunohistochemistry: Positive for CK7, CAM5.2, EMA, HNF-1β, napsin A, Leu M1, vimentin, BRCA1, WT1, TTF1. Negative for AFP, CK20, p53, CD10, CEA, ER, PR. The stroma is positive for type IV collagen and laminin [3].

Molecular: PIK3CA is the most common mutation, and while PTEN, CTNNB1, KRAS, BRAF, and p53 mutations may be present, however frequency is low [85, 86](Mayr, 2006). More recently, 17% of ovarian clear cell carcinomas showed microsatellite instability [87]. Hepatocyte nuclear factor-1 beta (HNF-1β) gene overexpression is specific for clear cell carcinoma [88].

Prognosis: Stage dependent, however clear cells have an adverse prognosis in the advanced stage [89]. Platinum-based chemotherapies are not as effective due to the low proliferative index.

CONSENT FOR PUBLICATION

Not applicable.

CONFLICT OF INTEREST

The author confirms that this chapter contents have no conflict of interest.

ACKNOWLEDGEMENTS

Declared none.

REFERENCES

[1]   American Cancer Society (ACS). What are the key statistics about ovarian cancer? 2014 [cited July 5, 2014]; Available from: http://www.cancer.org/cancer/ovariancancer/detailedguide/ ovarian-cancer-key-statistics

[2]   Surveillance, Epidemiology, End Results (SEER). http://www.seer.cancer.gov/statfacts/html/ovary.

html?statfacts_page=ovary.htmlx=15y=17

[3]   Seidman JD, Cho KR, Ronnett BM, Kurman RJ. Surface Epithelial Tumors of the Ovary.Blaustein's Pathology of the Female Genital Tract. 6th ed. New York, Dodrecht, Heidelberg, London: Springer 2011; pp. 679-784.
[http://dx.doi.org/10.1007/978-1-4419-0489-8_14]

[4]   Chen S, Parmigiani G. Meta-analysis of BRCA1 and BRCA2 penetrance. J Clin Oncol 2007; 25(11): 1329-33.
[http://dx.doi.org/10.1200/JCO.2006.09.1066] [PMID: 17416853]

[5]   Finch A, Beiner M, Lubinski J, *et al.* Hereditary Ovarian Cancer Clinical Study Group. Salpingo-oophorectomy and the risk of ovarian, fallopian tube, and peritoneal cancers in women with a BRCA1 or BRCA2 Mutation. JAMA 2006; 296(2): 185-92.
[http://dx.doi.org/10.1001/jama.296.2.185] [PMID: 16835424]

[6]   Russo A, Calò V, Bruno L, Rizzo S, Bazan V, Di Fede G. Hereditary ovarian cancer. Crit Rev Oncol Hematol 2009; 69(1): 28-44.
[http://dx.doi.org/10.1016/j.critrevonc.2008.06.003] [PMID: 18656380]

[7]   Prat J, Ribé A, Gallardo A. Hereditary ovarian cancer. Hum Pathol 2005; 36(8): 861-70.
[http://dx.doi.org/10.1016/j.humpath.2005.06.006] [PMID: 16112002]

[8]   Shaw PA, McLaughlin JR, Zweemer RP, *et al.* Histopathologic features of genetically determined ovarian cancer. Int J Gynecol Pathol 2002; 21(4): 407-11.
[http://dx.doi.org/10.1097/00004347-200210000-00011] [PMID: 12352190]

[9]   du Bois A, Reuss A, Pujade-Lauraine E, Harter P, Ray-Coquard I, Pfisterer J. Role of surgical outcome as prognostic factor in advanced epithelial ovarian cancer: a combined exploratory analysis of 3 prospectively randomized phase 3 multicenter trials: by the Arbeitsgemeinschaft Gynaekologische Onkologie Studiengruppe Ovarialkarzinom (AGO-OVAR) and the Groupe d'Investigateurs Nationaux Pour les Etudes des Cancers de l'Ovaire (GINECO). Cancer 2009; 115(6): 1234-44.
[http://dx.doi.org/10.1002/cncr.24149] [PMID: 19189349]

[10]   Wimberger P, Lehmann N, Kimmig R, *et al.* AGO-OVAR. Impact of age on outcome in patients with advanced ovarian cancer treated within a prospectively randomized phase III study of the Arbeitsgemeinschaft Gynaekologische Onkologie Ovarian Cancer Study Group (AGO-OVAR). Gynecol Oncol 2006; 100(2): 300-7.
[http://dx.doi.org/10.1016/j.ygyno.2005.08.029] [PMID: 16199079]

[11]   Gilks CB, Ionescu DN, Kalloger SE, *et al.* Cheryl Brown Ovarian Cancer Outcomes Unit of the British Columbia Cancer Agency. Tumor cell type can be reproducibly diagnosed and is of independent prognostic significance in patients with maximally debulked ovarian carcinoma. Hum Pathol 2008; 39(8): 1239-51.
[http://dx.doi.org/10.1016/j.humpath.2008.01.003] [PMID: 18602670]

[12]   Seidman JD, Yemelyanova A, Zaino RJ, Kurman RJ. The fallopian tube-peritoneal junction: a potential site of carcinogenesis. Int J Gynecol Pathol 2011; 30(1): 4-11.
[http://dx.doi.org/10.1097/PGP.0b013e3181f29d2a] [PMID: 21131840]

[13]   Kurman RJ, Shih IeM. The origin and pathogenesis of epithelial ovarian cancer: a proposed unifying theory. Am J Surg Pathol 2010; 34(3): 433-43.
[http://dx.doi.org/10.1097/PAS.0b013e3181cf3d79] [PMID: 20154587]

[14]   Kindelberger DW, Lee Y, Miron A, *et al.* Intraepithelial carcinoma of the fimbria and pelvic serous carcinoma: Evidence for a causal relationship. Am J Surg Pathol 2007; 31(2): 161-9.
[http://dx.doi.org/10.1097/01.pas.0000213335.40358.47] [PMID: 17255760]

[15]   Demopoulos RI, Aronov R, Mesia A. Clues to the pathogenesis of fallopian tube carcinoma: a morphological and immunohistochemical case control study. Int J Gynecol Pathol 2001; 20(2): 128-32.
[http://dx.doi.org/10.1097/00004347-200104000-00003] [PMID: 11293157]

[16]   Piek JMJ, Kenemans P, Verheijen RHM. Intraperitoneal serous adenocarcinoma: a critical appraisal of three hypotheses on its cause. Am J Obstet Gynecol 2004; 191(3): 718-32.
[http://dx.doi.org/10.1016/j.ajog.2004.02.067] [PMID: 15467531]

[17]   Salvador S, Gilks B, Köbel M, Huntsman D, Rosen B, Miller D. The fallopian tube: primary site of most pelvic high-grade serous carcinomas. Int J Gynecol Cancer 2009; 19(1): 58-64.
[http://dx.doi.org/10.1111/IGC.0b013e318199009c] [PMID: 19258943]

[18]   Seidman JD, Sherman ME, Bell KA, Katabuchi H, O'Leary TJ, Kurman RJ. Salpingitis, salpingoliths, and serous tumors of the ovaries: is there a connection? Int J Gynecol Pathol 2002; 21(2): 101-7.
[http://dx.doi.org/10.1097/00004347-200204000-00001] [PMID: 11917218]

[19]   Crum CP, Drapkin R, Miron A, *et al.* The distal fallopian tube: a new model for pelvic serous carcinogenesis. Curr Opin Obstet Gynecol 2007; 19(1): 3-9.
[http://dx.doi.org/10.1097/GCO.0b013e328011a21f] [PMID: 17218844]

[20]   Storey DJ, Rush R, Stewart M, *et al.* Endometrioid epithelial ovarian cancer : 20 years of prospectively collected data from a single center. Cancer 2008; 112(10): 2211-20.
[http://dx.doi.org/10.1002/cncr.23438] [PMID: 18344211]

[21]   Korner M, Burckhardt E, Mazzucchelli L. Higher frequency of chromosomal aberrations in ovarian endometriosis: a possible link to endometrioid adenocarcinoma. Mod Pathol 2006; 19: 1615-23.
[http://dx.doi.org/10.1038/modpathol.3800699] [PMID: 16980942]

[22]   Yoshikawa H, Jimbo H, Okada S, *et al.* Prevalence of endometriosis in ovarian cancer. Gynecol Obstet Invest 2000; 50 (Suppl. 1): 11-7.
[http://dx.doi.org/10.1159/000052873] [PMID: 11093056]

[23]   Kobayashi H, Sumimoto K, Moniwa N, *et al.* Risk of developing ovarian cancer among women with ovarian endometrioma: a cohort study in Shizuoka, Japan. Int J Gynecol Cancer 2007; 17(1): 37-43.
[http://dx.doi.org/10.1111/j.1525-1438.2006.00754.x] [PMID: 17291229]

[24]   Stern RC, Dash R, Bentley RC, Snyder MJ, Haney AF, Robboy SJ. Malignancy in endometriosis: frequency and comparison of ovarian and extraovarian types. Int J Gynecol Pathol 2001; 20(2): 133-9.
[http://dx.doi.org/10.1097/00004347-200104000-00004] [PMID: 11293158]

[25]   Ali-Fehmi R, Khalifeh I, Bandyopadhyay S, *et al.* Patterns of loss of heterozygosity at 10q23.3 and microsatellite instability in endometriosis, atypical endometriosis, and ovarian carcinoma arising in association with endometriosis. Int J Gynecol Pathol 2006; 25(3): 223-9.
[http://dx.doi.org/10.1097/01.pgp.0000192274.44061.36] [PMID: 16810057]

[26]   Cheng EJ, Kurman RJ, Wang M, *et al.* Molecular genetic analysis of ovarian serous cystadenomas. Lab Invest 2004; 84(6): 778-84.
[http://dx.doi.org/10.1038/labinvest.3700103] [PMID: 15077125]

[27]   Seidman JD, Mehrotra A. Benign ovarian serous tumors: a re-evaluation and proposed reclassification of serous "cystadenomas" and "cystadenofibromas". Gynecol Oncol 2005; 96(2): 395-401.
[http://dx.doi.org/10.1016/j.ygyno.2004.10.014] [PMID: 15661227]

[28]   Bell KA, Kurman RJ. A clinicopathologic analysis of atypical proliferative (borderline) tumors and well-differentiated endometrioid adenocarcinomas of the ovary. Am J Surg Pathol 2000; 24(11): 1465-79.
[http://dx.doi.org/10.1097/00000478-200011000-00002] [PMID: 11075848]

[29]   Longacre TA, McKenney JK, Tazelaar HD, Kempson RL, Hendrickson MR. Ovarian serous tumors of low malignant potential (borderline tumors): outcome-based study of 276 patients with long-term (or =5-year) follow-up. Am J Surg Pathol 2005; 29(6): 707-23.
[http://dx.doi.org/10.1097/01.pas.0000164030.82810.db] [PMID: 15897738]

[30]   Smith Sehdev AE, Sehdev PS, Kurman RJ. Noninvasive and invasive micropapillary (low-grade) serous carcinoma of the ovary: a clinicopathologic analysis of 135 cases. Am J Surg Pathol 2003; 27(6): 725-36.

[http://dx.doi.org/10.1097/00000478-200306000-00003] [PMID: 12766576]

[31]   Bell KA, Smith Sehdev AE, Kurman RJ. Refined diagnostic criteria for implants associated with ovarian atypical proliferative serous tumors (borderline) and micropapillary serous carcinomas. Am J Surg Pathol 2001; 25(4): 419-32.
[http://dx.doi.org/10.1097/00000478-200104000-00001] [PMID: 11257616]

[32]   Chang SJ, Ryu HS, Chang KH, Yoo SC, Yoon JH. Prognostic significance of the micropapillary pattern in patients with serous borderline ovarian tumors. Acta Obstet Gynecol Scand 2008; 87(4): 476-81.
[http://dx.doi.org/10.1080/00016340801995640] [PMID: 18382877]

[33]   Bell KA, Kurman RJ. A clinicopathologic analysis of atypical proliferative (borderline) tumors and well-differentiated endometrioid adenocarcinomas of the ovary. Am J Surg Pathol 2000; 24(11): 1465-79.
[http://dx.doi.org/10.1097/00000478-200011000-00002] [PMID: 11075848]

[34]   Rollins SE, Young RH, Bell DA. Autoimplants in serous borderline tumors of the ovary: a clinicopathologic study of 30 cases of a process to be distinguished from serous adenocarcinoma. Am J Surg Pathol 2006; 30(4): 457-62.
[http://dx.doi.org/10.1097/00000478-200604000-00005] [PMID: 16625091]

[35]   Singer G, Stöhr R, Cope L, *et al.* Patterns of p53 mutations separate ovarian serous borderline tumors and low- and high-grade carcinomas and provide support for a new model of ovarian carcinogenesis: a mutational analysis with immunohistochemical correlation. Am J Surg Pathol 2005; 29(2): 218-24.
[http://dx.doi.org/10.1097/01.pas.0000146025.91953.8d] [PMID: 15644779]

[36]   Seidman JD, Yemelyanova AV, Khedmati F, *et al.* Prognostic factors for stage I ovarian carcinoma. Int J Gynecol Pathol 2010; 29(1): 1-7.
[http://dx.doi.org/10.1097/PGP.0b013e3181af2372] [PMID: 19952945]

[37]   Smith Sehdev AE, Sehdev PS, Kurman RJ. Noninvasive and invasive micropapillary (low-grade) serous carcinoma of the ovary: a clinicopathologic analysis of 135 cases. Am J Surg Pathol 2003; 27(6): 725-36.
[http://dx.doi.org/10.1097/00000478-200306000-00003] [PMID: 12766576]

[38]   Bell KA, Smith Sehdev AE, Kurman RJ. Refined diagnostic criteria for implants associated with ovarian atypical proliferative serous tumors (borderline) and micropapillary serous carcinomas. Am J Surg Pathol 2001; 25(4): 419-32.
[http://dx.doi.org/10.1097/00000478-200104000-00001] [PMID: 11257616]

[39]   Gilks CB, Bell DA, Scully RE. Serous psammocarcinoma of the ovary and peritoneum. Int J Gynecol Pathol 1990; 9(2): 110-21.
[http://dx.doi.org/10.1097/00004347-199004000-00002] [PMID: 2332269]

[40]   Gershenson DM, Sun CC, Lu KH, *et al.* Clinical behavior of stage II-IV low-grade serous carcinoma of the ovary. Obstet Gynecol 2006; 108(2): 361-8.
[http://dx.doi.org/10.1097/01.AOG.0000227787.24587.d1] [PMID: 16880307]

[41]   Sangoi AR, McKenney JK, Dadras SS, Longacre TA. Lymphatic vascular invasion in ovarian serous tumors of low malignant potential with stromal microinvasion: a case control study. Am J Surg Pathol 2008; 32(2): 261-8.
[http://dx.doi.org/10.1097/PAS.0b013e318141fc7a] [PMID: 18223329]

[42]   Bell KA, Smith Sehdev AE, Kurman RJ. Refined diagnostic criteria for implants associated with ovarian atypical proliferative serous tumors (borderline) and micropapillary serous carcinomas. Am J Surg Pathol 2001; 25(4): 419-32.
[http://dx.doi.org/10.1097/00000478-200104000-00001] [PMID: 11257616]

[43]   Hsu C-Y, Kurman RJ, Vang R, Wang TL, Baak J, Shih IeM. Nuclear size distinguishes low- from high-grade ovarian serous carcinoma and predicts outcome. Hum Pathol 2005; 36(10): 1049-54.
[http://dx.doi.org/10.1016/j.humpath.2005.07.014] [PMID: 16226103]

[44]   Singer G, Stöhr R, Cope L, *et al.* Patterns of p53 mutations separate ovarian serous borderline tumors and low- and high-grade carcinomas and provide support for a new model of ovarian carcinogenesis: a mutational analysis with immunohistochemical correlation. Am J Surg Pathol 2005; 29(2): 218-24.
[http://dx.doi.org/10.1097/01.pas.0000146025.91953.8d] [PMID: 15644779]

[45]   Gilks CB. Subclassification of ovarian surface epithelial tumors based on correlation of histologic and molecular pathologic data. Int J Gynecol Pathol 2004; 23(3): 200-5.
[http://dx.doi.org/10.1097/01.pgp.0000130446.84670.93] [PMID: 15213595]

[46]   Gershenson DM, Sun CC, Lu KH, *et al.* Clinical behavior of stage II-IV low-grade serous carcinoma of the ovary. Obstet Gynecol 2006; 108(2): 361-8.
[http://dx.doi.org/10.1097/01.AOG.0000227787.24587.d1] [PMID: 16880307]

[47]   Bristow RE, Gossett DR, Shook DR, *et al.* Recurrent micropapillary serous carcinoma: the role of secondary cytoreductive surgery. Cancer 2002; 95: 791-800.
[http://dx.doi.org/10.1002/cncr.10789] [PMID: 12209723]

[48]   Garg R, Zahurak ML, Trimble EL, Armstrong DK, Bristow RE. Abdominal carcinomatosis in women with a history of breast cancer. Gynecol Oncol 2005; 99(1): 65-70.
[http://dx.doi.org/10.1016/j.ygyno.2005.05.013] [PMID: 15979132]

[49]   Salani R, Kurman RJ, Giuntoli R II, *et al.* Assessment of TP53 mutation using purified tissue samples of ovarian serous carcinomas reveals a higher mutation rate than previously reported and does not correlate with drug resistance. Int J Gynecol Cancer 2008; 18(3): 487-91.
[http://dx.doi.org/10.1111/j.1525-1438.2007.01039.x] [PMID: 17692090]

[50]   Willner J, Wurz K, Allison KH, *et al.* Alternate molecular genetic pathways in ovarian carcinomas of common histological types. Hum Pathol 2007; 38(4): 607-13.
[http://dx.doi.org/10.1016/j.humpath.2006.10.007] [PMID: 17258789]

[51]   Seidman JD, Kurman RJ, Ronnett BM. Primary and metastatic mucinous adenocarcinomas in the ovaries: incidence in routine practice with a new approach to improve intraoperative diagnosis. Am J Surg Pathol 2003; 27(7): 985-93.
[http://dx.doi.org/10.1097/00000478-200307000-00014] [PMID: 12826891]

[52]   Ronnett BM, Kajdacsy-Balla A, Gilks CB, *et al.* Mucinous borderline ovarian tumors: points of general agreement and persistent controversies regarding nomenclature, diagnostic criteria, and behavior. Hum Pathol 2004; 35(8): 949-60.
[http://dx.doi.org/10.1016/j.humpath.2004.03.006] [PMID: 15297962]

[53]   Seidman JD, Khedmati F. Exploring the histogenesis of ovarian mucinous and transitional cell (Brenner) tumors: a study of 120 tumors. Arch Pathol Lab Med 2008; 132: 1753-60.
[PMID: 18976011]

[54]   Riopel MA, Ronnett BM, Kurman RJ. Evaluation of diagnostic criteria and behavior of ovarian intestinal-type mucinous tumors: atypical proliferative (borderline) tumors and intraepithelial, microinvasive, invasive, and metastatic carcinomas. Am J Surg Pathol 1999; 23(6): 617-35.
[http://dx.doi.org/10.1097/00000478-199906000-00001] [PMID: 10366144]

[55]   Yemelyanova AV, Vang R, Judson K, Wu LS, Ronnett BM. Distinction of primary and metastatic mucinous tumors involving the ovary: analysis of size and laterality data by primary site with reevaluation of an algorithm for tumor classification. Am J Surg Pathol 2008; 32(1): 128-38.
[http://dx.doi.org/10.1097/PAS.0b013e3180690d2d] [PMID: 18162780]

[56]   Vang R, Gown AM, Barry TS, Wheeler DT, Ronnett BM. Ovarian atypical proliferative (borderline) mucinous tumors: gastrointestinal and seromucinous (endocervical-like) types are immunophenotypically distinctive. Int J Gynecol Pathol 2006; 25(1): 83-9.
[http://dx.doi.org/10.1097/01.pgp.0000177125.31046.fd] [PMID: 16306790]

[57]   Lee KR, Nucci MR. Ovarian mucinous and mixed epithelial carcinomas of mullerian (endocervical-like) type: a clinicopathologic analysis of four cases of an uncommon variant associated with

endometriosis. Int J Gynecol Pathol 2003; 22(1): 42-51.
[http://dx.doi.org/10.1097/00004347-200301000-00010] [PMID: 12496697]

[58]   Vang R, Gown AM, Barry TS, *et al.* Cytokeratins 7 and 20 in primary and secondary mucinous tumors of the ovary: analysis of coordinate immunohistochemical expression profiles and staining distribution in 179 cases. Am J Surg Pathol 2006; 30(9): 1130-9.
[http://dx.doi.org/10.1097/01.pas.0000213281.43036.bb] [PMID: 16931958]

[59]   Seidman JD, Kurman RJ, Ronnett BM. Primary and metastatic mucinous adenocarcinomas in the ovaries: incidence in routine practice with a new approach to improve intraoperative diagnosis. Am J Surg Pathol 2003; 27(7): 985-93.
[http://dx.doi.org/10.1097/00000478-200307000-00014] [PMID: 12826891]

[60]   Yemelyanova AV, Cosin JA, Bidus MA, Boice CR, Seidman JD. Pathology of stage I *versus* stage III ovarian carcinoma with implications for pathogenesis and screening. Int J Gynecol Cancer 2008; 18(3): 465-9.
[http://dx.doi.org/10.1111/j.1525-1438.2007.01058.x] [PMID: 17868343]

[61]   Chen S, Leitao MM, Tornos C, Soslow RA. Invasion patterns in stage I endometrioid and mucinous ovarian carcinomas: a clinicopathologic analysis emphasizing favorable outcomes in carcinomas without destructive stromal invasion and the occasional malignant course of carcinomas with limited destructive stromal invasion. Mod Pathol 2005; 18(7): 903-11.
[http://dx.doi.org/10.1038/modpathol.3800366] [PMID: 15696121]

[62]   Tabrizi AD, Kalloger SE, Köbel M, *et al.* Primary ovarian mucinous carcinoma of intestinal type: significance of pattern of invasion and immunohistochemical expression profile in a series of 31 cases. Int J Gynecol Pathol 2010; 29(2): 99-107.
[http://dx.doi.org/10.1097/PGP.0b013e3181bbbcc1] [PMID: 20173494]

[63]   Vang R, Gown AM, Barry TS, *et al.* Cytokeratins 7 and 20 in primary and secondary mucinous tumors of the ovary: analysis of coordinate immunohistochemical expression profiles and staining distribution in 179 cases. Am J Surg Pathol 2006; 30(9): 1130-9.
[http://dx.doi.org/10.1097/01.pas.0000213281.43036.bb] [PMID: 16931958]

[64]   McKenney JK, Soslow RA, Longacre TA. Ovarian mature teratomas with mucinous epithelial neoplasms: morphologic heterogeneity and association with pseudomyxoma peritonei. Am J Surg Pathol 2008; 32(5): 645-55.
[http://dx.doi.org/10.1097/PAS.0b013e31815b486d] [PMID: 18344868]

[65]   Cuatrecasas M, Villanueva A, Matias-Guiu X, Prat J. K-ras mutations in mucinous ovarian tumors: a clinicopathologic and molecular study of 95 cases. Cancer 1997; 79(8): 1581-6.
[http://dx.doi.org/10.1002/(SICI)1097-0142(19970415)79:8<1581::AID-CNCR2>3.0.CO;2-T] [PMID: 9118042]

[66]   Heinzelmann-Schwarz VA, Gardiner-Garden M, Henshall SM, *et al.* A distinct molecular profile associated with mucinous epithelial ovarian cancer. Br J Cancer 2006; 94(6): 904-13.
[http://dx.doi.org/10.1038/sj.bjc.6603003] [PMID: 16508639]

[67]   Wells M. Recent advances in endometriosis with emphasis on pathogenesis, molecular pathology, and neoplastic transformation. Int J Gynecol Pathol 2004; 23(4): 316-20.
[http://dx.doi.org/10.1097/01.pgp.0000139636.94352.89] [PMID: 15381900]

[68]   Sato N, Tsunoda H, Nishida M, *et al.* Loss of heterozygosity on 10q23.3 and mutation of the tumor suppressor gene PTEN in benign endometrial cyst of the ovary: possible sequence progression from benign endometrial cyst to endometrioid carcinoma and clear cell carcinoma of the ovary. Cancer Res 2000; 60(24): 7052-6.
[PMID: 11156411]

[69]   Roth LM, Emerson RE, Ulbright TM. Ovarian endometrioid tumors of low malignant potential: a clinicopathologic study of 30 cases with comparison to well-differentiated endometrioid adenocarcinoma. Am J Surg Pathol 2003; 27(9): 1253-9.

[http://dx.doi.org/10.1097/00000478-200309000-00009] [PMID: 12960810]

[70] Bell KA, Kurman RJ. A clinicopathologic analysis of atypical proliferative (borderline) tumors and well-differentiated endometrioid adenocarcinomas of the ovary. Am J Surg Pathol 2000; 24(11): 1465-79.
[http://dx.doi.org/10.1097/00000478-200011000-00002] [PMID: 11075848]

[71] Vang R, Gown AM, Farinola M, *et al.* p16 expression in primary ovarian mucinous and endometrioid tumors and metastatic adenocarcinomas in the ovary: utility for identification of metastatic HPV-related endocervical adenocarcinomas. Am J Surg Pathol 2007; 31(5): 653-63.
[http://dx.doi.org/10.1097/01.pas.0000213369.71676.25] [PMID: 17460447]

[72] Sato N, Tsunoda H, Nishida M, *et al.* Loss of heterozygosity on 10q23.3 and mutation of the tumor suppressor gene PTEN in benign endometrial cyst of the ovary: possible sequence progression from benign endometrial cyst to endometrioid carcinoma and clear cell carcinoma of the ovary. Cancer Res 2000; 60(24): 7052-6.
[PMID: 11156411]

[73] Storey DJ, Rush R, Stewart M, *et al.* Endometrioid epithelial ovarian cancer : 20 years of prospectively collected data from a single center. Cancer 2008; 112(10): 2211-20.
[http://dx.doi.org/10.1002/cncr.23438] [PMID: 18344211]

[74] Chen S, Leitao MM, Tornos C, Soslow RA. Invasion patterns in stage I endometrioid and mucinous ovarian carcinomas: a clinicopathologic analysis emphasizing favorable outcomes in carcinomas without destructive stromal invasion and the occasional malignant course of carcinomas with limited destructive stromal invasion. Mod Pathol 2005; 18(7): 903-11.
[http://dx.doi.org/10.1038/modpathol.3800366] [PMID: 15696121]

[75] Köbel M, Kalloger SE, Baker PM, *et al.* Diagnosis of ovarian carcinoma cell type is highly reproducible: a transcanadian study. Am J Surg Pathol 2010; 34(7): 984-93.
[http://dx.doi.org/10.1097/PAS.0b013e3181e1a3bb] [PMID: 20505499]

[76] Vang R, Gown AM, Farinola M, *et al.* p16 expression in primary ovarian mucinous and endometrioid tumors and metastatic adenocarcinomas in the ovary: utility for identification of metastatic HPV-related endocervical adenocarcinomas. Am J Surg Pathol 2007; 31(5): 653-63.
[http://dx.doi.org/10.1097/01.pas.0000213369.71676.25] [PMID: 17460447]

[77] Di Cristofano A, Ellenson LH. Endometrial carcinoma. Annu Rev Pathol 2007; 2: 57-85.
[http://dx.doi.org/10.1146/annurev.pathol.2.010506.091905] [PMID: 18039093]

[78] Liu J, Albarracin CT, Chang K-H, *et al.* Microsatellite instability and expression of hMLH1 and hMSH2 proteins in ovarian endometrioid cancer. Mod Pathol 2004; 17(1): 75-80.
[http://dx.doi.org/10.1038/modpathol.3800017] [PMID: 14631366]

[79] Storey DJ, Rush R, Stewart M, *et al.* Endometrioid epithelial ovarian cancer : 20 years of prospectively collected data from a single center. Cancer 2008; 112(10): 2211-20.
[http://dx.doi.org/10.1002/cncr.23438] [PMID: 18344211]

[80] Seidman JD, Soslow RA, Vang R, *et al.* Borderline ovarian tumors: diverse contemporary viewpoints on terminology and diagnostic criteria with illustrative images. Hum Pathol 2004; 35(8): 918-33.
[http://dx.doi.org/10.1016/j.humpath.2004.03.004] [PMID: 15297960]

[81] Seidman JD. Prognostic importance of hyperplasia and atypia in endometriosis. Int J Gynecol Pathol 1996; 15(1): 1-9.
[http://dx.doi.org/10.1097/00004347-199601000-00001] [PMID: 8852439]

[82] Pather S, Quinn MA. Clear-cell cancer of the ovary-is it chemosensitive? Int J Gynecol Cancer 2005; 15(3): 432-7.
[PMID: 15882166]

[83] Tan DSP, Kaye S. Ovarian clear cell adenocarcinoma: a continuing enigma. J Clin Pathol 2007; 60(4): 355-60.

[http://dx.doi.org/10.1136/jcp.2006.040030] [PMID: 17018684]

[84]   Veras E, Mao T-L, Ayhan A, *et al*. Cystic and adenofibromatous clear cell carcinomas of the ovary: distinctive tumors that differ in their pathogenesis and behavior: a clinicopathologic analysis of 122 cases. Am J Surg Pathol 2009; 33(6): 844-53.
[http://dx.doi.org/10.1097/PAS.0b013e31819c4271] [PMID: 19342944]

[85]   Mayr D, Hirschmann A, Löhrs U, Diebold J. KRAS and BRAF mutations in ovarian tumors: a comprehensive study of invasive carcinomas, borderline tumors and extraovarian implants. Gynecol Oncol 2006; 103(3): 883-7.
[http://dx.doi.org/10.1016/j.ygyno.2006.05.029] [PMID: 16806438]

[86]   Willner J, Wurz K, Allison KH, *et al*. Alternate molecular genetic pathways in ovarian carcinomas of common histological types. Hum Pathol 2007; 38(4): 607-13.
[http://dx.doi.org/10.1016/j.humpath.2006.10.007] [PMID: 17258789]

[87]   Jensen KC, Mariappan MR, Putcha GV, *et al*. Microsatellite instability and mismatch repair protein defects in ovarian epithelial neoplasms in patients 50 years of age and younger. Am J Surg Pathol 2008; 32(7): 1029-37.
[http://dx.doi.org/10.1097/PAS.0b013e31816380c4] [PMID: 18469706]

[88]   Tsuchiya A, Sakamoto M, Yasuda J, *et al*. Expression profiling in ovarian clear cell carcinoma: identification of hepatocyte nuclear factor-1 beta as a molecular marker and a possible molecular target for therapy of ovarian clear cell carcinoma. Am J Pathol 2003; 163(6): 2503-12.
[http://dx.doi.org/10.1016/S0002-9440(10)63605-X] [PMID: 14633622]

[89]   Chan JK, Teoh D, Hu JM, Shin JY, Osann K, Kapp DS. Do clear cell ovarian carcinomas have poorer prognosis compared to other epithelial cell types? A study of 1411 clear cell ovarian cancers. Gynecol Oncol 2008; 109(3): 370-6.
[http://dx.doi.org/10.1016/j.ygyno.2008.02.006] [PMID: 18395777]

CHAPTER 3

Dualistic Typing of Epithelial Ovarian Cancers: Emerging Paradigms for Oncogenic Progression and Cancer Treatment

D. Stave Kohtz[*]

Foundational Sciences, Central Michigan University College of Medicine, USA

Abstract: Dualistic classifications assign tumors arising from one tissue into two broad types based on differences in histology or grade, growth parameters (*e.g.*, hormone dependence or independence), prognosis, or expression of specific markers. Genomic analyses have allowed a more mechanistic expression of dualistic classification, so that tumor types may be founded on functional differences in the genetics of their development. This review considers the dualistic model of ovarian cancer, which is based primarily on whether or not mutations in the TP53 gene appear in the chronology of tumor progression. Type I ovarian cancers generally do not display mutations in the TP53 gene, and, according to several criteria, they have developed in the context of a relatively stable genome. In contrast, Type II ovarian cancers develop mutations in the TP53 gene early in tumorigenesis, and the resulting genome destabilization becomes a primary driver in tumorigenesis. Type I ovarian cancers generally are of lower grade and display a less malignant phenotype than Type II ovarian cancers, despite the better response of Type II ovarian cancers to certain chemotherapeutic regimens. Some reports have shown that mutation of TP53 can occur, albeit rarely late in a putative Type I progression, giving rise to an ovarian cancer with growth and survival properties similar to a Type II cancer. Future work should apply principles of dualistic cancer lineages acquired from ovarian and some other cancers (*e.g.*, sporadic and inflammatory bowel disease-associated colorectal cancer) to produce a unified model applicable to the prognostication and development of therapeutics for all cancers.

Keywords: Dualistic tumor classification, Genomic destabilization, Type I ovarian cancer, Type II ovarian cancer, TP53, Tumor progression.

INTRODUCTION

The dualistic distinction of Type I and Type II ovarian carcinomas (OvCas) aligns with the general observation that genetically divergent pathways of oncogenic

---
[*] **Corresponding author D. Stave Kohtz:** Foundational Sciences, Central Michigan University College of Medicine, USA; Tel: 989 774 3614; E-mail: kohtz1d@cmich.edu

Tamara L. Kalir (Ed.)

progression often arise within related tissue types [1, 2]. The precursor lesions for Type I tumors commonly occur on or within the ovary, whereas those for Type II tumors are thought to arise from the tubal or ovarian surface epithelium. The inception of oncogenic progenitors for Type I or Type II lineages is considered a deterministic fork in tumor development, and the potential for developing Type I lesions to provide precursors for Type II OvCas is discounted in the dualistic model. The key molecular difference between Type I and Type II molecular lineages in OvCas is the acquisition of defects in gene structure or regulation of TP53 during the early ontogeny of Type II neoplasms.

Precursor lesions for Type II ovarian neoplasms, including dysplastic cells in the fallopian tube epithelium and/or tubal intraepithelial carcinomas [3], have been identified with *TP53* mutations that are characteristic of serous carcinomas [4]. Defects in TP53 function are the early drivers in sporadic Type II neoplastic lineages, while familial forms are predisposed towards generating defects in *TP53* by the loss of function mutations in genes responsible for maintaining DNA integrity such as *BRCA1/2* [5]. Consistent with defects with *TP53*, Type II OvCas display chromosome instability, extensive copy number variations (CNVs), and other chromosomal defects [6]. In contrast, Type I OvCas do not commonly display defects in *TP53* or overt manifestations of genomic instability at a level consistent with Type II neoplasms [6]. Most Type I OvCas are thought to undergo stepwise progression from adenomas or low malignant potential growths to carcinoma, accumulating mutations in a subset of genes that, depending on histological type, can include *KRAS, NRAS, PIK3CA, PTEN, BRAF, CTNNB1, ERBB2, ARID1A, AKT,* or *PPP2R1A* [7]. Transitions of Type I to Type II neoplasms through later forming defects in *TP53* have been observed in specific instances [8, 9], with at least one reported case of high grade endometrioid OvCa generated through this pathway [10]. Defects in *TP53* or *BCL2* have been associated with malignant transformation of endometriotic cysts [11]. A murine model of endometrioid ovarian cancer has suggested that defects in *TP53* or *PIK3CA* arising late in tumor progression are responsible for generation of high grade endometrioid OvCa, a mechanism consistent with rare lineage conversions from Type I to Type II [12]. A large fraction of mucinous neoplasms classified as carcinomas also display mutations in *TP53* [13], and it is possible that all or a subset of these arose though late conversion of benign or borderline neoplasms.

Type I ovarian neoplasms are generally low grade, relatively indolent, and display endometrioid, clear cell, mucinous, low grade serous, or transitional cell histologies. In contrast to the relative indolence of most Type I neoplasms, clear cell carcinomas display a poor prognosis [14, 15]. Type II neoplasms are generally more aggressive and less well differentiated than Type I neoplasms, and present mostly as high grade serous ovarian carcinomas (HGOSCs), but also may appear as undifferentiated carcinomas and carcinosarcomas. The distinction between low and high grade ovarian cancers is frequently equated with Type I and Type II cancers, with the caveats that low grade and high grade serous OvCAs represent two distinct tumor types rather than low and high grade variants of the same neoplasm, and that some type I neoplasms, particularly clear cell carcinoma, may display high grade characteristics [16]. In addition, pathologists may preferentially identify most high grade OvCas as serous OvCas, and less commonly distinguish high grade endometrioid OvCas [16]. Analyses from the Cancer Genome Atlas Network revealed defects in *TP53* in 96% of Type II neoplasms [17]. Alternative mechanisms of *TP53* inactivation, including increased expression of *MDM2* or *MDM4* through copy-number gain, may account for *TP53* functional defects in Type II neoplasms without *TP53* mutations or changes in *TP53* methylation [5].

Ontogeny of Type I Ovarian Carcinomas

Risk analyses for ovarian cancer, including the role of prior surgery, hormone use, and use of non-steroidal anti-inflammatory drugs has supported the view that the oncogenic pathways driving progression of Type I and Type II OvCas are distinct [18]. A classification scheme for Type I ovarian carcinomas has been proposed to include three groups: i) endometriosis-related (endometrioid, clear cell, and seromucinous or mixed Müellerian), ii) low grade serous carcinomas, and iii) mucinous carcinomas and malignant Brenner tumors [2]. Most evidence supports a classic stepwise progressive model for Type I ovarian neoplasms. Type II neoplasia, because of the ubiquitous defects in the *TP53* gene as well as other defects that have been observed in genes involved in DNA repair [19], is driven primarily by genomic destabilization resulting in extensive copy number and other chromosomal defects. In contrast, the development of Type I OvCas proceeds through intermediate lesions or borderline tumors and can extend over several years. The rate limiting step for Type II OvCas is thought be mutation of *TP53,* a process that is accelerated by familial defects in *BRCA1/2*, and is followed by progression to carcinoma that is thought to be more rapid process than progression of Type I carcinomas [2]. There is evidence that genomic destabilization through loss of mismatch or homologous recombination repair gene function may also contribute to progression of endometrial and clear cell and clear cell carcinoma [20, 21], but these mutations occur later and function less prominently in progression than do mutations in *TP53* or *BRCA1/2* in Type II carcinomas.

Many Type I ovarian neoplasms are diagnosed while still confined to the ovary, suggesting that some tumors of this type arise directly from epithelium of the ovary. A positive association between endometriosis and the occurrence of ovarian clear cell and endometrioid carcinomas suggests that released cytokines or other factors may induce the growth and transformation of cells with endometrioid or clear cell phenotypes from the ovarian epithelium. Alternatively, the ovary may provide a substrate for the growth of precursors of these cells that are released from the inflamed endometrium [22]. Mutations in *PTEN* and *KRAS* are frequently observed in ovarian endometrioid carcinomas, with *KRAS* mutations being preferentially associated with endometriosis-associated neoplasms [23, 24]. In contrast, enhanced accumulation of β-catenin appears in ovarian endometrioid neoplasms lacking *KRAS* mutations [23]. Mutations in *CTNNB1* (β-catenin gene), are observed in ovarian endometrioid carcinomas, but are rarely observed in other Type I neoplasms [25, 26]. Detection of *PTEN* mutations, which are observed in ovarian endometrioid neoplasm arising in either the presence or absence of endometriosis, have been observed in benign endometrial lesions adjacent to ovarian endometrioid or clear cell carcinomas. Similarly, inactivating mutations and/or loss of expression of *ARID1A*, a tumor suppressor involved in SWI/SNF chromatin remodeling, have been reported in a majority of ovarian endometrioid and clear cell carcinomas, as well as in endometriotic cyst epithelium in the vicinity of the carcinoma [27]. Ovarian undifferentiated carcinomas are often associated with low-grade endometrioid tumors, and somatic mutations found in the low-grade neoplasms were shared by the carcinomas. Mutations in *PIK3CA*, *CTNNB1*, *TP53*, *FBXW7*, and/or *PPP2R1A* are observed mostly in the undifferentiated carcinomas, suggesting these mutations arise later in progression and contribute to the transition from benign to malignant neoplasia [28].

Most observations support an endometrial origin for the precursor cells of a large subset of ovarian endometrioid or clear cell carcinomas [29, 30]. Although endometriosis has been associated with a large fraction of ovarian endometrioid, clear cell, and seromucinous tumors, it is not clear that these tumors are exclusively derived from endometrial cells or induced by factors released by endometriosis. Seromucinous ovarian tumors are rare borderline or malignant tumors that are associated with endometriosis in ~23% of cases and that appear microscopically to have varied cellular composition. The medullary/paraovarian/ tubal or deeply cortical localization that is frequently observed suggests that seromucinous tumors originate from the secondary Müellerian system or vestigial structures [31].

Low grade serous are less common than high grade serous OvCas, and consistent with other Type I OvCas, are thought to progress in a stepwise fashion from benign lesions. The latter include serous cystadenomas or more advanced ovarian lesions such as atypical proliferative serous or borderline serous tumors [32]. Serous tumors with micropapillary architecture have been proposed to represent an intermediate between borderline tumors and low grade serous carcinomas [33 - 35]. Low grade serous OvCas generally lack *TP53* defects and are genetically stable. Mutations in *KRAS* are observed in one third of serous borderline tumors and 33% of low grade serous carcinomas, and mutations in *BRAF* are observed in 28% of serous borderline tumors and 30% of low grade serous OvCas [36 - 39]. The presence of *KRAS/BRAF* mutation is a favorable prognostic factor for women with low grade serous ovarian carcinoma [40]. In addition, *KRAS* and *BRAF* mutations are also observed in cystadenomas adjacent to serous borderline tumors [41]. Together, these observations indicate that *KRAS* and *BRAF* mutations occur early in low grade serous tumorigenesis and promote progression by constitutively activating downstream MAPK signaling pathways. Similar to high grade serous OvCas, low grade serous OvCas are thought to arise from fallopian tube epithelium, and gene expression profiles of low grade serous OvCas align better with fallopian tube epithelium than with expression profiles of cells from ovarian surface epithelium [42].

The phenotype of mucinous carcinomas is anomalous as it is not reflective of Müellerian tissues, but rather resembles cells of the gastrointestinal tract [43]. It is likely that many or most mucinous carcinomas in ovary are metastatic in origin, and primary mucinous ovarian carcinomas derived from structures such as the fallopian tube are rare [44]. The coincident appearance of some mucinous ovarian carcinomas with mature cystic teratomas has suggested that the associated mucinous neoplasms may derive from germ cells or teratomas, a conclusion supported by DNA genotyping and other investigations [45, 46]. Ovarian neoplasms bearing mucinous histology are classified as benign, borderline (including endocervical-like or Müellerian), intestinal, or most rarely, as carcinomas [47]. Mutations in the *KRAS* gene have been observed in Type I mucinous OvCas of Müellerian and gastrointestinal types [48]. The mutational landscape of mucinous neoplasms includes genes that are typical Type I drivers (*KRAS*, *BRAF*, ERBB3), as well as frequent appearance of mutation in *RNF43*, *ELF3*, *GNAS*, *CDKN2A*, and *KLF5* [13]. In some studies, approximately half of mucinous carcinomas have mutations in *TP53* [13]. It is possible that *TP53* mutations arise late in mucinous tumor progression during conversion from low to high grade forms as may be observed rarely with other Type I neoplasms. Alternatively, *TP53* mutations appear more frequently in mucinous than in other Type I histotypes and may play a role different from that in Type II ovarian neoplasms, perhaps more akin to the role of late *TP53* mutations in sporadic colon cancers.

Brenner tumors are the rarest form of ovarian neoplasm, and although most are benign, Brenner tumors can appear in benign, borderline (atypical proliferative), or malignant forms. Brenner tumors and some ovarian mucinous tumors may derive from metaplastic transitional cells at the tuboperitoneal junction [49]. Comprehensive molecular analyses of Brenner tumors have been hindered by their rarity. The tumors consist of transitional-appearing epithelium surrounded by a fibromatous stroma, and mutations have been detected in both cellular components. Rare mutations in *PIK3CA* have been detected specifically in the stromal components and not shared by the epithelial component, while mutations in *CDKN2A* appear to be associated with progression from benign to atypical proliferative forms [50]. Isoforms of *TP63* are commonly expressed in benign and borderline Brenner tumors, and may be used to distinguish them from other ovarian neoplasms [51]. Only a fraction of malignant Brenner tumors express *TP63,* and TP63 immunoreactivity is absent from ovarian transitional cell carcinomas [51]. As *TP63* is expressed in urinary bladder transition cell carcinomas, cervical transitional cell metaplasia, and Walthard cell rests, it is possible that the cellular origin of benign and borderline Brenner tumors may differ from some malignant Brenner tumors, and the metastatic forms may not derive from these sites. Brenner tumors are commonly associated with adjacent mucinous tumors; however, expression of the phenotypic markers *PAX2*, *PAX8*, *GATA3*, and *SALL4*, which are observed in Brenner tumors, is absent from the mucinous tumor cells [52].

Ontogeny of Type II Ovarian Carcinomas

Most Type II ovarian malignancies are high grade serous malignancies, but also included in this class are undifferentiated carcinomas, and carcinosarcomas. Germline *BRCA1/2* defects manifest in the ovary most often as high grade serous ovarian carcinomas [53, 54], but also have been associated with endometrioid, clear cell, and carcinosarcomas [55, 56]. High grade ovarian serous carcinomas (HGOSC) most closely represent the paradigm for development of Type II ovarian neoplasms, and account for ~75% of ovarian carcinomas [6, 17, 57]. High grade endometrioid and other putatively "converted" neoplasms are generated by progression through a series of mutations in a specific subset of genes and by the appearance of precursor or intermediate neoplasms. In these cancers, defects in *TP53* accompany late conversion to a carcinoma or malignant phenotype. This contrasts the early appearance of *TP53* defects in ovarian high grade serous carcinomas, which lead to profound genomic destabilization, rapid tumor progression, accumulation of copy number changes, and only a weak consensus in the mutations or genetic changes observed between individual tumors.

The classical view of the origin of high grade ovarian serous neoplasms suggested that they were derived from ovarian surface epithelium, a view that was supported by reports of increased TP53 protein observed focally in ovarian inclusion cysts in women with serous carcinomas [58]. These lesions were not observed, however, in ovaries of women with germ line *BRCA1/2* mutations [59]. Dysplastic lesions were reported in prophylactically removed ovaries from women with presumptive germ line *BRCA* mutations, and these were thought to represent preneoplastic transformation events [60]. The involvement of the ovarian surface epithelium in the genesis of HGOSC was support by the proposed relationship between repeated ovulations and the frequency of development of ovarian neoplasms [61]. The incessant ovulation hypothesis proposed that the stress and inflammation caused by ovulation on the surface of the ovary promotes oncogenesis; the gonadotropin hypothesis suggests that gonadotropins promote cellular transformation by stimulating the ovarian surface epithelium [62]. Both hypotheses have gained support from the observation that use of oral contraceptives reduces the risk of ovarian neoplasms, and both have prompted questions about the safety of fertility drugs [63]. In addition, the incidence of ovarian cancer increases after menopause along with increased gonadotropin levels, supporting the gonadotropin hypothesis [62]. Progression of epithelial cells derived from the fimbria of the fallopian tube towards ovarian cancer could also be promoted by ovulation, as inflammation and proliferation at the ovarian surface may promote trapping of sloughed fimbrial cells [64].

Development of high grade serous carcinomas from a precursor lesion in the fimbriae of the fallopian was first suggested by the presence of serous tubal in situ carcinoma in prophylactically removed fallopian tubes of women with germ line mutations in *BRCA1/2* [65, 66]. These lesions are the likely precursors of serous tubal intraepithelial carcinoma (STIC). Enhanced expression of *H2AX* and the presence of shorter telomeres indicated that DNA damage signaling is enhanced in STICs [67]. A tubal abnormality referred to as a secretory cell outgrowths (SCOUTs) has been reported as the earliest evidence of transformation in the fallopian tube [68]. The link to HGOSC is tenuous, as these lesions are characterized by a lack of *TP53* mutations, low PTEN and low Ki67, and they present as an array of secretory cells with a pseudostratified appearance [69]. The earliest veritable precursor lesion, referred to as the "p53 signature" [70], has been detected as a strongly TP53-positive strand of single cell deep, non-proliferative epithelium in the fimbriae of fallopian tubes that were removed as part of prophylactic surgery [66, 71]. Intermediate lesions have been referred to as serous tubal intraepithelial lesions or transitional intraepithelial lesion of the tube, and display p53 signatures, proliferative characteristics, tubal dysplasia and atypia [72, 73].

The consistency of PAX8 staining in most epithelial ovarian cancers (except mucinous) and in fallopian tube lesions supports the fallopian tube as an origin for high and low grade serous ovarian neoplasms [74 - 76]. Recent genomic evolutionary analyses have provided strong evidence that p53 signatures and serous tubal in situ carcinoma are precursors of HGOSCs, and progression from these lesions to *HGOSC* is thought to take approximately seven years [77]. In a genetically engineered murine model of HGOSC (Dicer-Pten double knockout), removal of the fallopian tube at an early age prevents cancer, whereas removal of the ovaries does not prevent cancer, strongly implicating the fallopian tubes as the tissue origin of HGOSC [78]. However, when these animals are further modified to express a p53 mutation (p53(R172H), similar to human HGOSCs), they develop HGOSCs from their ovaries after removal of the fallopian tubes [79]. Further, p53(R172H)-Pten double mutant mice also develop HGOSC from both fallopian tube and ovarian surface epithelium. Together, these observations indicate that while fallopian tube, in particularly fimbrial epithelial cells, is an established source of precursors for HGOSC, a role for the ovarian surface epithelium in some cases has not been ruled out. Determination of the cellular origin(s) of HGOSC is important for directing prophylactic surgery in women at risk for ovarian cancer [80].

Genetic Divergence in Type I and II Ovarian Neoplasms

The progression of Type I and Type II OvCas diverges at inception: primary genetic changes in nascent Type I lesions alter MAPK growth signaling pathways to deregulate growth control, while the primary changes in Type II lesions negatively impact *BRCA1/2* and/or *TP53* surveillance of DNA integrity and thereby promote the accumulation of mutations, chromosomal abnormalities and copy number variations. The totality of genomic changes in Type II OvCas greatly exceeds that of Type I OvCas, although the specific role of individual changes as drivers or passengers in the oncogenic process is less clear for Type II than for Type I OvCas. Type II OvCas display profound instability over the entire genome, but confounding genetic analyses of Type II OvCas is a dearth of significantly mutated genes present in at least 5% of cases. Significantly mutated genes are identified statistically in a tumor type as genes with mutations that are positively associated with tumor progression [81]. An analysis of 12 different cancer types including HGOSCs revealed 127 significantly mutated genes, and the number of significantly mutated gene occurring in at least 5% of cases examined varied significantly [82]. A cluster analysis of *TP53*-driven tumors revealed the lowest number of significantly mutated genes appearing in certain breast, head and neck, and ovarian cancers [82]. Type II OvCa displayed the lowest number of non-synonymous point mutations in significantly mutated genes of any of the cancer types examined (<2), with the prevailing mutation found in *TP53*. Median total mutation frequencies (number of mutations per Mb) for Type II OvCas were below the average for the 12 tumor type examined (although not the lowest); however, these studies considered transversions and transitions, but did not incorporate copy number variations [82]. Analyses of seven tumorigenic amplicons revealed wide-spread copy number changes in Type II tumor compared to a relatively flat chromosomal landscape observed in Type I tumors [83]. Other analyses at higher resolution revealed numerous and frequent microdeletions and amplifications within the genomes of Type II OvCas, and copy number variations common to Type II OvCas as well as those linked to patient outcome or metastatic potential have been identified [57, 84 - 87].

Outside of mutations in *TP53* and, less frequently, mutations in *BRCA* genes, different Type II OvCas display few common driver point mutations, and progress instead through accumulation of DNA copy number aberrations and chromosomal abnormalities [88]. In addition to germ line mutations in *BRCA1 and BRCA2* (14-16% frequency), other lower frequency germ line mutations (6% or less) have been observed in massive parallel sequencing studies of women with primary ovarian, peritoneal, or fallopian tube carcinoma [19]. Although a study from The Cancer Genome Atlas (TCGA) Research Network [17]) did not identify germ line mutations among ovarian cancer patients in any genes other than *BRCA1* or *BRCA2*, this may be due to low depth of coverage and lack of intronic coverage in that study. A consistent theme among the identified germ line mutations arises from their functions in maintaining DNA integrity and in DNA repair [19]. Germ line mutations appeared in all of the Fanconi anemia pathway genes that were tested in the Walsh study (*NBN, MRE11, RAD50, RAD51C, PALB2, BARD1,* and *BRIP1*) as well as in *TP53* (Li-Fraumeni syndrome type 1), *MSH6* (Lynch syndrome), or *CHK2* (Li-Fraumeni syndrome type 2). Loss of the normal allele for these genes was usually observed in the tumor cells [19].

Statistically significant recurrent somatic mutations (other than *TP53* or *BRCA 1/2*) were found at low frequency in the TCGA study in the *RB1, NF1, FAT3, CSMD3, GABRA6,* and *CDK12* genes [17]. In addition, epigenetic alterations resulting in reduced expression of BRCA and other genes are observed with low frequency in Type II OvCas [89]. Global analyses of amplified genes in HGSOCs revealed low frequency increases in the copy number of *CCNE1, NOTCH3, HBXAP, AKT2, PIK3CA* or chr12p13, but increased copy numbers of *ERBB2* were not observed in Type II cancers [83]. The Cancer Genome Atlas project identified four HGOSC Type II ovarian cancer transcriptional subtypes [17], while the Australian Ovarian Cancer study identified five transcriptional subtypes [88]. These subtypes arise through analyses of affected molecular pathways, and the relationship between Type II ovarian cancer subtypes and specific genetic changes is under investigation. The Cancer Genome Atlas project identified four subtypes based on promoter methylation, and three based on miRNA subtypes. Frequent disruptions of the RB, PI3K, NOTCH, and FOXM1 pathways were noted as independent of the Type II molecular subtype [17].

Low grade Type I ovarian tumors arise from progressive transformation of premalignant neoplasms, and in contrast to Type II neoplasms, development of Type I neoplasms occurs in the context of a relatively stable genome. In contrast to Type II ovarian neoplasms, Type I neoplasms display a consensus of high frequency gene mutations that are associated with specific histological forms (discussed above). Low grade serous cancers (Type I) frequently display activating mutations in genes that function in the RAS pathway (*KRAS*, *BRAF*) and increased copy number of *ERBB2*, while low grade endometrioid cancers frequently display activating mutations in the WNT-β-catenin (*CTNNB1*) pathway [90] and loss of function mutations in *PTEN* [1, 25, 26]. The mutational landscape of low grade mucinous neoplasms frequently includes members of the RAS pathway (*KRAS*, *BRAF*, or *ERBB3*), along with frequent mutations in other genes including *CDKN2A* [13]. Clear cell and endometrial cancers frequently display mutations in *ARID1A* [27]. The pathways leading to malignant neoplasms for Type I and II ovarian tumors are distinct; a question remains, however, regarding the rare appearance or absence in Type II neoplasms of defects in certain genes that are frequently found to be defective in Type I neoplasms. Increases in *ERBB2* copy number, frequently observed in low grade serous type I neoplasms, are rarely observed and not associated with malignant potential in HGOSCs [83, 91, 92]. Genetic changes or mutations commonly observed in Type I neoplasms, such as in *KRAS* and/or *BRAF* in low grade serous tumors, *KRAS* in mucinous tumors, *CTNNB1* and/or *PTEN* in endometrioid tumors, and *ARID1A* and/or *PIK3CA* in clear cell or endometrioid tumors are rarely or not found in Type II ovarian tumors [1, 93, 94]. Pathway analyses have shown that despite infrequent or the absence of physical aberrations in these genes Type II ovarian neoplasms, activation or suppression of signaling through the pathways that involve these genes is frequently observed. Thus, in the context of proliferating Type II tumor cells, these genes and their products appear to operate under normal regulatory and functional rules, but intrinsic defects in them are not driving neoplasia [17].

An analysis of the co-occurrence or exclusivity of mutations or small insertions or deletions in 127 significantly mutated genes revealed a set of 12 genes that show strong exclusivity or co-occurrence in over 3,000 tumors from 12 different tumor types [82]. From this study, tumors that possess mutations in *TP53* show strong exclusion of mutations in *PTEN*, *VHL*, *ARID1A*, *PBRM1*, *PIK3CA*, *PIK3R1*, *GATA3*, and/or *CTNNB1*, moderate exclusion of mutations in *KRAS* and/or *DNMT3A*, and strong co-occurrence of mutations in *APC* and *CDKN2A*. These results are consistent with the divergence of mutated genes observed between Type I and Type II ovarian tumors: Type II neoplasms are characterized by mutations in *TP53* and display an absence or low frequency of mutations in *KRAS*, *BRAF*, *PTEN*, *ARID1A*, *PIK3CA*, and *CTNNB1*. Mutations in subsets of the latter genes are observed frequently in different Type I ovarian neoplasms.

DNMT3A mutations have not been observed in any form of ovarian cancer [95]. Mucinous tumors, which display the highest frequency *TP53* mutations of the Type I ovarian tumors, also display frequent mutations in *CDKN2A*. Consistent with this, the analysis of 12 different tumor types revealed that *CDKN2A* mutations frequently co-occur with *TP53* mutations [82]. Finally, *K-RAS* or *BRAF* mutations are observed frequently in borderline tumors but not in invasive serous carcinoma and very rarely in other invasive subtype, supporting distinct rather than serial oncogenic pathways [39]. In reciprocal analyses, Nakayama the most frequently amplified sub-chromosomal regions in Type II ovarian tumors harbor the *CCNE1, AKT2, NOTCH3, RSF1*, and *PIK3CA* loci, and are not found to be amplified in Type I tumors [83]. Somatic mutations in *PIK3CA* are not observed in Type II cancers but they are in some Type I neoplasms. An ovarian tumor with defective *TP53* has been reported in which *PIK3CA* is mutated; this tumor displayed endometrioid histology, and thus may represent a transition of low grade Type I endometrioid cancer to high grade *via* late somatic mutation of *TP53* [96].

Genomic comparisons have revealed the presence of exclusive or co-occurring genetic defects among different types of neoplasms. Mutually exclusive mutations in genes are also observed when differentiating subsets of individual neoplasms of a certain type. The progression of Type I ovarian neoplasms is marked by mutations that occur in a specific panel of genes and in a certain order. The co-occurrence of certain genetic defects is not hard to understand when considering the different "hallmarks" of cancers and how an evolving tumor might be selected for mutations that meet these criteria for unrestrained growth [97]. In contrast, mutual exclusion of mutations in certain genes suggests that the combination of mutations is either toxic or growth restraining, despite the growth-promoting properties of either mutation in different genetic versions of the same tumor type. A well-documented example of mutual exclusion is the absence of co-existing mutations of *KRAS* and *EGFR* in lung adenocarcinomas, despite the high frequency of mutations in these genes individually in the same tumor type [98]. A potential explanation is that synthetic lethality results from "too much of a good thing," that is, activating mutations in more than one component of a shared RAS pathway. The exclusion of certain mutations frequently observed in Type I ovarian cancers from *TP53*-mutant positive Type II ovarian cancers is more challenging to explain. Mutations in *TP53* occur early in the ontogeny of Type II ovarian cancers, resulting in genomic destabilization and a greater probability of generating oncogenic genetic defects. Certain mutations that are frequently observed in Type 1 tumors are apparently toxic or growth suppressive to the developing Type II tumor cells, although a mechanism is not immediately apparent. Nonetheless, the observation of excluded gene mutations points towards pathways that may be useful as targets for development of treatments for Type II ovarian cancers.

Prognosis and Therapeutic Responses of Type I and II Ovarian Carcinomas

The overall prognosis and therapeutic responses of Type I and Type II OvCas are different. The five-year survival for Type I OvCas at ~55%, and for Type II OvCas it is ~30% [12]. The long-term prognosis of most Type I ovarian carcinomas is better than that of Type II cancers, primarily because many Type I tumors are detected prior to metastasis and can be fully removed by surgery. Murine models of ovarian cancer have suggested that metastasis occurs late in the course of Type I disease, supporting the success of surgical and other interventions in Type I disease. On the other hand, when reached, late stage Type I ovarian carcinoma is deadly [12]. In contrast, most Type II carcinomas are initially detected at later stages, but actually respond better than Type I neoplasms to treatment with platinum or PARP inhibitors. Current treatment for advanced stage Type II ovarian cancers includes surgical debulking and platinum/paclitaxel chemotherapy, and while the majority of patients achieve complete remission after six cycles of chemotherapy, the rate of relapse exceeds 50% [99]. Ironically, the inactivation of genes involved in DNA damage responses, including *TP53*, *BRCA1*, or *BRCA2,* and others, contributes to the enhanced sensitivity of Type II to DNA damage from chemotherapeutic agents [88]. TP53-dependent mechanisms of platinum toxicity are prevalent in normal cells and are responsible for the cytotoxic effects of platinum drugs in the kidney [100, 101]. The mechanism of platinum toxicity in Type II ovarian cancer cells is apparently TP53-independent and differs significantly from the less sensitive toxic responses of normal and Type I ovarian tumor cells. The greater sensitivity of *TP53*-defective tumor cells to cytotoxic agents such as platinum drugs suggests that TP53 may have a protective role (at least at lower doses) in Type I and normal cells. Defects in *BRCA1* or *BRCA2* are observed in approximately 10% of all ovarian cancer cases. Patient with germline mutations in BRCA1 or BRCA2 show higher response rates to chemotherapy and longer progression-free survival [17, 102, 103]. Defects in *BRCA 2* are associated with better survival and therapeutic responses than defects in *BRCA 1* or than wild-type *BRCA* genes. The importance of loss of BRCA function in enhancing platinum sensitivity in Type II ovarian cancers is further demonstrated by the selective emergence of drug-resistant *BRCA* reversion mutations after platinum-based chemotherapy [104].

Associating gene expression profiles with prognosis in HGOSC has proven challenging. The expression patterns of a panel of eleven genes was shown to have predictive value in determining survival of patients with high grade serous treated with carboplatin and paclitaxel. Further, an analysis of clinical endpoints and genetic alterations in HGOSCs noted eight regions of amplification or deletion on five chromosomes that clustered into subgroups, suggesting that HGOSCs may be segregated into clinically distinct subgroups. An earlier expression analysis of more than 300 HGOSCs identified five distinct molecular subtypes, four of these subtypes overlap with subgroup identified by a Cancer Genome Atlas Research network study [17]. These four subgroups were associated with specific clinical outcomes in another study [105]. The Cancer Genome Atlas Research Network study also delineated in HGOSCs three microRNA subtypes, four promoter methylation subtypes and a transcriptional signature associated with survival duration [17]. This study also confirmed the impact of *BRCA1* or *BRCA2* and *CCNE1* gene aberrations on survival. Another study employed high resolution copy number analysis and considered the association between copy number variation and prognosis in 118 cases of ovarian cancer. Newly identified genes or chromosomal regions, as well some that had been previously reported to have frequent copy number increases or deletions, were considered. This study found that increase copy number of *CCNE1* or enhanced extracellular matrix deposition and stromal responses were associated with poor therapeutic outcome [84]. Further studies have shown that amplification of *CCNE1* is critical for survival of ovarian cancer cells challenged by platinum and have suggested that the subgroup of HGOSC displaying amplified *CCNE1* may be "addicted" to this gene [106]. These properties may make CCNE1 suitable as a therapeutic target, either alone or in combination with platinum chemotherapy (see below).

MicroRNAs (miRNAs) are short non-coding RNAs that negatively regulate expression of target genes at the post-transcriptional level. The operant mechanisms of miRNA function include interference with mRNA translation and stability [107]. MicroRNA expression impacts both normal development and the differentiation of tumor cell phenotypes. A study of 489 HGOSCs by The Cancer Genome Atlas Research Network identified three tumor subtypes based on miRNA expression and found that high expression of miR-181a is associated with shorter disease-free interval [17]. Further studies revealed that miR-181a functions in induction of epithelial-mesenchymal transitions (EMTs) by TGF-β *via* suppression of Smad7 [108]. An integrated analysis of 459 cases from the TCGA and 560 cases from independent cohorts revealed an miRNA regulatory network associated with poor overall survival and promotion of the mesenchymal phenotype [109]. Differential expression of eight miRNAs was tightly associated with this network, which functioned in regulation of E-cadherin expression, migration and invasion during EMTs. Aberrant expression of the miR-200 family has been implicated in the control of metastasis and invasion of ovarian cancers, primarily *via* its role in regulating EMTs [110 - 112]. EMT is associated with drug resistance and growth of cancer stem cells, and the list of miRNAs involved in regulation of EMT continues to grow. Testing expression of characterized panels of miRNAs could provide important prognostic indicators for ovarian cancer, and specific miRNAs may be leveraged as targets for development of disease-modifying therapeutic agents.

Progress in advancing treatment of ovarian carcinomas beyond cytoreduction surgery and platinum/paclitaxel combination chemotherapy, which was introduced over 40 years ago [113], has been slow. As the treatment paradigms for ovarian carcinomas change, so shall the analyses employed to predict patient outcomes and prognosis. Amplification of *CCNE1* is observed in approximately 20% of HGOSCs and has been associated with chemo-resistance and overall poor prognosis [114]. A recent study has suggested that dinaciclib, a potent inhibitor of CDK 1, 2, 5, and 9, may be effective in combination with other chemotherapeutic drugs such as platinum or PARP inhibitors [115]. While treatment of cancer cells with CDK2 inhibitors alone results in resistance being acquired through upregulation of receptor-tyrosine kinase signaling, dinaciclib treatment of ovarian cancer cells with amplified *CCNE1* sensitizes the cells to platinum drugs [115]. Defects in *BRCA* genes make ovarian cancer patients good candidates for induction or maintenance therapies with PARP inhibitors [116]. The use of pegylated liposomal doxorubicin has shown efficacy in patients with *BRCA* defects and platinum resistance (recurrence within 6 months of prior therapy) [117]. Other potential combination therapeutic strategies for treatment of ovarian cancers with PARP inhibitors that so far have been considered for breast cancer regimens include phosphoinositide 3-kinase (PI3K) inhibitors and antiangiogenic agents (VEGFR2 inhibitors). Inhibition of PI3K results in sensitization to PARP inhibitors [118, 119]. The use of PARP inhibitors appears to increase phosphorylation of VEGFR2 and promote endothelial cell survival, an effect that is countered by VEGFR2 inhibitors [120]. In addition, inhibition of VEGFR2 leads to hypoxia in the tumors, making the neoplastic cells more sensitive to PARP inhibitors [121]. The folate receptor is overexpressed in more than 90% of ovarian cancers, and anti-folate receptor strategies are being tested for use in treatment of platinum-resistant ovarian cancer [122].

The stable genomes and linear progression pathways of Type I neoplasms makes these neoplasms more likely to be addicted to specific oncogenes and therefore more responsive to targeted therapies than the Type II ovarian cancers. Clinical trials with EGFR inhibitors or HER-2 targeted therapies found no benefit in unselected cases of ovarian cancer [123 - 125]. Amplification of HER2 is frequently observed (18%) in mucinous ovarian carcinomas, and evidence has been reported that HER2-targeted therapy may be an effective treatment for this population of advanced or recurrent cancers [126]. Low grade ovarian serous carcinomas frequently show activating mutations in *KRAS* or *BRAF*, and trials with MAPK pathways inhibitors have shown promising results with these tumors

[37, 127, 128]. Activating mutations of *PIK3CA* or *AKT*, or suppressor mutations in *PTEN*, result in activation of the PI3K survival pathways and are observed in up to 30% of clear cell and endometrioid ovarian carcinomas [122]. Development of small molecules to inhibit this pathway may yield appropriate treatments for these Type I ovarian cancers.

Numerous antibodies to tumor associated antigens, tumor-promoting molecules, and immune checkpoint molecules as well as small molecules are being considered for therapeutic applications in ovarian cancers (reviewed in [129]). For Type II ovarian carcinomas, the initial response to cytotoxic therapies is frequently quite strong; it is the prevention of recurrence, mediated by dormant cancer cells that presumably derive from drug resistant cancer stem cells, that is an important goal for future therapeutics. A favorable strategy of attack may include targeting signaling pathways that "wake up" the dormant cells and cause a relapse. Such therapeutic agents would increase the disease-free interval by hitting the snooze button on the alarm that awakens dormant ovarian cancer cells.

CONSENT FOR PUBLICATION

Not applicable.

CONFLICT OF INTEREST

The author confirms that this chapter contents have no conflict of interest.

ACKNOWLEDGEMENTS

Declared none.

REFERENCES

[1]   Shih IeM, Kurman RJ. Ovarian tumorigenesis: a proposed model based on morphological and molecular genetic analysis. Am J Pathol 2004; 164(5): 1511-8.
        [http://dx.doi.org/10.1016/S0002-9440(10)63708-X] [PMID: 15111296]

[2]   Kurman RJ, Shih IeM. The Dualistic Model of Ovarian Carcinogenesis: Revisited, Revised, and Expanded. Am J Pathol 2016; 186(4): 733-47.
        [http://dx.doi.org/10.1016/j.ajpath.2015.11.011] [PMID: 27012190]

[3]   Li HX, Lu ZH, Shen K, *et al.* Advances in serous tubal intraepithelial carcinoma: correlation with high grade serous carcinoma and ovarian carcinogenesis. Int J Clin Exp Pathol 2014; 7(3): 848-57.
        [PMID: 24696706]

[4]   Jarboe EA, Pizer ES, Miron A, Monte N, Mutter GL, Crum CP. Evidence for a latent precursor (p53 signature) that may precede serous endometrial intraepithelial carcinoma. Mod Pathol 2009; 22(3): 345-50.
        [http://dx.doi.org/10.1038/modpathol.2008.197] [PMID: 19151662]

[5]   Ahmed AA, Etemadmoghadam D, Temple J, *et al.* Driver mutations in TP53 are ubiquitous in high grade serous carcinoma of the ovary. J Pathol 2010; 221(1): 49-56.
        [http://dx.doi.org/10.1002/path.2696] [PMID: 20229506]

[6]   Bowtell DD. The genesis and evolution of high-grade serous ovarian cancer. Nat Rev Cancer 2010; 10(11): 803-8.
[http://dx.doi.org/10.1038/nrc2946] [PMID: 20944665]

[7]   Spreafico A, Oza AM, Clarke BA, *et al.* Genotype-matched treatment for patients with advanced type I epithelial ovarian cancer (EOC). Gynecol Oncol 2017; 144(2): 250-5.
[http://dx.doi.org/10.1016/j.ygyno.2016.12.002] [PMID: 28062115]

[8]   Quddus MR, Rashid LB, Hansen K, Sung CJ, Lawrence WD. High-grade serous carcinoma arising in a low-grade serous carcinoma and micropapillary serous borderline tumour of the ovary in a 23-yea--old woman. Histopathology 2009; 54(6): 771-3.
[http://dx.doi.org/10.1111/j.1365-2559.2009.03283.x] [PMID: 19438755]

[9]   Boyd C, McCluggage WG. Low-grade ovarian serous neoplasms (low-grade serous carcinoma and serous borderline tumor) associated with high-grade serous carcinoma or undifferentiated carcinoma: report of a series of cases of an unusual phenomenon. Am J Surg Pathol 2012; 36(3): 368-75.
[http://dx.doi.org/10.1097/PAS.0b013e31823732a9] [PMID: 22082603]

[10]   Provencher DM, Lounis H, Champoux L, *et al.* Characterization of four novel epithelial ovarian cancer cell lines. In Vitro Cell Dev Biol Anim 2000; 36(6): 357-61.
[http://dx.doi.org/10.1290/1071-2690(2000)036<0357:COFNEO>2.0.CO;2] [PMID: 10949993]

[11]   Nezhat F, Cohen C, Rahaman J, Gretz H, Cole P, Kalir T. Comparative immunohistochemical studies of bcl-2 and p53 proteins in benign and malignant ovarian endometriotic cysts. Cancer 2002; 94(11): 2935-40.
[http://dx.doi.org/10.1002/cncr.10566] [PMID: 12115382]

[12]   Wu R, Baker SJ, Hu TC, Norman KM, Fearon ER, Cho KR. Type I to type II ovarian carcinoma progression: mutant Trp53 or Pik3ca confers a more aggressive tumor phenotype in a mouse model of ovarian cancer. Am J Pathol 2013; 182(4): 1391-9.
[http://dx.doi.org/10.1016/j.ajpath.2012.12.031] [PMID: 23499052]

[13]   Ryland GL, Hunter SM, Doyle MA, *et al.* Australian Ovarian Cancer Study Group Mutational landscape of mucinous ovarian carcinoma and its neoplastic precursors. Genome Med 2015; 7(1): 87.
[http://dx.doi.org/10.1186/s13073-015-0210-y] [PMID: 26257827]

[14]   Chan JK, Teoh D, Hu JM, Shin JY, Osann K, Kapp DS. Do clear cell ovarian carcinomas have poorer prognosis compared to other epithelial cell types? A study of 1411 clear cell ovarian cancers. Gynecol Oncol 2008; 109(3): 370-6.
[http://dx.doi.org/10.1016/j.ygyno.2008.02.006] [PMID: 18395777]

[15]   Seidman JD, Cho KR, Ronnett RM, *et al.* Surface epithelial tumors of the ovary.Blaustein's pathology of the female genital tract. 6th ed. New York: Springer 2011; pp. 679-784.
[http://dx.doi.org/10.1007/978-1-4419-0489-8_14]

[16]   McCluggage WG. My approach to and thoughts on the typing of ovarian carcinomas. J Clin Pathol 2008; 61(2): 152-63.
[http://dx.doi.org/10.1136/jcp.2007.049478] [PMID: 17704261]

[17]   Network CGAR. Cancer Genome Atlas Research Network Integrated genomic analyses of ovarian carcinoma. Nature 2011; 474(7353): 609-15.
[http://dx.doi.org/10.1038/nature10166] [PMID: 21720365]

[18]   Terada KY, Ahn HJ, Kessel B. Differences in risk for type 1 and type 2 ovarian cancer in a large cancer screening trial. J Gynecol Oncol 2016; 27(3)e25
[http://dx.doi.org/10.3802/jgo.2016.27.e25] [PMID: 27029746]

[19]   Walsh T, Casadei S, Lee MK, *et al.* Mutations in 12 genes for inherited ovarian, fallopian tube, and peritoneal carcinoma identified by massively parallel sequencing. Proc Natl Acad Sci USA 2011; 108(44): 18032-7.
[http://dx.doi.org/10.1073/pnas.1115052108] [PMID: 22006311]

[20] Mills AM, Liou S, Ford JM, Berek JS, Pai RK, Longacre TA. Lynch syndrome screening should be considered for all patients with newly diagnosed endometrial cancer. Am J Surg Pathol 2014; 38(11): 1501-9.
[http://dx.doi.org/10.1097/PAS.0000000000000321] [PMID: 25229768]

[21] Lack of MRE11-RAD50-NBS1 (MRN) complex detection occurs frequently in low-grade epithelial ovarian cancer, 17. 2017.

[22] Nezhat F, Datta MS, Hanson V, Pejovic T, Nezhat C, Nezhat C. The relationship of endometriosis and ovarian malignancy: a review. Fertil Steril 2008; 90(5): 1559-70.
[http://dx.doi.org/10.1016/j.fertnstert.2008.08.007] [PMID: 18993168]

[23] Stewart CJ, Walsh MD, Budgeon CA, Crook ML, Buchanan DB. Immunophenotypic analysis of ovarian endometrioid adenocarcinoma: correlation with KRAS mutation and the presence of endometriosis. Pathology 2013; 45(6): 559-66.
[http://dx.doi.org/10.1097/PAT.0b013e3283650ad7] [PMID: 24018808]

[24] Stewart CJ, Leung Y, Walsh MD, Walters RJ, Young JP, Buchanan DD. KRAS mutations in ovarian low-grade endometrioid adenocarcinoma: association with concurrent endometriosis. Hum Pathol 2012; 43(8): 1177-83.
[http://dx.doi.org/10.1016/j.humpath.2011.10.009] [PMID: 22305241]

[25] Palacios J, Gamallo C. Mutations in the beta-catenin gene (CTNNB1) in endometrioid ovarian carcinomas. Cancer Res 1998; 58(7): 1344-7.
[PMID: 9537226]

[26] Kobayashi H, Kajiwara H, Kanayama S, *et al.* Molecular pathogenesis of endometriosis-associated clear cell carcinoma of the ovary (review). Oncol Rep 2009; 22(2): 233-40.
[http://dx.doi.org/10.3892/or_00000429] [PMID: 19578761]

[27] Ayhan A, Mao TL, Seckin T, *et al.* Loss of ARID1A expression is an early molecular event in tumor progression from ovarian endometriotic cyst to clear cell and endometrioid carcinoma. Int J Gynecol Cancer 2012; 22(8): 1310-5.
[http://dx.doi.org/10.1097/IGC.0b013e31826b5dcc] [PMID: 22976498]

[28] Kuhn E, Ayhan A, Bahadirli-Talbott A, Zhao C, Shih IeM. Molecular characterization of undifferentiated carcinoma associated with endometrioid carcinoma. Am J Surg Pathol 2014; 38(5): 660-5.
[http://dx.doi.org/10.1097/PAS.0000000000000166] [PMID: 24451280]

[29] Obata K, Morland SJ, Watson RH, *et al.* Frequent PTEN/MMAC mutations in endometrioid but not serous or mucinous epithelial ovarian tumors. Cancer Res 1998; 58(10): 2095-7.
[PMID: 9605750]

[30] Sato N, Tsunoda H, Nishida M, *et al.* Loss of heterozygosity on 10q23.3 and mutation of the tumor suppressor gene PTEN in benign endometrial cyst of the ovary: possible sequence progression from benign endometrial cyst to endometrioid carcinoma and clear cell carcinoma of the ovary. Cancer Res 2000; 60(24): 7052-6.
[PMID: 11156411]

[31] Karpathiou G, Chauleur C, Corsini T, *et al.* Seromucinous ovarian tumor A comparison with the rest of ovarian epithelial tumors. Ann Diagn Pathol 2017; 27: 28-33.
[http://dx.doi.org/10.1016/j.anndiagpath.2017.01.002] [PMID: 28325358]

[32] Fischerova D, Zikan M, Dundr P, Cibula D. Diagnosis, treatment, and follow-up of borderline ovarian tumors. Oncologist 2012; 17(12): 1515-33.
[http://dx.doi.org/10.1634/theoncologist.2012-0139] [PMID: 23024155]

[33] Seidman JD, Kurman RJ. Subclassification of serous borderline tumors of the ovary into benign and malignant types. A clinicopathologic study of 65 advanced stage cases. Am J Surg Pathol 1996; 20(11): 1331-45.

[http://dx.doi.org/10.1097/00000478-199611000-00004] [PMID: 8898837]

[34]   Vang R, Shih IeM, Kurman RJ. Ovarian low-grade and high-grade serous carcinoma: pathogenesis, clinicopathologic and molecular biologic features, and diagnostic problems. Adv Anat Pathol 2009; 16(5): 267-82.
[http://dx.doi.org/10.1097/PAP.0b013e3181b4fffa] [PMID: 19700937]

[35]   McCluggage WG. The pathology of and controversial aspects of ovarian borderline tumours. Curr Opin Oncol 2010; 22(5): 462-72.
[http://dx.doi.org/10.1097/CCO.0b013e32833b0dc1] [PMID: 20531187]

[36]   Haas CJ, Diebold J, Hirschmann A, Rohrbach H, Löhrs U. In serous ovarian neoplasms the frequency of Ki-ras mutations correlates with their malignant potential. Virchows Arch 1999; 434(2): 117-20.
[http://dx.doi.org/10.1007/s004280050314] [PMID: 10071245]

[37]   Singer G, Oldt R III, Cohen Y, *et al.* Mutations in BRAF and KRAS characterize the development of low-grade ovarian serous carcinoma. J Natl Cancer Inst 2003; 95(6): 484-6.
[http://dx.doi.org/10.1093/jnci/95.6.484] [PMID: 12644542]

[38]   Sieben NL, Macropoulos P, Roemen GM, *et al.* In ovarian neoplasms, BRAF, but not KRAS, mutations are restricted to low-grade serous tumours. J Pathol 2004; 202(3): 336-40.
[http://dx.doi.org/10.1002/path.1521] [PMID: 14991899]

[39]   Mayr D, Hirschmann A, Löhrs U, Diebold J. KRAS and BRAF mutations in ovarian tumors: a comprehensive study of invasive carcinomas, borderline tumors and extraovarian implants. Gynecol Oncol 2006; 103(3): 883-7.
[http://dx.doi.org/10.1016/j.ygyno.2006.05.029] [PMID: 16806438]

[40]   Kaldawy A, Segev Y, Lavie O, Auslender R, Sopik V, Narod SA. Low-grade serous ovarian cancer: A review. Gynecol Oncol 2016; 143(2): 433-8.
[http://dx.doi.org/10.1016/j.ygyno.2016.08.320] [PMID: 27581327]

[41]   Ho CL, Kurman RJ, Dehari R, Wang TL, Shih IeM. Mutations of BRAF and KRAS precede the development of ovarian serous borderline tumors. Cancer Res 2004; 64(19): 6915-8.
[http://dx.doi.org/10.1158/0008-5472.CAN-04-2067] [PMID: 15466181]

[42]   Qiu C, Lu N, Wang X, *et al.* Gene expression profiles of ovarian low-grade serous carcinoma resemble those of fallopian tube epithelium. Gynecol Oncol 2017; 147(3): 634-41.
[http://dx.doi.org/10.1016/j.ygyno.2017.09.029] [PMID: 28965696]

[43]   Seidman JD, Cho KR, Ronnett BM, *et al.* Surface epithelial tumors of the ovary.New York: Springer-Verlag: Blaustein's Pathology of the Female Genital Tract 6th 2011; pp. 679-784.
[http://dx.doi.org/10.1007/978-1-4419-0489-8_14]

[44]   Wheal A, Jenkins R, Mikami Y, Das N, Hirschowitz L. Primary Mucinous Carcinoma of the Fallopian Tube: Case Report and Review of Literature. Int J Gynecol Pathol 2017; 36(4): 393-9.
[http://dx.doi.org/10.1097/PGP.0000000000000330] [PMID: 27662036]

[45]   Wang Y, Schwartz LE, Anderson D, *et al.* Molecular analysis of ovarian mucinous carcinoma reveals different cell of origins. Oncotarget 2015; 6(26): 22949-58.
[http://dx.doi.org/10.18632/oncotarget.5146] [PMID: 26355245]

[46]   Snir OL, Buza N, Hui P. Mucinous epithelial tumours arising from ovarian mature teratomas: a tissue genotyping study. Histopathology 2016; 69(3): 383-92.
[http://dx.doi.org/10.1111/his.12959] [PMID: 26952875]

[47]   Lee KR, Scully RE. Mucinous tumors of the ovary: a clinicopathologic study of 196 borderline tumors (of intestinal type) and carcinomas, including an evaluation of 11 cases with 'pseudomyxoma peritonei'. Am J Surg Pathol 2000; 24(11): 1447-64.
[http://dx.doi.org/10.1097/00000478-200011000-00001] [PMID: 11075847]

[48]   Gemignani ML, Schlaerth AC, Bogomolniy F, *et al.* Role of KRAS and BRAF gene mutations in mucinous ovarian carcinoma. Gynecol Oncol 2003; 90(2): 378-81.

[http://dx.doi.org/10.1016/S0090-8258(03)00264-6] [PMID: 12893203]

[49] Gadducci A, Guerrieri ME, Genazzani AR. New insights on the pathogenesis of ovarian carcinoma: molecular basis and clinical implications. Gynecol Endocrinol 2012; 28(8): 582-6.
[http://dx.doi.org/10.3109/09513590.2011.649595] [PMID: 22304686]

[50] Kuhn E, Ayhan A, Shih IeM, Seidman JD, Kurman RJ. The pathogenesis of atypical proliferative Brenner tumor: an immunohistochemical and molecular genetic analysis. Mod Pathol 2014; 27(2): 231-7.
[http://dx.doi.org/10.1038/modpathol.2013.142] [PMID: 23887305]

[51] Liao XY, Xue WC, Shen DH, Ngan HY, Siu MK, Cheung AN. p63 expression in ovarian tumours: a marker for Brenner tumours but not transitional cell carcinomas. Histopathology 2007; 51(4): 477-83.
[http://dx.doi.org/10.1111/j.1365-2559.2007.02804.x] [PMID: 17880529]

[52] Roma AA, Masand RP. Different staining patterns of ovarian Brenner tumor and the associated mucinous tumor. Ann Diagn Pathol 2015; 19(1): 29-32.
[http://dx.doi.org/10.1016/j.anndiagpath.2014.12.002] [PMID: 25596159]

[53] Risch HA, McLaughlin JR, Cole DE, *et al.* Prevalence and penetrance of germline BRCA1 and BRCA2 mutations in a population series of 649 women with ovarian cancer. Am J Hum Genet 2001; 68(3): 700-10.
[http://dx.doi.org/10.1086/318787] [PMID: 11179017]

[54] Pal T, Permuth-Wey J, Betts JA, *et al.* BRCA1 and BRCA2 mutations account for a large proportion of ovarian carcinoma cases. Cancer 2005; 104(12): 2807-16.
[http://dx.doi.org/10.1002/cncr.21536] [PMID: 16284991]

[55] Zhang S, Royer R, Li S, *et al.* Frequencies of BRCA1 and BRCA2 mutations among 1,342 unselected patients with invasive ovarian cancer. Gynecol Oncol 2011; 121(2): 353-7.
[http://dx.doi.org/10.1016/j.ygyno.2011.01.020] [PMID: 21324516]

[56] Germline and somatic mutations in homologous recombination genes predict platinum response and survival in ovarian, fallopian tube, and peritoneal carcinomas, 20. 2014.

[57] Patch AM, Christie EL, Etemadmoghadam D, *et al.* Australian Ovarian Cancer Study Group Whole-genome characterization of chemoresistant ovarian cancer. Nature 2015; 521(7553): 489-94.
[http://dx.doi.org/10.1038/nature14410] [PMID: 26017449]

[58] Hutson R, Ramsdale J, Wells M. p53 protein expression in putative precursor lesions of epithelial ovarian cancer. Histopathology 1995; 27(4): 367-71.
[http://dx.doi.org/10.1111/j.1365-2559.1995.tb01528.x] [PMID: 8847068]

[59] Barakat RR, Federici MG, Saigo PE, Robson ME, Offit K, Boyd J. Absence of premalignant histologic, molecular, or cell biologic alterations in prophylactic oophorectomy specimens from BRCA1 heterozygotes. Cancer 2000; 89(2): 383-90.
[http://dx.doi.org/10.1002/1097-0142(20000715)89:2<383::AID-CNCR25>3.0.CO;2-T] [PMID: 10918170]

[60] Deligdisch L, Gil J, Kerner H, Wu HS, Beck D, Gershoni-Baruch R. Ovarian dysplasia in prophylactic oophorectomy specimens: cytogenetic and morphometric correlations. Cancer 1999; 86(8): 1544-50.
[http://dx.doi.org/10.1002/(SICI)1097-0142(19991015)86:8<1544::AID-CNCR22>3.0.CO;2-I] [PMID: 10526284]

[61] Fathalla MF. Incessant ovulation and ovarian cancer - a hypothesis re-visited. Facts Views Vis Obgyn 2013; 5(4): 292-7.
[PMID: 24753957]

[62] Mok SC, Kwong J, Welch WR, *et al.* Etiology and pathogenesis of epithelial ovarian cancer. Dis Markers 2007; 23(5-6): 367-76.
[http://dx.doi.org/10.1155/2007/474320] [PMID: 18057520]

[63] Riman T, Persson I, Nilsson S. Hormonal aspects of epithelial ovarian cancer: review of

epidemiological evidence. Clin Endocrinol (Oxf) 1998; 49(6): 695-707.
[http://dx.doi.org/10.1046/j.1365-2265.1998.00577.x] [PMID: 10209555]

[64] Kalir TA, Kohtz DS. Chemoresistance, Dormancy and Recurrence in Platinum Drug Theraapy of Ovarian Cancers In:Tumor Dormancy, Quiescence, and Senescence, Vol 3: Aging, Cancer, and Noncancer Pathologies Tumor Dormancy and Cellular Quiescence and Senescence. Springer Netherlands: Dordrecht 2014; pp. 79-97.

[65] Medeiros F, Muto MG, Lee Y, *et al.* The tubal fimbria is a preferred site for early adenocarcinoma in women with familial ovarian cancer syndrome. Am J Surg Pathol 2006; 30(2): 230-6.
[http://dx.doi.org/10.1097/01.pas.0000180854.28831.77] [PMID: 16434898]

[66] Lee Y, Miron A, Drapkin R, *et al.* A candidate precursor to serous carcinoma that originates in the distal fallopian tube. J Pathol 2007; 211(1): 26-35.
[http://dx.doi.org/10.1002/path.2091] [PMID: 17117391]

[67] Kuhn E, Meeker A, Wang TL, Sehdev AS, Kurman RJ, Shih IeM. Shortened telomeres in serous tubal intraepithelial carcinoma: an early event in ovarian high-grade serous carcinogenesis. Am J Surg Pathol 2010; 34(6): 829-36.
[http://dx.doi.org/10.1097/PAS.0b013e3181dcede7] [PMID: 20431479]

[68] Chen EY, Mehra K, Mehrad M, *et al.* Secretory cell outgrowth, PAX2 and serous carcinogenesis in the Fallopian tube. J Pathol 2010; 222(1): 110-6.
[http://dx.doi.org/10.1002/path.2739] [PMID: 20597068]

[69] Roh MH, Yassin Y, Miron A, *et al.* High-grade fimbrial-ovarian carcinomas are unified by altered p53, PTEN and PAX2 expression. Mod Pathol 2010; 23(10): 1316-24.
[http://dx.doi.org/10.1038/modpathol.2010.119] [PMID: 20562848]

[70] Saleemuddin A, Folkins AK, Garrett L, *et al.* Risk factors for a serous cancer precursor ("p53 signature") in women with inherited BRCA mutations. Gynecol Oncol 2008; 111(2): 226-32.
[http://dx.doi.org/10.1016/j.ygyno.2008.07.018] [PMID: 18718648]

[71] Kindelberger DW, Lee Y, Miron A, *et al.* Intraepithelial carcinoma of the fimbria and pelvic serous carcinoma: Evidence for a causal relationship. Am J Surg Pathol 2007; 31(2): 161-9.
[http://dx.doi.org/10.1097/01.pas.0000213335.40358.47] [PMID: 17255760]

[72] Carcangiu ML, Radice P, Manoukian S, *et al.* Atypical epithelial proliferation in fallopian tubes in prophylactic salpingo-oophorectomy specimens from BRCA1 and BRCA2 germline mutation carriers. Int J Gynecol Pathol 2004; 23(1): 35-40.
[http://dx.doi.org/10.1097/01.pgp.0000101082.35393.84] [PMID: 14668548]

[73] Gross AL, Kurman RJ, Vang R, Shih IeM, Visvanathan K. Precursor lesions of high-grade serous ovarian carcinoma: morphological and molecular characteristics. J Oncol 2010; 2010(126295)126295
[http://dx.doi.org/10.1155/2010/126295] [PMID: 20445756]

[74] Ozcan A, Liles N, Coffey D, Shen SS, Truong LD. PAX2 and PAX8 expression in primary and metastatic müllerian epithelial tumors: a comprehensive comparison. Am J Surg Pathol 2011; 35(12): 1837-47.
[http://dx.doi.org/10.1097/PAS.0b013e31822d787c] [PMID: 21989345]

[75] Tong GX, Hamele-Bena D. The differential expression of PAX2 and PAX8 in the ovarian surface epithelium and fallopian tubal epithelium is an important issue. Am J Surg Pathol 2012; 36(7): 1099-100.
[http://dx.doi.org/10.1097/PAS.0b013e3182500c1b] [PMID: 22472954]

[76] Xiang L, Kong B. PAX8 is a novel marker for differentiating between various types of tumor, particularly ovarian epithelial carcinomas. Oncol Lett 2013; 5(3): 735-8.
[http://dx.doi.org/10.3892/ol.2013.1121] [PMID: 23425942]

[77] Labidi-Galy SI, Papp E, Hallberg D, *et al.* High grade serous ovarian carcinomas originate in the fallopian tube. Nat Commun 2017; 8(1): 1093.

[http://dx.doi.org/10.1038/s41467-017-00962-1] [PMID: 29061967]

[78] Kim J, Coffey DM, Creighton CJ, Yu Z, Hawkins SM, Matzuk MM. High-grade serous ovarian cancer arises from fallopian tube in a mouse model. Proc Natl Acad Sci USA 2012; 109(10): 3921-6.
[http://dx.doi.org/10.1073/pnas.1117135109] [PMID: 22331912]

[79] Kim J, Coffey DM, Ma L, Matzuk MM. The ovary is an alternative site of origin for high-grade serous ovarian cancer in mice. Endocrinology 2015; 156(6): 1975-81.
[http://dx.doi.org/10.1210/en.2014-1977] [PMID: 25815421]

[80] Dietl J, Wischhusen J. The forgotten fallopian tube. Nat Rev Cancer 2011; 11(3): 227. [author reply].
[http://dx.doi.org/10.1038/nrc2946-c1] [PMID: 21326326]

[81] Dees ND, Zhang Q, Kandoth C, *et al.* MuSiC: identifying mutational significance in cancer genomes. Genome Res 2012; 22(8): 1589-98.
[http://dx.doi.org/10.1101/gr.134635.111] [PMID: 22759861]

[82] Kandoth C, McLellan MD, Vandin F, *et al.* Mutational landscape and significance across 12 major cancer types. Nature 2013; 502(7471): 333-9.
[http://dx.doi.org/10.1038/nature12634] [PMID: 24132290]

[83] Nakayama K, Nakayama N, Jinawath N, *et al.* Amplicon profiles in ovarian serous carcinomas. Int J Cancer 2007; 120(12): 2613-7.
[http://dx.doi.org/10.1002/ijc.22609] [PMID: 17351921]

[84] Etemadmoghadam D, deFazio A, Beroukhim R, *et al.* AOCS Study Group Integrated genome-wide DNA copy number and expression analysis identifies distinct mechanisms of primary chemoresistance in ovarian carcinomas. Clin Cancer Res 2009; 15(4): 1417-27.
[http://dx.doi.org/10.1158/1078-0432.CCR-08-1564] [PMID: 19193619]

[85] Malek JA, Mery E, Mahmoud YA, *et al.* Copy number variation analysis of matched ovarian primary tumors and peritoneal metastasis. PLoS One 2011; 6(12)e28561
[http://dx.doi.org/10.1371/journal.pone.0028561] [PMID: 22194851]

[86] Sung CO, Song IH, Sohn I. A distinctive ovarian cancer molecular subgroup characterized by poor prognosis and somatic focal copy number amplifications at chromosome 19. Gynecol Oncol 2014; 132(2): 343-50.
[http://dx.doi.org/10.1016/j.ygyno.2013.11.036] [PMID: 24321399]

[87] Despierre E, Moisse M, Yesilyurt B, *et al.* Somatic copy number alterations predict response to platinum therapy in epithelial ovarian cancer. Gynecol Oncol 2014; 135(3): 415-22.
[http://dx.doi.org/10.1016/j.ygyno.2014.09.014] [PMID: 25281495]

[88] Berns EM, Bowtell DD. The changing view of high-grade serous ovarian cancer. Cancer Res 2012; 72(11): 2701-4.
[http://dx.doi.org/10.1158/0008-5472.CAN-11-3911] [PMID: 22593197]

[89] Cho KR, Shih IeM. Ovarian cancer. Annu Rev Pathol 2009; 4: 287-313.
[http://dx.doi.org/10.1146/annurev.pathol.4.110807.092246] [PMID: 18842102]

[90] Schwartz DR, Wu R, Kardia SL, *et al.* Novel candidate targets of beta-catenin/T-cell factor signaling identified by gene expression profiling of ovarian endometrioid adenocarcinomas. Cancer Res 2003; 63(11): 2913-22.
[PMID: 12782598]

[91] Dimova I, Zaharieva B, Raitcheva S, Dimitrov R, Doganov N, Toncheva D. Tissue microarray analysis of EGFR and erbB2 copy number changes in ovarian tumors. Int J Gynecol Cancer 2006; 16(1): 145-51.
[http://dx.doi.org/10.1111/j.1525-1438.2006.00286.x] [PMID: 16445625]

[92] Farley J, Fuchiuji S, Darcy KM, *et al.* Associations between ERBB2 amplification and progression-free survival and overall survival in advanced stage, suboptimally-resected epithelial ovarian cancers: a Gynecologic Oncology Group Study. Gynecol Oncol 2009; 113(3): 341-7.

[http://dx.doi.org/10.1016/j.ygyno.2009.02.009] [PMID: 19272639]

[93]   Kuo KT, Mao TL, Jones S, *et al.* Frequent activating mutations of PIK3CA in ovarian clear cell carcinoma. Am J Pathol 2009; 174(5): 1597-601.
[http://dx.doi.org/10.2353/ajpath.2009.081000] [PMID: 19349352]

[94]   Teer JK, Yoder S, Gjyshi A, Nicosia SV, Zhang C, Monteiro ANA. Mutational heterogeneity in non-serous ovarian cancers. Sci Rep 2017; 7(1): 9728.
[http://dx.doi.org/10.1038/s41598-017-10432-9] [PMID: 28852190]

[95]   Zou Y, Huang MZ, Liu FY, *et al.* Absence of *DICER1, CTCF, RPL22, DNMT3A, TRRAP, IDH1* and *IDH2* hotspot mutations in patients with various subtypes of ovarian carcinomas. Biomed Rep 2015; 3(1): 33-7.
[http://dx.doi.org/10.3892/br.2014.378] [PMID: 25469243]

[96]   Kolasa IK, Rembiszewska A, Felisiak A, *et al.* PIK3CA amplification associates with resistance to chemotherapy in ovarian cancer patients. Cancer Biol Ther 2009; 8(1): 21-6.
[http://dx.doi.org/10.4161/cbt.8.1.7209] [PMID: 19029838]

[97]   Hanahan D, Weinberg RA. Hallmarks of cancer: the next generation. Cell 2011; 144(5): 646-74.
[http://dx.doi.org/10.1016/j.cell.2011.02.013] [PMID: 21376230]

[98]   Varmus H, Unni AM, Lockwood WW. How Cancer Genomics Drives Cancer Biology: Does Synthetic Lethality Explain Mutually Exclusive Oncogenic Mutations? Cold Spring Harb Symp Quant Biol 2016; 81: 247-55.
[http://dx.doi.org/10.1101/sqb.2016.81.030866] [PMID: 28123049]

[99]   Ozols RF. Systemic therapy for ovarian cancer: current status and new treatments. Semin Oncol 2006; 33(2) (Suppl. 6): S3-S11.
[http://dx.doi.org/10.1053/j.seminoncol.2006.03.011] [PMID: 16716797]

[100] Wei Q, Dong G, Yang T, Megyesi J, Price PM, Dong Z. Activation and involvement of p53 in cisplatin-induced nephrotoxicity. Am J Physiol Renal Physiol 2007; 293(4): F1282-91.
[http://dx.doi.org/10.1152/ajprenal.00230.2007] [PMID: 17670903]

[101] Molitoris BA, Dagher PC, Sandoval RM, *et al.* siRNA targeted to p53 attenuates ischemic and cisplatin-induced acute kidney injury. J Am Soc Nephrol 2009; 20(8): 1754-64.
[http://dx.doi.org/10.1681/ASN.2008111204] [PMID: 19470675]

[102] Yang D, Khan S, Sun Y, *et al.* Association of BRCA1 and BRCA2 mutations with survival, chemotherapy sensitivity, and gene mutator phenotype in patients with ovarian cancer. JAMA 2011; 306(14): 1557-65.
[http://dx.doi.org/10.1001/jama.2011.1456] [PMID: 21990299]

[103] Vencken PM, Kriege M, Hoogwerf D, *et al.* Chemosensitivity and outcome of BRCA1- and BRCA2-associated ovarian cancer patients after first-line chemotherapy compared with sporadic ovarian cancer patients. Ann Oncol 2011; 22(6): 1346-52.
[http://dx.doi.org/10.1093/annonc/mdq628] [PMID: 21228333]

[104] Norquist B, Wurz KA, Pennil CC, *et al.* Secondary somatic mutations restoring BRCA1/2 predict chemotherapy resistance in hereditary ovarian carcinomas. J Clin Oncol 2011; 29(22): 3008-15.
[http://dx.doi.org/10.1200/JCO.2010.34.2980] [PMID: 21709188]

[105] Gorringe KL, George J, Anglesio MS, *et al.* Australian Ovarian Cancer Study Copy number analysis identifies novel interactions between genomic loci in ovarian cancer. PLoS One 2010; 5(9)0011408
[http://dx.doi.org/10.1371/journal.pone.0011408] [PMID: 20844748]

[106] Etemadmoghadam D, George J, Cowin PA, *et al.* Australian Ovarian Cancer Study Group Amplicon-dependent CCNE1 expression is critical for clonogenic survival after cisplatin treatment and is correlated with 20q11 gain in ovarian cancer. PLoS One 2010; 5(11)e15498
[http://dx.doi.org/10.1371/journal.pone.0015498] [PMID: 21103391]

[107] Hu W, Coller J. What comes first: translational repression or mRNA degradation? The deepening

mystery of microRNA function. Cell Res 2012; 22(9): 1322-4.
[http://dx.doi.org/10.1038/cr.2012.80] [PMID: 22613951]

[108]   Parikh A, Lee C, Joseph P, *et al.* microRNA-181a has a critical role in ovarian cancer progression through the regulation of the epithelial-mesenchymal transition. Nat Commun 2014; 5(2977): 2977.
[http://dx.doi.org/10.1038/ncomms3977] [PMID: 24394555]

[109]   Yang D, Sun Y, Hu L, *et al.* Integrated analyses identify a master microRNA regulatory network for the mesenchymal subtype in serous ovarian cancer. Cancer Cell 2013; 23(2): 186-99.
[http://dx.doi.org/10.1016/j.ccr.2012.12.020] [PMID: 23410973]

[110]   Koutsaki M, Spandidos DA, Zaravinos A. Epithelial-mesenchymal transition-associated miRNAs in ovarian carcinoma, with highlight on the miR-200 family: prognostic value and prospective role in ovarian cancer therapeutics. Cancer Lett 2014; 351(2): 173-81.
[http://dx.doi.org/10.1016/j.canlet.2014.05.022] [PMID: 24952258]

[111]   Sulaiman SA, Ab Mutalib NS, Jamal R. miR-200c Regulation of Metastases in Ovarian Cancer: Potential Role in Epithelial and Mesenchymal Transition. Front Pharmacol 2016; 7(271): 271.
[http://dx.doi.org/10.3389/fphar.2016.00271] [PMID: 27601996]

[112]   Koutsaki M, Libra M, Spandidos DA, Zaravinos A. The miR-200 family in ovarian cancer. Oncotarget 2017; 8(39): 66629-40.
[http://dx.doi.org/10.18632/oncotarget.18343] [PMID: 29029543]

[113]   Vaughan S, Coward JI, Bast RC Jr, *et al.* Rethinking ovarian cancer: recommendations for improving outcomes. Nat Rev Cancer 2011; 11(10): 719-25.
[http://dx.doi.org/10.1038/nrc3144] [PMID: 21941283]

[114]   Kanska J, Zakhour M, Taylor-Harding B, Karlan BY, Wiedemeyer WR. Cyclin E as a potential therapeutic target in high grade serous ovarian cancer. Gynecol Oncol 2016; 143(1): 152-8.
[http://dx.doi.org/10.1016/j.ygyno.2016.07.111] [PMID: 27461360]

[115]   Taylor-Harding B, Aspuria PJ, Agadjanian H, *et al.* Cyclin E1 and RTK/RAS signaling drive CDK inhibitor resistance *via* activation of E2F and ETS. Oncotarget 2015; 6(2): 696-714.
[http://dx.doi.org/10.18632/oncotarget.2673] [PMID: 25557169]

[116]   Banerjee S, Kaye SB, Ashworth A. Making the best of PARP inhibitors in ovarian cancer. Nat Rev Clin Oncol 2010; 7(9): 508-19.
[http://dx.doi.org/10.1038/nrclinonc.2010.116] [PMID: 20700108]

[117]   Kaye SB, Lubinski J, Matulonis U, *et al.* Phase II, open-label, randomized, multicenter study comparing the efficacy and safety of olaparib, a poly (ADP-ribose) polymerase inhibitor, and pegylated liposomal doxorubicin in patients with BRCA1 or BRCA2 mutations and recurrent ovarian cancer. J Clin Oncol 2012; 30(4): 372-9.
[http://dx.doi.org/10.1200/JCO.2011.36.9215] [PMID: 22203755]

[118]   Ibrahim YH, García-García C, Serra V, *et al.* PI3K inhibition impairs BRCA1/2 expression and sensitizes BRCA-proficient triple-negative breast cancer to PARP inhibition. Cancer Discov 2012; 2(11): 1036-47.
[http://dx.doi.org/10.1158/2159-8290.CD-11-0348] [PMID: 22915752]

[119]   Juvekar A, Burga LN, Hu H, *et al.* Combining a PI3K inhibitor with a PARP inhibitor provides an effective therapy for BRCA1-related breast cancer. Cancer Discov 2012; 2(11): 1048-63.
[http://dx.doi.org/10.1158/2159-8290.CD-11-0336] [PMID: 22915751]

[120]   Mathews MT, Berk BC. PARP-1 inhibition prevents oxidative and nitrosative stress-induced endothelial cell death *via* transactivation of the VEGF receptor 2. Arterioscler Thromb Vasc Biol 2008; 28(4): 711-7.
[http://dx.doi.org/10.1161/ATVBAHA.107.156406] [PMID: 18239155]

[121]   Hegan DC, Lu Y, Stachelek GC, Crosby ME, Bindra RS, Glazer PM. Inhibition of poly(ADP-ribose) polymerase down-regulates BRCA1 and RAD51 in a pathway mediated by E2F4 and p130. Proc Natl

Acad Sci USA 2010; 107(5): 2201-6.
[http://dx.doi.org/10.1073/pnas.0904783107] [PMID: 20133863]

[122] Banerjee S, Kaye SB. New strategies in the treatment of ovarian cancer: current clinical perspectives and future potential. Clin Cancer Res 2013; 19(5): 961-8.
[http://dx.doi.org/10.1158/1078-0432.CCR-12-2243] [PMID: 23307860]

[123] Schilder RJ, Sill MW, Chen X, *et al.* Phase II study of gefitinib in patients with relapsed or persistent ovarian or primary peritoneal carcinoma and evaluation of epidermal growth factor receptor mutations and immunohistochemical expression: a Gynecologic Oncology Group Study. Clin Cancer Res 2005; 11(15): 5539-48.
[http://dx.doi.org/10.1158/1078-0432.CCR-05-0462] [PMID: 16061871]

[124] Gordon MS, Matei D, Aghajanian C, *et al.* Clinical activity of pertuzumab (rhuMAb 2C4), a HER dimerization inhibitor, in advanced ovarian cancer: potential predictive relationship with tumor HER2 activation status. J Clin Oncol 2006; 24(26): 4324-32.
[http://dx.doi.org/10.1200/JCO.2005.05.4221] [PMID: 16896006]

[125] Kaye SB, Poole CJ, Dańska-Bidzińska A, *et al.* A randomized phase II study evaluating the combination of carboplatin-based chemotherapy with pertuzumab *versus* carboplatin-based therapy alone in patients with relapsed, platinum-sensitive ovarian cancer. Ann Oncol 2013; 24(1): 145-52.
[http://dx.doi.org/10.1093/annonc/mds282] [PMID: 23002282]

[126] Anglesio MS, Kommoss S, Tolcher MC, *et al.* Molecular characterization of mucinous ovarian tumours supports a stratified treatment approach with HER2 targeting in 19% of carcinomas. J Pathol 2013; 229(1): 111-20.
[http://dx.doi.org/10.1002/path.4088] [PMID: 22899400]

[127] Wong KK, Tsang YT, Deavers MT, *et al.* BRAF mutation is rare in advanced-stage low-grade ovarian serous carcinomas. Am J Pathol 2010; 177(4): 1611-7.
[http://dx.doi.org/10.2353/ajpath.2010.100212] [PMID: 20802181]

[128] Farley J, Brady WE, Vathipadiekal V, *et al.* Selumetinib in women with recurrent low-grade serous carcinoma of the ovary or peritoneum: an open-label, single-arm, phase 2 study. Lancet Oncol 2013; 14(2): 134-40.
[http://dx.doi.org/10.1016/S1470-2045(12)70572-7] [PMID: 23261356]

[129] Bax HJ, Josephs DH, Pellizzari G, Spicer JF, Montes A, Karagiannis SN. Therapeutic targets and new directions for antibodies developed for ovarian cancer. MAbs 2016; 8(8): 1437-55.
[http://dx.doi.org/10.1080/19420862.2016.1219005] [PMID: 27494775]

CHAPTER 4

Genomic Analysis of Epithelial Ovarian Cancer

Gonzalo Carrasco-Avino[1,*], Benjamin Greenbaum[2], Mireia Castillo-Martin[3], Adolfo Firpo[4], Carlos Cordon-Cardo[5] and Tamara Kalir[6]

[1] *Departments of Pathology, Clinica las Condes and Hospital Clínico Universidad de Chile, and Adjunct Assistant Professor of Pathology, Department of Pathology, The Icahn School of Medicine at Mount Sinai, N.Y.C, USA*

[2] *Assistant Professor of Medicine and Pathology, The Icahn School of Medicine at Mount Sinai, NYC, USA*

[3] *Molecular and Experimental Pathology Laboratory, Champalimaud Centre for the Unknown, Lisbon, Portugal; and Assistant Professor of Research, Department of Pathology, The Icahn School of Medicine at Mount Sinai, USA*

[4] *Professor of Pathology, The Icahn School of Medicine at Mount Sinai, USA*

[5] *Professor and System Chair, The Icahn School of Medicine at Mount Sinai, USA*

[6] *Associate Professor of Pathology, The Icahn School of Medicine at Mount Sinai, USA*

Abstract: High-grade serous carcinoma (HGSC) is the most common epithelial ovarian cancer (EOC) accounting for 60% to 80% of ovarian cancers. Its main molecular alterations are 1) mutation or non-function of TP53, 2) BRCA1 or BRCA2 germline mutations and 3) alterations in the EGFR/HER2 pathway with Her2 overexpression. Despite these well-known genetic alterations, our understanding of gene interactions in canonical pathways remains fairly rudimentary. One approach to better understand gene-biopathway interplay is using *in-silico* analyses of gene expression microarray databases available in the public data repositories. Minimum information about a microarray experiment (MIAME) guidelines established, as a pre-requisite for the publication of microarray data, that data supporting published conclusions are made available for further analyses by other researchers. However, in spite of the availability of large, responsibly generated datasets to the public, secondary analyses are rarely performed. The purpose of this chapter is to show an example of this approach by undertaking an *in-silico* analysis of Public Gene Expression Omnibus (GEO) datasets comparing the gene expression between HGSC and Fallopian Tube Epithelium (FTE) and between HGSC and Ovarian Surface Epithelium (OSE), to then apply a Functional Genomics approach to study the gene interaction of HGSC in canonical pathways, *in-silico* activation of these pathways, and how chemotherapeutic drugs potentially affect them. We will explain step by step the methodology and results, including the datasets selection, data filtering and normalization, comparison of

* Corresponding author Gonzalo Carrasco-Avino: Departments of Pathology, Clinica las Condes and Hospital Clínico Universidad de Chile, and Adjunct Assistant Professor of Pathology, Department of Pathology, The Icahn School of Medicine at Mount Sinai, N.Y.C, USA; Tel: +56995321208; E-mail: gcarrasa@me.com

the gene expression between the samples using a class comparison analysis, validation by immunohistochemistry (IHC) and Functional Genomics Analysis using Ingenuity Pathway Analysis (IPA).

Keywords: Canonical pathways, Epithelial ovarian cancer, Functional genomics, Gene interaction, *In-silico* analysis, Ingenuity Pathway Analysis, Mutations.

INTRODUCTION

The World Health Organization classifies ovarian neoplasms according to the most likely tissue of origin: surface epithelium (65%), germ cell (15%), sex cord-stromal (10%), metastases (5%), and miscellaneous (5%) [1]. Surface epithelial ovarian cancer (EOC) is further classified by cell type (serous, mucinous, endometrioid, *etc.*) and grade of atypia (benign, atypical proliferative, or malignant) [2]. The great majority of the malignant ovarian tumors are EOC (90%) corresponding to the most important cause of gynecologic cancer mortality in developed countries. Most cases are diagnosed at advanced stage, mainly due to lacking of screening programs, which turns into an overall 5-years survival rate of 30% [3]. Surgery is the treatment of choice to achieve optimal tumor debulking and subsequent histopathology analysis and FIGO staging [4]. High-grade pelvic-type serous carcinoma (HGSC) is the most common EOC accounting for 60% to 80% of ovarian cancers. The origin of pelvic-type HGSC is a subject of debate, although evidence is rapidly accumulating in support of a malignant transformation of the fallopian tube mucosal epithelial cells [5].

The main pathways and/or mutations described in HGSC are: 1) TP53 pathway, which either by mutation or non-function in up to 50% to 80% of tumors, distinguishes HGSC from other ovarian cancer subtypes. Furthermore, a "p53 signature", defined as morphologically normal epithelium containing p53-positive secretory cells is a current proposed precursor [6 - 9] Fig. (**1**), taken and modified from [8]); 2) BRCA1 or BRCA2 germline mutations, which are observed in approximately 18% of the patients with pelvic-type HGSC [10]; 3) EGFR/HER2 pathway, with Her2 over-expression being observed in 20% to 30% of the epithelial ovarian cancers [7, 11]. Despite these well-known genetic alterations in HGSC, our understanding of gene interactions and signaling molecules in canonical pathways remains fairly rudimentary.

One approach to better understand gene-biopathway interplay is using *in-silico* analysis of gene expression microarray databases available in the public data repositories. Some of these databases are The Cancer Genome Atlas (TCGA), DNA Data Bank of Japan, European Bioinformatics Institute, the National Center for Biotechnology Information (NCBI), and ArrayExpress [12]. Coupling *in-silico* analysis with high-throughput genomic technology has enabled the identification of therapeutic targets and risk factors for specific diseases, an important application in this newly emerging era of personalized medicine [13]. Minimum information about a microarray experiment (MIAME) guidelines has been established, and a pre-requisite for the publication of microarray data is that data supporting published conclusions are made available to researchers, rendering their data useful for further analyses by others [14, 15]. However in spite of the availability of large, responsibly generated datasets to the public, secondary analyses are rarely performed [16, 17]. Along this line, we'll show an example of one potential approach by undertaking an *in-silico* analysis of Public Gene Expression Omnibus (GEO) datasets comparing the gene expression between HGSC and Fallopian Tube Epithelium (FTE) and between HGSC and Ovarian Surface Epithelium (OSE), to then apply a Functional Genomics approach to

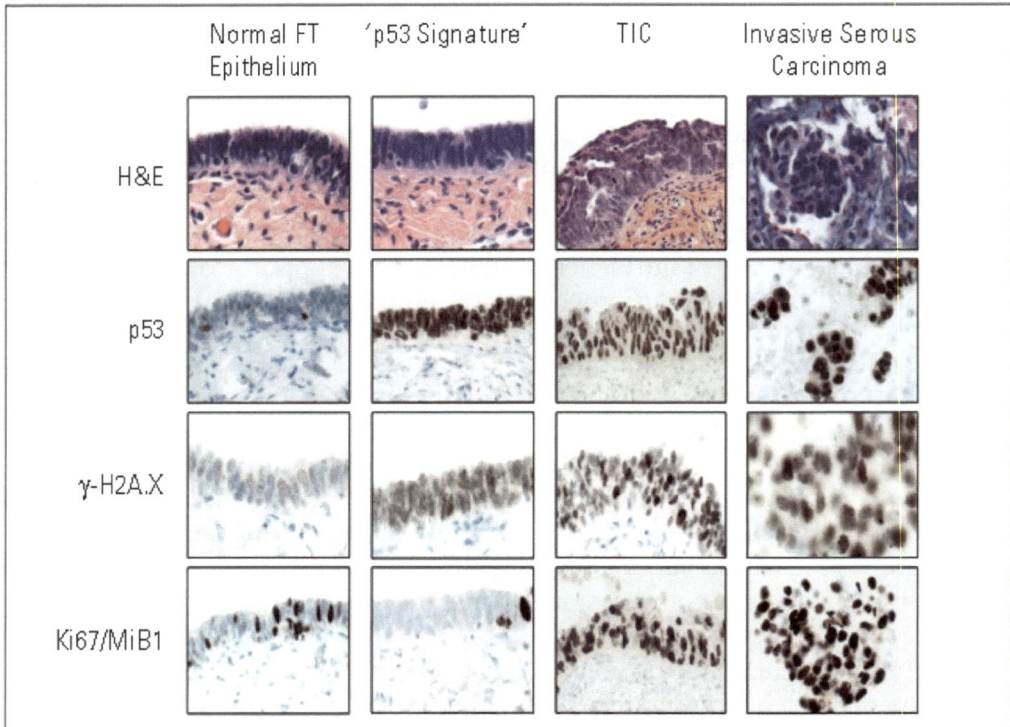

Fig. (1). Pathologic features of the fallopian tube (FT) carcinogenesis spectrum. While normal FT epithelium contains both ciliated and secretory cells, p53 signature—the proposed precursor lesion— is characterized by normal tissue morphology with p53-positive secretory cells harboring DNA damage (H2A.X staining). Tubal intraepithelial carcinoma (TIC) shares these features but has acquired a proliferative advantage (increased Ki-67/MiB1 staining). Invasive serous carcinoma shows increased proliferation and disruption of the basement membrane (Taken from Levanon *et al.*, 2008).

study the gene interaction of HGSC in canonical pathways, *in-silico* activation of these pathways, and how chemotherapeutic drugs potentially affect them. We will explain step by step the methodology and results, including the datasets selection, data filtering and normalization, comparison of the gene expression between the samples using a class comparison analysis, validation by immunohistochemistry and Functional Genomics Analysis using Ingenuity Pathway Analysis (IPA).

DATASETS SELECTION

We downloaded the raw data (CEL files) from GSE10971 and GSE14407 datasets (Affymetrix Human Genome U133 Plus 2.0 Array). GSE10971 contains the gene expression of 24 laser capture microdissected non-malignant distal Fallopian tube epithelium (FTE), as well as 13 high grade serous carcinoma either tubal or ovarian in origin, as previously described by Tone *et al.* [18]. GSE14407 contains the gene expression of 12 OSE collected by a Cytobrush® Plus and 12 laser capture microdissected HGSC as previously described by Bowen *et al.* [19].

DATA NORMALIZATION AND FILTERING

The data were normalized using the robust multiarray average method (RMA) and a log2-based transformation using the "median" array as a reference array [20]. (BrB-ArrayTools v4.3.2). Probes were filtered-out if: 1.- less than 20% of the expression data values were at least 1.5 minimum fold-change in either direction from the gene's median value (minimum fold-change filter); 2.- the variance of their log-expression values across arrays was in the bottom 50th percentile (Variance filter) and 3.- the percentage of missing values exceeded 50%. Gene annotations were obtained from Bioconductor packages. Normalized, filtered data were stored as Excel® files. Data filtering and normalization yielded 13,756 gene probes from GSE10971 dataset and 13,566 gene probes from GSE14407 dataset out of the original 54,675, which were subsequently used in Class Comparison Analysis.

CLASS COMPARISON ANALYSIS

Two-class Significance Analysis of Microarrays (SAM) (1000 permutations [21]; Tusher *et al.* method; median FDR = 0; 90th %ile FDR < 0.05%) and T-test (Welch approximation; 1000 permutations; Adjusted Bonferroni correction; p<0.01) were applied to identify differentially expressed gene probes between HGSC and FTE and between HGSC and OSE samples. Hierarchical clustering (HCL) support trees (re-sampling method: Bootstrap Genes; Iterations: 1000) were constructed considering significant gene probes only [22]. (MultiExperiment Viewer (MeV)). The comparison of HGSC and FTE (GSE10971) with SAM Fig. (**2A**) identified 2,097 significant probes (15%), 610 (4%) over-expressed in

HGSC and 1,487 (11%) over-expressed in FTE. The support tree, constructed based on these significantly expressed gene probes, showed distinct clusters of HGSC and FTE samples with 100% support (Fig. **2B**). In the same way, the comparison of HGSC and OSE (GSE14407), indentified 3,052 significant probes (23%), 145 (1%) over-expressed in HGSC and 2,907 (21%) in OSE (Fig. **2C**). The support tree also showed distinct clusters of HGSC and OSE with a 100% of support (Fig. **2D**). This demonstrated a true biological difference based on gene expression profile and a strong correlation with morphology.

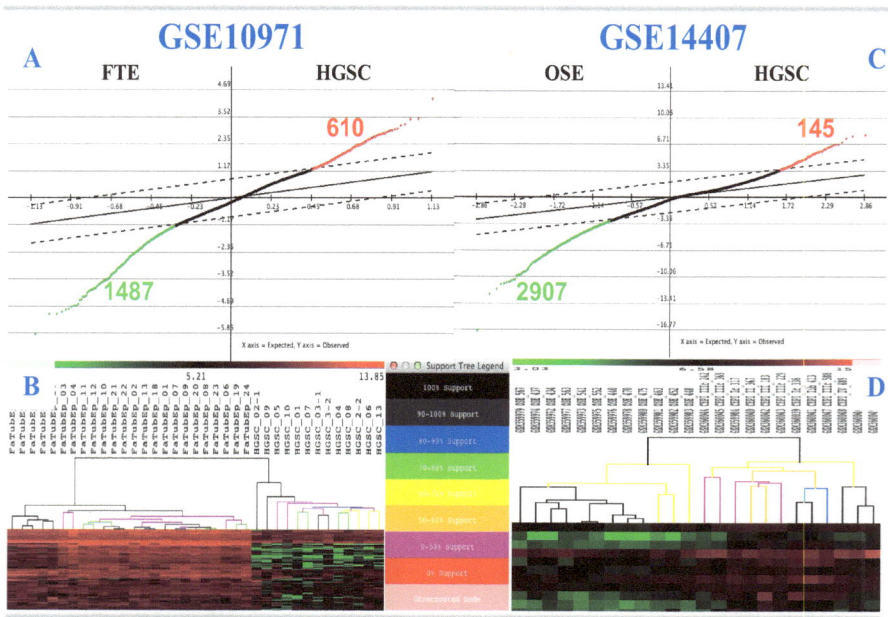

Fig. (2). (**A** and **C**) Significance Analysis of Microarrays (SAM) comparing gene expression profile of 24 FTE with 13 HGSC (GSE10971), and 12 OSE with 12 HGSC (GSE14407) (90th %ile FDR = 0.08%). Genes outside the doted lines in green are significantly over-expressed in FTE and OSE ("negative significant") when compared with HGSC and the ones in red are significantly over-expressed in HGSC ("positive significant") when compared with FTE and OSE. (**B** and **D**) Support Trees constructed with significant genes previously identified with SAM. In each case, two distinct groups were formed, in **B** one formed exclusively by FTE and the second by HGSC cases and in **C**, one formed exclusively by OSE and the second by HGSC cases; both **B** and **C** with a 100% of support.

Confirmation of Clustering

In parallel with the above method, we generated Hierarchical Support trees using an alternate procedure. This was done to ensure that the significant clusters found appeared when different normalization methods were applied. For this procedure the data were normalized by RMA and probes were collapsed to their mean value for the gene they represent, using the Bioinformatics Toolbox in Matlab 2010b.

Again, a 50% variance threshold was applied to the data, as well as lower variance thresholds for comparison. Significant differentially expressed genes between HGSC and FTE were assessed using the nonparametric Two-Sample Kolmogorov Smirnov Test, using the full Bonferroni correction. Trees were then constructed using agglomerative HCL with the average Euclidean distance between clusters. The same distinct clustering of HGSC *vs.* FTE and HGSC *vs.* OSE was also found using our second method for confirmation.

VALIDATION BY IMMUNOHISTOCHEMISTRY

We chose 5 primary immunohistochemistry (IHC) antibodies available in our laboratory routinely used in research and clinical basis to confirm the above-mentioned *in-silico* results. IHC was conducted on formalin-fixed and paraffin-embedded whole tissue sections from our own collection from the Pathology Department, Icahn School of Medicine at Mount Sinai, corresponding to 19 HGSC, with adjacent normal fallopian tube, 7 OSE cases as well as 12 fallopian tube sections from 6 patients with no history of gynecological neoplasm. Standard avidin-biotin protocol was used. Briefly, 5μm sections were deparaffinized and submitted to antigen retrieval for 20 min in EDTA buffer at pH 8.0. Subsequently, slides were incubated in 10% normal serum for 30 min, followed by primary antibody incubation overnight at 4°C. Then, slides were incubated with biotinylated secondary antibodies at a 1:1000 dilution for 30 min (Vector Laboratories, Inc.) followed by avidin-biotin peroxidase complexes at a 1:25 dilution (Vector Laboratories, Inc.) for 30 min. Diaminobenzidine was used as chromogen and hematoxylin as the nuclear counterstain. Primary antibodies used in this study included Stathmin rabbit polyclonal (Cell Signaling, cat# 3352), PAX-2 rabbit polyclonal (Prestige Antibodies, Sigma, cat# HPA047704), cdc2 mouse monoclonal (clone P0H1, Cell signaling, cat# 9116), VEGF rabbit monoclonal (clone EP1176Y, Abcam, cat# ab52917) and PAX8 (clone MRQ-50, Ventana Roche, cat# 7604618). To confirm the sensitivity and specificity of the different antibodies, positive and negative controls were run in parallel with the cases. Immunoreactivity was scored by determining the percentage of cells that displayed a positive immunostain from undetectable (0%) to homogeneous expression (100%), as well as the intensity, from negative (0) to high intensity (2+) and it was compared with the expression values obtained in the *in-silico* analysis. The expression values and fold changes are summarized in Table **1**. Comparing FTE and HGSC (GSE10971), CDK1 (CDC2), VEGF-A and Stathmin-1 are significantly overexpressed in HGSC compared with FTE; on the contrary, PAX2 is significantly overexpressed in FTE compared with HGSC and PAX8 is equally expressed in FTE and HGSC. Comparing HGSC and OSE (GSE14407), PAX8, CDK1 (CDC2) and VEGF-A are overexpressed in HGSC; PAX2 and Stathmin-1 are equally expressed in HGSC and OSE. IHC confirmed overexpression of PAX8 in both HGSC and FTE (adjacent and healthy controls), but showed negative reaction in OSE; PAX2 showed strong and diffuse positivity in FTE, but negative reaction in HGSC and OSE; despite high expression values of VEGF-A in HGSC, IHC was negative in tumor cells and positive in small capillaries immediate adjacent to them. Stathmin-1 showed strong and medium intensity positivity in HGSC and OSE respectively and it was negative in FTE (Fig. (3) and Table 2). These results validate the previous *in-silico* analysis.

Table 1. Expression values and fold changes of markers used for protein validation.

	Dataset GSE10971			Dataset GSE14407		
	FTE	HGSC		OSE	HGSC	
Gene	Exp value	Exp value	Fold change	Exp value	Exp value	Fold change
PAX8	8.8	7.33	-1.48 (ns)	6.68	8.17	1.49
PAX2	6.3	3.97	-2.33	5.86	6.33	0.47 (ns)
CDK1 (CDC2)	3.18	5.75	2.57	6.69	8.78	2.09
VEGF-A	6.07	8.13	2.07	5.1	6.26	1.16
Stathmin-1	5.22	8.53	3.31	8.51	8.88	0.37 (ns)

Table 2. Comparison of Group Immunoscores (Mean +/- S.D).

	Group		
Marker	HGSC	Adjacent FTE	FTE Control
Stathmin	171.17 +/- 65.28*	6.29 +/- 3.76	0.64 +/- 0.64
Cdc2	95.58 +/- 55.09	2.56 +/- 7.26	3.75 +/- 4.33
VEGF	Negative in tumor cells.**	Negligible staining.***	Negligible staining.***
PAX2	8.47 +/- 13.04	111.77 +/- 65.80	92.44 +/- 53.47
PAX8	253.79 +/- 48.86	209.54 +/- 55.71	122.73 +/- 14.12

* Positive in subepithelial cortical stromal cells
** Positive in tumor-associated mesenchyme especially vascular endothelial cells
*** Negative in epithelial cells and adjacent mesenchymal stromal cells and vasculature

FUNCTIONAL GENOMICS

Fold change (logged) of significantly differentially expressed gene probes from FTE and HGSC groups were loaded into Ingenuity Pathway Analysis (IPA; Ingenuity Systems® [23],); a core analysis using IPA default settings and filtering parameters was performed; a cut-off or fold change filter was not used at this point since it was applied during data normalization. The mapped gene probes were analyzed; unmapped and duplicated gene probes were excluded.

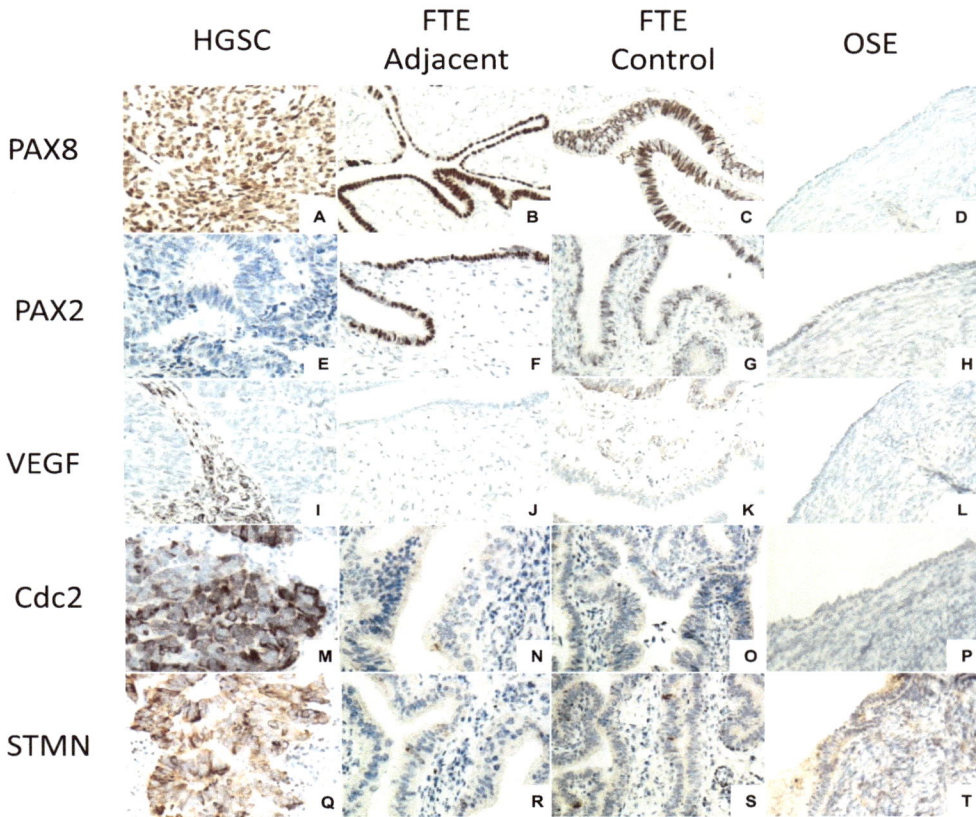

Fig. (3). Representative immunohistochemistry results of selected markers. Müllerian markers PAX8 and PAX2 were positive in both adjacent and control FTE but negative in OSE. PAX8 expression was retained in HGSC but PAX2 was lost. VEGF was negative in tumor cells, FTE and OSE and positive in intra-tumoral blood vessels. Cdc2 and Stathmin were positive in HGSC and negative in adjacent and control FTE. Cdc2 is negative in OSE. Stathmin was positive in OSE and ovarian stroma cells.

Canonical Pathways

IPA assigned the significantly differentially expressed genes into canonical pathways from the IPA library by two ways: 1.- Right-tailed Fisher's exact test ($p < 0.05$; Benjamini-Hochberg multiple testing correction was applied) [24] and 2.- A ratio between the number of genes in a given pathway that meet cut-off criteria, divided by the total number of genes that make up that pathway. Core analysis identified 23 significant canonical pathways in HGSC, functionally related mainly to cell cycle control, DNA strand breaks signaling response, genotoxic stress, mismatch repair and also pathways related to specific types of tumors like ovary, breast and pancreas. Ovarian Cancer Signaling pathway was not significant, probably because of the stringency of our analysis (Benjamini-Hochberg multiple testing correction [24]).

The most relevant canonical pathway was Cell Cycle: G2/M DNA Damage Checkpoint Regulation (p= 1.81E-10; ratio 13/49 (0.265)), represented in Fig. (4); over and under-expressed genes/molecules that mapped to the pathway are colored in red and green respectively.

Fig. (4). Cell Cycle: G2/M DNA Damage Checkpoint Regulation Canonical Pathway. Mapped molecules from FTE (green, under-expressed) and HGSC (red, over-expressed) (B).

The following four canonical pathways were Mitotic Roles of Polo-Like Kinase (p= 2.53E-09; ratio 14/74), Estrogen-mediated S-phase Entry (p= 1.41E-08; ratio 9/28), Cell Cycle Control of Chromosomal Replication (p= 4.65E-08; ratio 9/34) and Role of BRCA1 in DNA Damage Response (p= 1.49E-07; ratio 12/71).

The canonical pathways in FTE were related to metabolic functions such as Noradrenaline and Adrenaline Degradation (p= 7.05E-05; ratio 8/53), Serotonin Degradation (p= 8.56E-04; ratio 8/78), Dopamine Degradation (p= 1.32E-03; ratio 5/38), Pyrimidine Deoxyribonucleotides *De Novo* Biosynthesis I (p= 2.13E-03; ratio 5/44) and Fatty Acid Activation (p= 2.19E-03; ratio 4/19).

Similarly, when compared with OSE, HGSC canonical pathways were mainly related with cell cycle regulation. The five most relevant ones were Cell Cycle: G2/M DNA Damage Checkpoint Regulation (p= 2.07E-07; ratio 9/49 (0.184)), Mitotic Roles of Polo-Like Kinase (p= 5.73E-07; ratio 10/74 (0.135)), ATM Signaling (p= 3.44E-06; ratio 9/66 (0.136)), DNA damage-induced 14-3-3s Signaling (p= 3.55E-05; ratio 5/22 (0.227)) and Hereditary Breast Cancer

Signaling (p= 1.11E-04; ratio 10/134 (0.075)).

Molecule Activity Predictor (MAP)

MAP was applied to show the activation or inhibition of canonical pathways *in-silico*. The tool allows prediction of upstream and/or downstream effects of activation or inhibition of molecules in a network or pathway using the mapping genes that were included in our input data [25]. As an example, we analyzed the most relevant canonical pathway affected in HGSC according to our analysis: "Cell Cycle: G2/M DNA Damage Checkpoint Regulation" pathway. MAP showed the overall activation of Cdc2-Cyclin B complex mainly by Cdc25B/C and CKS1; furthermore, inactivation of p53 dependent genes Reprimo and p21 was also observed with subsequent loss of their Cdc25 inhibitory effect, contributing to its activation. The result of these interactions would be the theoretical abolishment of the G2/M DNA damage checkpoint, allowing the cells entry to M phase without appropriate DNA repair. On the contrary, in FTE, MAP showed activation of p53 dependent genes Reprimo and cyclin-dependent kinase inhibitor 1A (p21, Cip1), resulting in the inhibition of cyclin-dependent kinase 1 (Cdc2). This allowed us to conclude and predict that the delay in the mitotic entry from G2 to mitosis (M) is preserved. MAP analysis is showed in Fig. (**5**).

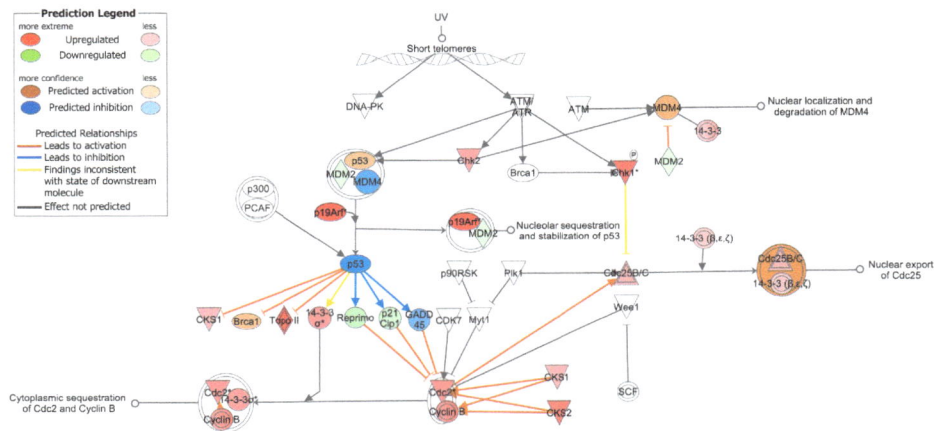

Fig. (5). Molecule activity predictor (MAP) based on mapped molecules, shows *in-silico* inactivation of p53 and activation of CdC2-Cyclin B complex, which in turn will activate M phase entry by the cell, abolishing the G2/M DNA damage checkpoint regulation.

Chemotherapeutic Drugs Overlay

Having identified the pathways and their activation, we explored how known chemotherapeutic drugs possibly affect them *in-silico* and if our findings correlated with literature. Continuing with the analysis of the "Cell Cycle: G2/M DNA Damage Checkpoint Regulation" pathway, several chemotherapeutic drugs may potentially affect it at different levels; one of the most promising ones is Alvocidib (Flavopiridol), which blocks CDC2, theoretically blocking the transition of G2 to M phases (Fig. **6**). A literature search yielded nine research articles showing the effectiveness of Alvocidib in ovarian carcinoma, increasing the therapeutic effect or suppressing ovarian cancer cell lines growth [26 - 34]. These articles validated our *in-silico* analysis, which was done blindly and following an exploratory approach.

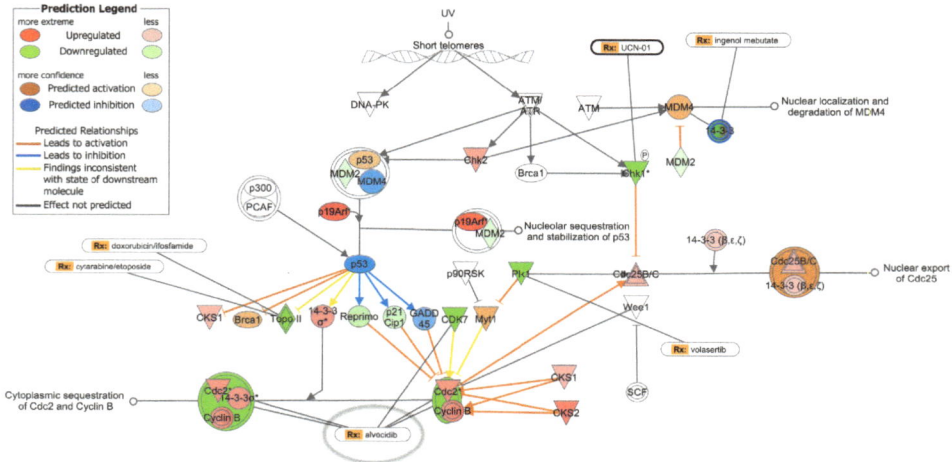

Fig. (6). Molecule activity predictor (MAP) and chemotherapeutic drugs overlay. Alvocidib, which blocks CDC2, theoretically blocking the transition of G2 to M phases, thus maintaining the G2/M DNA damage regulation checkpoint.

DISCUSSION

Secondary Analysis of Publicly Available Gene Expression Datasets

Minimum information about a microarray experiment (MIAME) ensures, as a pre-requisite for publication of microarray data, that data supporting published conclusions are made available to researchers, rendering their data useful for further analyses by others [14, 15]. However in spite of the availability of large, responsibly generated datasets to the public, secondary analysis of publically available gene expression datasets are rarely performed [16, 35]. We believe that secondary analyses are of great importance, not only to validate original analyses' results, but also to respond different questions, generating new hypotheses that can be answered in the lab. We showed an example of a secondary analysis to two GEO datasets following an exploratory approach. We downloaded and reanalyzed previously published gene expression profile datasets (GSE10971 and GSE14407) from a subset of HGSC, FTE and OSE cases. We validated our *in-silico* analysis on tissue samples by immunohistochemistry and then performed a Functional Genomics approach using Ingenuity Pathway Analysis (IPA), a next generation software not used in the original microarray analyses [18, 19].

The original microarray experiments from which these gene expression datasets were derived investigated, in one hand, the molecular signatures of FTE of BRCA1/2 mutation carriers potentially involved in predisposition to HGSC in the increased risk population, giving more and more evidence pointing out FTE as the most probable origin [6, 8, 18, 36 - 38] and, on the other hand, the molecular signatures of HGSC and OSE supporting the hypothesis that OSE are multipotent and capable of serving as the origin of HGSC, but without ruling out the possibility of other sources [39]. To test the congruence between the results of our analytical approach with the original experimental results, we systematically compared our key results with the published ones in the original study.

We first identified the differentially expressed genes between HGSC and FTE samples to perform a HCL support tree based only on these genes. The support tree clustered all HGSC samples in one distinct group irrespective of whether they presumably were of ovarian or tubal origin as Tone *et al.* described in their original analysis. However, the support tree also showed a distinct cluster of FTE samples and none of them clustered with HGSC samples as previously shown by Tone *et al.* [18]. One possible explanation for this discrepancy is the different methodological approach used by us, as we performed the HCL using only the differentially expressed genes previously identified by SAM. A second explanation is the usage of different HCL merging and linkage methods, which are not clearly specified by Tone *et al.* in the original analysis [18].

In the same way, we identified differentially expressed genes between HGSC and OSE. The HCL support tree showed distinct clusters of HGSC and OSE samples as previously shown by Bowen *et al.*. Our results differ in terms of the number and proportion of overexpressed genes in HGSC and OSE when compared to each other: 145 and 2,907 respectively, *versus* 1,210 and 1,110 genes found by Bowen *et al.* [19].

Our results were confirmed by a totally independent approach in terms of data normalization and filtering.

Validation by Immunohistochemistry

In order to validate our *in-silico* results, we chose five molecules differentially expressed in HGSC either compared with FTE or OSE. As shown in the *in-silico* analysis, immunostains for CDC2 and Stathmin-1 were positive in HGSC and negative in FTE.

Stathmin1 (STMN1) and CDC2 (CDK1) were shown to be overexpressed by both *in-silico* and IHC tissue validation. STMN1 is a multifunctional ubiquitous cytoplasmic phosphoprotein that depolymerizes microtubules, having a critical role both in entry and exit of M-phase. It has been described as a potential marker of Fallopian tube secretory cell transformation and serous carcinoma initiation, being immunohistochemically positive in serous tubal intraepithelial carcinoma (STIC) and invasive HGSC, but negative in normal Fallopian tube epithelial secretory cells and "p53 signatures" [5, 40]. STMN1 was unexpectedly positive in OSE and ovarian stroma, supporting the *in-silico* findings in which STMN1 was not differentially expressed when HGSC and OSE were compared. STMN1 positivity in OSE has not been previously described and it would be of interest to be studied and confirmed in the future. CDC2 is a member of the Ser/Thr protein kinase family presenting a catalytic subunit of the M-phase promoting factor protein kinase complex, essential for G1/S and G2/M phase transitions of the cell cycle. Immunostain positivity for CDC2 and p53 has been described in epithelial ovarian cancer and negatively correlated with the expression of p21 [41].

Paired box 8 (PAX8) was shown to be overexpressed in HGSC only when compared with OSE but not with FTE by our *in-silico* analysis; nevertheless, IHC showed that PAX8 is overexpressed in both HGSC as well as adjacent and normal FTE. This gene encodes a member of the paired box (PAX) family of transcription factors important in the embryogenesis of the thyroid, Müllerian, and renal/upper urinary tracts [42]. PAX8 IHC has been used to determine gynecologic, kidney or thyroid tumor origin in the routine pathology practice [43]. Our results showed that FTE and HGSC but not OSE, are both from müllerian origin and HGSC may be derived from a malignant transformation of the fallopian tube mucosal epithelial cell.

Paired box two (PAX2), another member of the paired box (PAX) family of transcription factors, was shown to be overexpressed in FTE but neither in HGSC nor in OSE (Table 1); these results were confirmed by IHC. PAX2 has been shown to be also expressed in müllerian and upper urinary tract but not in thyroid or thymus and it could be of utility as a complementary IHC to PAX8 for the diagnosis of non-mucinous epithelial ovarian tumors and renal cell carcinomas [44]. Nevertheless, in a review from Ordonez *et al.*, only 63 (48%) of 132 primary and 11 (40%) of 28 metastatic serous carcinomas were reported to be PAX2 positive [44].

Finally, our *in-silico* analysis showed VEGF to be overexpressed in HGSC when compared to FTE and OSE, but IHC was negative in tumor cells and positive in small capillaries immediate adjacent to them. VEGF-A is a member of the PDGF/VEGF growth factor family that induces proliferation and migration of vascular endothelial cells, and is essential for both physiological and pathological angiogenesis [45].

Functional Genomics

To gain further insights into the molecular genetic basis of the discriminatory power of HGSC and to better understand the interaction of the genes differentiating HGSC, FTE and OSE, we performed pathway/network enrichment analysis using the Ingenuity Pathway Analysis knowledge base to map the genes into canonical pathways and biological networks without bias. Not surprisingly, canonical pathways related to HGSC are those involving cell cycle regulation, which are expected to be affected in cancer. On the other hand, this also validates our *in-silico* analysis gene-cancer-related segregation. The IPA software is a web-delivered application that takes a set of genes as input and dynamically enriches a set of pathways and networks stored in a repository of expertly curated biological interactions and functional annotations created from millions of individually modeled relationships between proteins, genes, complexes, cells, tissues, drugs, and diseases [46] (The Ingenuity Knowledge Base; http://www.ingenuity.com/products/ireport), describes their inter-relationships and possible biological relevance [47]. This powerful tool gives us the opportunity to explore our data at the level of gene interaction in canonical pathways, biological networks, bio-functions and chemotherapeutic drug overlay that may generate new hypothesis to be tested in the lab or find key interaction points that could potentially be molecular targets for new treatments and translational research.

Weaknesses and Future Challenges

One of the main weaknesses of our analysis is the low number of cases in the datasets; thus, incorporation of more cases is critical. One possible solution is combining different datasets, but in order to do this, data must be further processed to eliminate non-biological differences or batch-effect. There are anecdotal reports of clusters being found that separate data based on the hospital in which the sample was collected, the technician who ran the microarray assay, or the day of the week on which the array was run. Unnecessary variability must be minimized and biological signal must be filtered from the noise [48]. Since we are working with publicly available data obtained by others, we cannot manage the conditions in which the experiments were performed, thus batch effect must be corrected using computational softwares (*e.g.* "R", Mathlab®). However, discussion on the detail of batch effect correction is beyond the scope of this chapter.

CONCLUSION

Nowadays, the new era of personalized medicine requires the identification of therapeutic targets and early detection biomarkers coupling *in-silico* analysis with high-throughput genomic technology. We believe that a secondary *in-silico* analysis of gene expression microarray databases available in public data repositories is one feasible approach to better understand gene-biopathway interplay. Secondary analyses are crucial for validating original results and for generating new hypotheses that can be answered in the lab. Minimum information about a microarray experiment (MIAME) ensures that data supporting published conclusions are made available to researchers, rendering their data useful for secondary analyses by others. However, in spite of the availability of large, responsibly generated datasets to the public, secondary analysis of publically available gene expression datasets are rarely performed. Here we showed an example of a secondary analysis of previously published gene expression profile GEO datasets (GSE10971 and GSE14407) from a subset of HGSC, FaTubEp and OSE cases, validating our results on tissue samples by immunohistochemistry and adding a pathway/network enrichment analysis using Ingenuity Pathway Analysis (IPA), a next generation software not used in the original microarray analyses.

CONSENT FOR PUBLICATION

Not applicable.

CONFLICT OF INTEREST

The author confirms that this chapter contents have no conflict of interest.

ACKNOWLEDGEMENTS

Analyses were performed using BRB-ArrayTools developed by Dr. Richard Simon and BRB-ArrayTools Development Team.

REFERENCES

[1]   Cancer IARo. WHO Classification of Tumours of the Female Reproductive Organs. IARC WHO Classification of Tumours 2014.

[2]   Sivridis E, Giatromanolaki A. Prognostic aspects on endometrial hyperplasia and neoplasia. Virchows Arch 2001; 439(2): 118-26.
      [http://dx.doi.org/10.1007/s004280100418] [PMID: 11561751]

[3]   Soslow RA, Tornos C, Eds. Diagnostic Pathology of Ovarian Tumors. New York: Springer 2011.

[4]   Staropoli N, Ciliberto D, Chiellino S, *et al.* Is ovarian cancer a targetable disease? A systematic review

and meta-analysis and genomic data investigation. Oncotarget 2016; 7(50): 82741-56.
[http://dx.doi.org/10.18632/oncotarget.12633] [PMID: 27764790]

[5]   Barlin JN, Levine DA. The evolving pathogenesis model of high-grade pelvic serous carcinoma. Gynecol Oncol 2011; 123(1): 1-2.
[http://dx.doi.org/10.1016/j.ygyno.2011.07.015] [PMID: 21807403]

[6]   Crum CP, Drapkin R, Miron A, *et al.* The distal fallopian tube: a new model for pelvic serous carcinogenesis. Curr Opin Obstet Gynecol 2007; 19(1): 3-9.
[http://dx.doi.org/10.1097/GCO.0b013e328011a21f] [PMID: 17218844]

[7]   Landen CN Jr, Birrer MJ, Sood AK. Early events in the pathogenesis of epithelial ovarian cancer. J Clin Oncol 2008; 26(6): 995-1005.
[http://dx.doi.org/10.1200/JCO.2006.07.9970] [PMID: 18195328]

[8]   Levanon K, Crum C, Drapkin R. New insights into the pathogenesis of serous ovarian cancer and its clinical impact. J Clin Oncol 2008; 26(32): 5284-93.
[http://dx.doi.org/10.1200/JCO.2008.18.1107] [PMID: 18854563]

[9]   Dietl J. Revisiting the pathogenesis of ovarian cancer: the central role of the fallopian tube. Arch Gynecol Obstet 2014; 289(2): 241-6.
[http://dx.doi.org/10.1007/s00404-013-3041-3] [PMID: 24100801]

[10]   McAlpine JN, Porter H, Köbel M, *et al.* BRCA1 and BRCA2 mutations correlate with TP53 abnormalities and presence of immune cell infiltrates in ovarian high-grade serous carcinoma. Mod Pathol 2012; 25(5): 740-50.
[http://dx.doi.org/10.1038/modpathol.2011.211] [PMID: 22282309]

[11]   Afify AM, Werness BA, Mark HF. HER-2/neu oncogene amplification in stage I and stage III ovarian papillary serous carcinoma. Exp Mol Pathol 1999; 66(2): 163-9.
[http://dx.doi.org/10.1006/exmp.1999.2255] [PMID: 10409445]

[12]   Barrett T, Troup DB, Wilhite SE, *et al.* NCBI GEO: archive for high-throughput functional genomic data. Nucleic Acids Res 2009; 37(Database issue): D885-90.
[http://dx.doi.org/10.1093/nar/gkn764] [PMID: 18940857]

[13]   Wray CJ, Ko TC, Tan FK. Secondary use of existing public microarray data to predict outcome for hepatocellular carcinoma. J Surg Res 2014; 188(1): 137-42.
[http://dx.doi.org/10.1016/j.jss.2013.12.013] [PMID: 24560427]

[14]   Brazma A. Minimum Information About a Microarray Experiment (MIAME)--successes, failures, challenges. ScientificWorldJournal 2009; 9: 420-3.
[http://dx.doi.org/10.1100/tsw.2009.57] [PMID: 19484163]

[15]   Brazma A, Hingamp P, Quackenbush J, *et al.* Minimum information about a microarray experiment (MIAME)-toward standards for microarray data. Nat Genet 2001; 29(4): 365-71.
[http://dx.doi.org/10.1038/ng1201-365] [PMID: 11726920]

[16]   Ventura B. Mandatory submission of microarray data to public repositories: how is it working? Physiol Genomics 2005; 20(2): 153-6.
[http://dx.doi.org/10.1152/physiolgenomics.00264.2004] [PMID: 15661852]

[17]   Mas VR, Maluf DG, Archer KJ, *et al.* Genes involved in viral carcinogenesis and tumor initiation in hepatitis C virus-induced hepatocellular carcinoma. Mol Med 2009; 15(3-4): 85-94.
[http://dx.doi.org/10.2119/molmed.2008.00110] [PMID: 19098997]

[18]   Tone AA, Begley H, Sharma M, *et al.* Gene expression profiles of luteal phase fallopian tube epithelium from BRCA mutation carriers resemble high-grade serous carcinoma. Clin Cancer Res 2008; 14(13): 4067-78.
[http://dx.doi.org/10.1158/1078-0432.CCR-07-4959] [PMID: 18593983]

[19]   Bowen NJ, Walker LD, Matyunina LV, *et al.* Gene expression profiling supports the hypothesis that human ovarian surface epithelia are multipotent and capable of serving as ovarian cancer initiating

cells. BMC Med Genomics 2009; 2: 71.
[http://dx.doi.org/10.1186/1755-8794-2-71] [PMID: 20040092]

[20]   BrB-ArrayTools v4.3.2; http://linus.nci.nih.gov/BRB-ArrayTools.html

[21]   Tusher VG, Tibshirani R, Chu G. Significance analysis of microarrays applied to the ionizing radiation response. Proc Natl Acad Sci USA 2001; 98(9): 5116-21.
[http://dx.doi.org/10.1073/pnas.091062498] [PMID: 11309499]

[22]   MultiExperiment Viewer (MeV); http://www.tm4.org

[23]   IPA; Ingenuity Systems®, [25] http://www.ingenuity.com

[24]   Benjamini Y, Hochberg Y. Controlling the False Discovery Rate: A Practical and Powerful Approach to Multiple Testing. J R Stat Soc Ser A Stat Soc 1995; (1): 289-300.

[25]   http://ingenuity.force.com/ipa/articles/Feature_Description/MAP-Molecule-Activity-Predictor

[26]   Raju U, Nakata E, Mason KA, Ang KK, Milas L. Flavopiridol, a cyclin-dependent kinase inhibitor, enhances radiosensitivity of ovarian carcinoma cells. Cancer Res 2003; 63(12): 3263-7.
[PMID: 12810657]

[27]   Mason KA, Hunter NR, Raju U, *et al.* Flavopiridol increases therapeutic ratio of radiotherapy by preferentially enhancing tumor radioresponse. Int J Radiat Oncol Biol Phys 2004; 59(4): 1181-9.
[http://dx.doi.org/10.1016/j.ijrobp.2004.03.003] [PMID: 15234054]

[28]   Song Y, Shen K, Tang PP. [Therapeutic effect of flavopiridol, a small molecular cyclin-dependent kinase inhibitor, in human ovarian carcinoma]. Zhonghua Fu Chan Ke Za Zhi 2007; 42(11): 761-4.
[PMID: 18307904]

[29]   Song Y, Shen K, Xu F. [Synergism of antitumor effects on ovarian carcinoma using autocatalytic caspase-3 combined with flavopiridol]. Zhonghua Fu Chan Ke Za Zhi 2010; 45(10): 781-6.
[PMID: 21176562]

[30]   Bible KC, Peethambaram PP, Oberg AL, *et al.* Mayo Phase 2 Consortium (P2C); North Central Cancer Treatment Group (NCCTG). A phase 2 trial of flavopiridol (Alvocidib) and cisplatin in platin-resistant ovarian and primary peritoneal carcinoma: MC0261. Gynecol Oncol 2012; 127(1): 55-62.
[http://dx.doi.org/10.1016/j.ygyno.2012.05.030] [PMID: 22664059]

[31]   Baumann KH, Kim H, Rinke J, Plaum T, Wagner U, Reinartz S. Effects of alvocidib and carboplatin on ovarian cancer cells *in vitro*. Exp Oncol 2013; 35(3): 168-73.
[PMID: 24084453]

[32]   Song Y, Xin X, Zhai X, Xia Z, Shen K. Sequential combination therapy with flavopiridol and autocatalytic caspase-3 driven by amplified hTERT promoter synergistically suppresses human ovarian carcinoma growth *in vitro* and in mice. J Ovarian Res 2014; 7: 121.
[http://dx.doi.org/10.1186/s13048-014-0121-3] [PMID: 25528169]

[33]   Yang G, Sun H, Kong Y, Hou G, Han J. Diversity of RGD radiotracers in monitoring antiangiogenesis of flavopiridol and paclitaxel in ovarian cancer xenograft-bearing mice. Nucl Med Biol 2014; 41(10): 856-62.
[http://dx.doi.org/10.1016/j.nucmedbio.2014.08.008] [PMID: 25195014]

[34]   Song Y, Xin X, Zhai X, Xia Z, Shen K. Sequential combination of flavopiridol with Taxol synergistically suppresses human ovarian carcinoma growth. Arch Gynecol Obstet 2015; 291(1): 143-50.
[http://dx.doi.org/10.1007/s00404-014-3408-0] [PMID: 25118834]

[35]   Mas VR, Maluf DG, Archer KJ, *et al.* Genes involved in viral carcinogenesis and tumor initiation in hepatitis C virus-induced hepatocellular carcinoma. Mol Med 2009; 15(3-4): 85-94.
[http://dx.doi.org/10.2119/molmed.2008.00110] [PMID: 19098997]

[36]   Piek JM, Kenemans P, Verheijen RH. Intraperitoneal serous adenocarcinoma: a critical appraisal of three hypotheses on its cause. Am J Obstet Gynecol 2004; 191(3): 718-32.

[http://dx.doi.org/10.1016/j.ajog.2004.02.067] [PMID: 15467531]

[37]   Medeiros F, Muto MG, Lee Y, *et al*. The tubal fimbria is a preferred site for early adenocarcinoma in women with familial ovarian cancer syndrome. Am J Surg Pathol 2006; 30(2): 230-6.
[http://dx.doi.org/10.1097/01.pas.0000180854.28831.77] [PMID: 16434898]

[38]   Kindelberger DW, Lee Y, Miron A, *et al*. Intraepithelial carcinoma of the fimbria and pelvic serous carcinoma: Evidence for a causal relationship. Am J Surg Pathol 2007; 31(2): 161-9.
[http://dx.doi.org/10.1097/01.pas.0000213335.40358.47] [PMID: 17255760]

[39]   Bowen NJ, Walker LD, Matyunina LV, *et al*. Gene expression profiling supports the hypothesis that human ovarian surface epithelia are multipotent and capable of serving as ovarian cancer initiating cells. BMC Med Genomics 2009; 2: 71.
[http://dx.doi.org/10.1186/1755-8794-2-71] [PMID: 20040092]

[40]   Karst AM, Levanon K, Duraisamy S, *et al*. Stathmin 1, a marker of PI3K pathway activation and regulator of microtubule dynamics, is expressed in early pelvic serous carcinomas. Gynecol Oncol 2011; 123(1): 5-12.
[http://dx.doi.org/10.1016/j.ygyno.2011.05.021] [PMID: 21683992]

[41]   Shi HR, Zhang RT. [Expression and significance of P53, P21WAF1 and CDK1 proteins in epithelial ovarian cancer]. Chin J Cancer 2009; 28(8): 882-5.
[http://dx.doi.org/10.5732/cjc.008.10417] [PMID: 19664338]

[42]   Laury AR, Perets R, Piao H, *et al*. A comprehensive analysis of PAX8 expression in human epithelial tumors. Am J Surg Pathol 2011; 35(6): 816-26.
[http://dx.doi.org/10.1097/PAS.0b013e318216c112] [PMID: 21552115]

[43]   Xiang L, Kong B. PAX8 is a novel marker for differentiating between various types of tumor, particularly ovarian epithelial carcinomas. Oncol Lett 2013; 5(3): 735-8.
[http://dx.doi.org/10.3892/ol.2013.1121] [PMID: 23425942]

[44]   Ordóñez NG. Value of PAX2 immunostaining in tumor diagnosis: a review and update. Adv Anat Pathol 2012; 19(6): 401-9.
[http://dx.doi.org/10.1097/PAP.0b013e318271a382] [PMID: 23060065]

[45]   Provided by RefSeq. 2015.

[46]   The Ingenuity Knowledge Base; http://www.ingenuity.com/products/ireport

[47]   Long F, Liu H, Hahn C, Sumazin P, Zhang MQ, Zilberstein A. Genome-wide prediction and analysis of function-specific transcription factor binding sites. In Silico Biol (Gedrukt) 2004; 4(4): 395-410.
[PMID: 15506990]

[48]   Quackenbush J. Computational approaches to analysis of DNA microarray data. Yearb Med Inform 2006; 91-103.
[http://dx.doi.org/10.1055/s-0038-1638484] [PMID: 17051302]

CHAPTER 5

Psychological Aspects of Ovarian Cancer Healing

Jacob M. Appel[*]

Psychiatry and Medical Education, Director of Ethics Education in Psychiatry, Icahn School of Medicine at Mount Sinai, USA

Abstract: This chapter explores the psychological aspects of healing from ovarian cancer. Topics discussed include: i) psychological status of the patient - those with psychiatric disorders and those with secondary anxiety or depression arising after the diagnosis of cancer, ii) communication – how much and when to communicate, iii) psychological distress and demoralization, iv) complicating factors including loss of fertility, pain, fatigue and cosmetic concerns, v) caregiver burnout, vi) treatments including: depression, anxiety and talk therapy, vii) end-of-life issues including palliative and hospice care, and aid-in-dying.

Keywords: Aid in dying, Anxiety, Caregiver burnout, Depression, Distress, Demoralization, End of life, Fatigue, Fertility, Hospice, Psychiatric, Pain, Palliative care, Talk therapy.

INTRODUCTION

Cancer is the second leading cause of death in the United States. In 2016, 1,685,210 patients received a new cancer diagnosis and 595,690 died of the disease [1]. More than fourteen million Americans currently carry such a diagnosis, living in various stages of illness, treatment and recovery [1]. In addition to its taxing physical burden, the disease takes a considerable psychological toll both on patients, their loved ones and their caregivers. Gynecological malignancies share many of the emotional and psychiatric sequelae of other neoplasms, but also raise distinctive mental health concerns. Fears related to prognosis and suffering, common in many cancer diagnoses, may be compounded by specific, gender-based questions in the areas of fertility, appearance and sexual relations. Ovarian cancer, with 21,161 new diagnoses and 14,195 deaths in the United States in 2014, causes the most loss of life among gynecological cancers [2]. Only the tenth leading cause of cancer, but the fifth leading cause of death, its relative infrequency and relatively high lethality raise

[*] **Corresponding author Jacob M. Appel:** Psychiatry and Medical Education, Director of Ethics Education in Psychiatry, Icahn School of Medicine at Mount Sinai, USA; Tel: 212-663-3643; E-mail: jacobmappel@gmail.com

issues less likely to arise in the treatment of more common and more easily treatable forms of cancer. Patients often face "aggressive abdominal surgeries, multiple chemotherapy regimens and relatively poor survival rates," as well as a high likelihood of recurrent disease, all of which prove emotionally wearing [3]. At the same time, the survival rate for epithelial ovarian cancer—it is most common form—now exceeds thirty percent at ten years, so a subset of women will experience the psychological symptoms of long-term cancer patients [4].

Unfortunately, limited data are available on the relationship between mental health and gynecological cancers. Women have historically been underrepresented as subjects of clinical research [5 - 8]. Minority women have a particularly poor record of representation [9, 10]. Research funding for ovarian, uterine and uterine cervix cancers lags behind expenditures for other forms of cancer [11, 12]. Psychological morbidity in ovarian cancer, including depression and anxiety, has been significantly understudied [13, 14]. However, what data are available-much of which comes from assessments of specific mental health symptoms—strongly suggests significant levels of psychological distress among ovarian cancer patients. Cancer patients more generally exhibit higher rates of anxiety disorders and depressive disorders than the at-large population [15, 16]. It is extremely likely that ovarian cancer patients do so as well. Assessing for psychological distress should be part of any effective treatment plan. Higher rates of psychological symptoms and psychiatric illness among patients affected by ovarian cancer argue for initial screenings at time of diagnosis and routine mental health assessments during the course of care [15].

Abbas and Sert advocate for a holistic approach to assessing the effectiveness of ovarian cancer therapies, contending there is "more to treatment of the disease than the disease itself" [17]. At a minimum, healthcare providers should be screening for psychiatric symptoms and referring patients with significant clinical distress to appropriate resources including psychiatrists, psychotherapists, and group therapy programs, as indicated.

Clinical Settings

Clinicians are likely to encounter patients suffering from ovarian cancer in varying settings. Initial diagnosis may occur either in the outpatient setting—either a private office or clinic—or after hospitalization for symptoms. Surgical recovery will require inpatient hospitalization and many patients return to the hospital during the course of chemotherapy or for worsening symptom of disease. In those patients whose disease ultimately progresses, patients may elect for palliative options including relocation to a hospice center or home-based hospice care. Each of these settings may require specialized approaches and skills, as well as support from trained mental health professionals. Patients suffering from significant psychological distress or psychiatric disorders in the inpatient setting should generally be followed by the hospital's consult-liaison service or psychiatrists trained in psychosocial medicine or psycho-oncology. Increasingly, tertiary cancer centers and outpatient clinics are including psychiatrists on their care teams. When such integrated care is not available, patients with psychiatric or psychological needs should be referred to an outpatient mental health provider. With the patient's permission, oncologists should remain in close contact with that outside psychiatrist or psychologist to ensure unified care and to prevent confusion over medications, including contraindications, and medication-induced side effects that may be mistaken for either medical or psychiatric symptoms.

Types of Patients

Psychiatric disorders in patients with ovarian cancer will fall into two distinct varieties with their own specific sets of treatment needs. One group of patients will carry a significant psychiatric diagnosis prior to their cancer diagnosis, such as the woman with schizophrenia or bipolar disorder who later presents with ovarian cancer. Another subset of patients will receive a psychiatric diagnosis (usually adjustment disorder, anxiety, depression or even PTSD) subsequent to their cancer diagnosis for symptoms arising *after* they have learned that they have cancer. A considerable gray area between these two phenomena also exists: Some patients who exhibit only mild psychological distress at baseline—such as chronic, low-level anxiety or frequent depressive moods—may develop full-blown clinical psychiatric disorders as a result of a cancer diagnosis and subsequent treatment.

Each of these groups of patients require psychiatric care specifically attuned to their conditions. For patients with pre-existing psychiatric comorbidities, finding ways to continue with existing mental health treatment is essential. These patients and their loved ones may raise concerns about cancer therapies interacting with psychotropic drugs or cancer symptoms impeding access to therapy programs. Newly diagnosed patients may fear the stigma of mental illness and may resist both diagnosis and treatment. Even patients who are accepting of their diagnosis and prognosis will often raise questions about the duration of mental health treatment. Some of these patients, if pharmacological treatment proves effective, will then discontinue medications on their own and relapse. Emphasizing to patients with a new diagnosis that they are not "crazy" and that psychological stress is a natural—if treatable—aspect of most serious medical illnesses may prove reassuring.

Capacity Assessment

The assessment of a patient's ability to consent to proposed interventions and therapies is a crucial aspect of ethical medical care and is a frequent concern in older cancer patients [18]. Since protecting autonomy is often an essential aspect of maintaining a patient's psychological wellbeing, the right to make medical decisions should only be impinged upon after systematic, formal evaluation. States vary as to whether such assessment must be done by a psychiatrist or can be performed by any licensed physician. Capacity issues often arise in the context of psychological distress or full-blown mental illness. Some general principles worth noting are 1) that capacity is specific to any individual medical decision, so a patient may have capacity to consent to one procedure (a blood draw) but not another (ablative surgery) and 2) that capacity may evolve over time and should be evaluated in as close chronological proximity to the proposed intervention as possible. The standard method for assessing decisional capacity in the United States is derived from a seminal article by Appelbaum and Grisso that outlines four criteria [19]: 1) communicating a clear, consistent choice; 2) understanding relevant information such as diagnosis and prognosis; 3) appreciating the current medical situation, including the risks and potential benefits of any proposed interventions (or the failure to intervene); and 4) an ability to rationally manipulate information [19]. Patients must meet all four criteria to make their own decisions. Another model, which may be used alongside Appelbaum and Grisso's, argues for a "sliding scale" in which the level of scrutiny imposed is determined by two factors: 1) whether the decision is high or low risk and 2) whether it comports with widely accepted medical practice [19]. So a patient who accepts having her vital signs measured in the morning will receive a low level of scrutiny regarding her capacity, while a patient who refuses a diagnostic biopsy of a potentially life-threatening tumor will face more scrutiny when determining her capacity to render a decision. When assessing capacity, providers should inform the patient that this is a part of regular hospital protocol so that the patient does not feel singled out and physician-patient trust is not undermined. If the patient's capacity is uncertain, repeat evaluation is indicated [20]. In the absence of capacity, providers should turn to the appropriate advance directive (*e.g.* living will, health care proxy) or statutorily-authorized third-party decision maker (*e.g.* surrogate, next of kin) for further guidance. Occasionally, usually in the absence of such guidance, a court order may be necessary to pursue diagnosis or treatment. Yet even patients who lack formal capacity often have an active role to play in shaping their own care. To the utmost degree possible, they should be kept informed about medical decisions and their affirmative assent should be obtained.

Communication

Women have reported finding communication with health care professionals during the diagnostic interval between the appearance of symptoms and a confirmatory diagnosis to be "confusing and difficult" [19]. When discussing treatment, it is essential to clarify the goals of a particular intervention—whether palliative or curative [21]. This will reduce both misunderstanding and the prospect for unnecessary disappointment; such clarity is also likely to foster trust and improve the provider-patient bond. Included in any discussion of both illness and treatment should be a clear discussion of survival information [22]. Honest disclosure of prognosis is essential to maintain autonomy in patient decision-making and to avoid paternalistic interference that may leave the patient feeling ignored or betrayed [22]. However, care should also be taken not to undermine the patient's optimism or to crush her hopes. Faith—even faith in "miracles" or statistically unlikely occurrences—can be of significant psychological value to some patients [22]. Denial, if it does not considerably impede care, can also prove psychologically protective.

One particularly challenging scenario that occasionally arises is a request by a close family member *not* to communicate all pertinent information to a patient because of an expressed belief that the patient would not want to know [23, 24]. Relatives may seek to withhold a cancer diagnosis, the severity of the disease, or its prognosis. As a general rule, such requests should not be honored without clear evidence that these were the patient's wishes [25]. However, in cases where the patient's cultural or religious values may differ significantly from the American norm—such as an elderly, recent immigrant—oblique means may be used to ascertain the patient's underlying preferences [26]. For obvious reasons, a provider should not ask the patient: "If you had cancer, would you want to know?" (The question conveys the answer—much like asking one's spouse, "If I were having an extramarital affair, would you want me to tell you?") Instead, a provider might ask the patient what caused the deaths of each of her deceased relatives, ideally until the patients mentions deaths from cancer, and whether the those relatives were told of their conditions. If a patient responds by saying, "Of course we didn't tell her she had cancer," that may provide enough circumstantial evidence to withhold information. Whether or not revealing the diagnosis is necessary for the patient to make future medical decisions is also a relevant factor. A patient with untreatable disease, for example, might not require the same detail of information as one who must choose between various therapies. On the other hand, prognosis may be relevant to patient's non-medical decisions, such as whether to write a will or how to allocate time between work and family. These cases often require the involvement of a hospital's ethics consultant or ethics committee.

PSYCHIATRIC CONDITIONS

Psychiatric symptoms may arise as a result of medical symptoms that precede the diagnosis of cancer or may follow diagnosis [27]. S. A. Payne reports that depression and anxiety are the most significant determinants in subjective quality of life among advanced breast and ovarian cancer patients [28]. A striking 82% of variance in quality of life was attributable to anxiety and another 10% to depression [29]. Abbas and Sert argue that "social wellbeing and comfort" are a crucial part of any assessment of the efficacy and cost effectiveness or treatment in ovarian cancer [17]. Poor social support and intrusive thoughts have been linked to increased psychiatric illness, and Hipkins *et al.* found that these factors appear to play a larger role than physical symptoms in predicting psychiatric morbidity [30]. Similarly, Ersek *et al.* did not find a direct connection between physical symptoms and overall quality of life, while noting that fatigue remains a major concern of many patients [23]. However, Borduka-Bevers *et al.* reported that higher rates of depression and anxiety coincided with poor medical performance [3]. Norton, Mann *et al.* found that perceived levels of control and self-esteem were significantly correlated with psychological distress in ovarian cancer patients [31].

Assessments of the frequency of psychological distress in ovarian cancer patients vary widely. For example, Kornblith *et al.* found that one third of such patients reported significant psychological distress [32]. Yet the percentage who reported specific symptoms of distress proved far higher. Seventy-two percent reported worrying, 64% feeling sad, 62% feeling nervous, and 46% feeling irritable, while a majority (55%) described their worrying as moderate to severe and one in four reported that it caused them quite a bit of distress [32]. One challenge in studying psychiatric illness in cancer is that many sub-clinical symptoms may not trigger DSM diagnoses, yet they still contribute significantly to patient distress. Wide ranging estimates on the prevalence of depression and anxiety may stem from the failure of studies to distinguish between symptoms and full-blown disorders that meet the criteria of the Diagnostic Statistical Manual (DSM) [32]. Adjustment disorders—a DSM-V diagnosis that requires symptoms to arise within three months of a psychological stressor—are common in cancer patients [33]. However, the diagnosis is poorly studied and highly controversial [34]. Distinguishing appropriate, short-term reactions to negative social stressors from serious disorders like major depressive disorder (MDD) or generalized anxiety disorder (GAD) can prove challenging in the setting of a recent cancer diagnosis. Sellick and Crook observe saliently that, "Many individuals have symptoms of depression that do not meet the criteria for MDD or even Dysthymic Disorder for that matter, and yet suffer tremendously, often in silence and without intervention. These people cannot be forgotten" [35].

Another challenge reflects the reluctance of some patients to report their psychological symptoms to physicians [36, 37]. A comparison of patient's self-reported symptoms with those documented in medical charts found that only 31% of cases of depression and 14% of anxiety were recorded, suggesting that patients are withholding reports of these symptoms from their providers [38]. Patients may not wish to be perceived as complaining or ungrateful, or may not want to bother their oncologists. Finally, the DSM may prove a poor tool for measuring distress levels in ovarian cancer patients, as changes in appetite, decreased libido, poor sleep and fatigue are features of both the underlying illness and potential psychiatric disorders [39].

Depression

Cancer diagnoses are significantly associated with elevated rates of clinical depression [40, 41]. Neuroendocrine receptors tied to depression have been implicated in the disease progression of ovarian cancer [42, 43]. Lutgendorf *et al.* found that patients reporting higher depressive symptoms and less social support show higher concentrations of intra-tumor norepinephrine and increased activity of several beta-adrenergic transcription pathways, suggesting a link between psychosocial status and the spread of disease [44]. Huang *et al.*, using data from the Nurses' Health Study and Nurses' Health Study II, found evidence that depression itself may be a risk factor for ovarian cancer, with evidence of clinical depression 2-4 years before a cancer diagnosis most predictive of a future ovarian cancer diagnosis [45]. Such findings are consistent with the view that psychosocial stress may play a role in promoting the disease [45].

Limited data available for ovarian cancer patients suggests higher rates of depressive symptoms—and presumably, clinical depressive disorders—than encountered in healthy populations. Borduka-Bevers *et al.* found that 21% of patients recorded depression scores above 16 on the Center for Epidemiological Studies-Depression (CES-D) scale, a good screening cut-off for a likelihood of clinical depression [3]. Portenoy *et al.* found that 70% of ovarian cancer patients evaluated on the Memorial System Assessment Scale reported "sadness" [46]. A study by Mielcarek *et al.* of 106 patients in Poland with advanced ovarian cancer reported a prevalence of 20.8% for clinical depression (measured by the Hospital and Anxiety Depression Scale) prior to surgery [16]. Rates of depression were significantly associated directly with a past history of abortion and with elevated levels of tumor marker Ca125 after surgery but before a second course of adjuvant chemotherapy, and inversely with the number of previous deliveries [16]. No correlation was associated with marital status, social status, education level, age, presence of residual disease after surgery, intestinal stoma, blood transfusion, time since diagnosis, FIGO stage, or length of post-surgical hospital stay [16].

Borduka-Bevers reported younger patients are more likely to be depressed than older patients [3]. Certain chemotherapy agents have been tied to depression, and there is at least one case report of suicidality highly correlated to a regimen of paclitaxel and carboplatin for ovarian cancer [47]. Overall prevalence rates for depression in ovarian cancer patients, according to a meta-analysis by Watts *et al.* were 25.34% prior to undergoing cancer treatment, 22.99% for patients currently undergoing treatment, and 12.71% for those who had completed treatment [48].

These higher rates of depression appear to endure through the course of the illness. They do abate with time for a subset of patients. Hipkins *et al.* found that 33% of patients reported depression at the conclusion of chemotherapy, this number decreased to 19% at three month follow-up [30]. In contrast, Mielcarek found some fluctuation in rates of depression over the course of treatment in advanced cancer patients, but no consistent trend [16].

Anxiety

Anxiety is a very common psychological sequela of both cancer diagnosis and treatment, frequently rising to levels of clinical concern. Anxiety appears to occur at higher rates than depression in cancer patients [49]. Distinguishing between adjustment disorders secondary to diagnosis and full-blown anxiety disorders may prove challenging in retrospect, but both are likely widespread and significantly elevated over rates in the general population. Sukegawa *et al.* reported high levels of adjustment disorders (33.3%) in patients awaiting surgery for ovarian cancer [49]. Portenoy *et al.* found that 72% of ovarian cancer patients evaluated on the Memorial System Assessment Scale complained of "worrying" [46]. Borduka-Bevers *et al.* found that 29% of patients reported anxiety scores above the 75th percentile on the Spielberger State-Trait Anxiety Inventory [3]. Mielcarek *et al.* report significant anxiety in 48.1% of ovarian cancer patients at time of diagnosis [16]. Overall prevalence rates for anxiety in ovarian cancer patients, according to a meta-analysis by Watts *et al.*, were 19.12% prior to undergoing cancer treatment, 26.23% for patients currently undergoing treatment, and 27.09% for those who had completed treatment [48].

One exception to the general pattern of higher rates of anxiety than depression are those patients who have terminal prognoses, who appear to suffer higher rates of depression than anxiety [48]. Unlike depression, anxiety appears to ameliorate considerably with the passage of time [29]. Mielcarek *et al.* identified three likely causes for anxiety at time of diagnosis: fears related to the disease itself (such as disability and death), concerns related to the potential for long term treatment, and the prospect of impending surgery [16]. Serum levels of the tumor marker CA-125 become a source of obsessive anxiety in some patients [50]. Fitch *et al.*

surveyed 315 Canadian ovarian cancer patients and found that among those over sixty-one, 45% reported fears of recurrence [51]. Among women under forty-five, 64% reported a significant fear of recurrence [52]. Hipkins *et al.* found that 38% of patients reported anxiety at the conclusion of chemotherapy, and that this number increased to 47% at three month follow-up; this increase contrasted with cases of depression, which saw a decline over time [30]. Borduka-Bevers *et al.* found that those patients who require bed rest experience considerably higher levels of anxiety than those who do not [3].

Other Psychiatric Conditions

Cancer patients report significant rates of post-traumatic stress disorder (PTSD). Limited data suggests that this is true of ovarian cancer patients. Matulonis *et al.* reported that 26% of such patients met the clinical criteria for PTSD [53]. A prospective study by Goncalves *et al.*, measuring PTSD symptoms at four time intervals following diagnosis, found a prevalence as high as 45% for all patients; 13% of patients reported PTSD at all four assessments, and only 30% never qualified for a diagnosis of PTSD [54]. Younger age and previous use of antidepressants were predictive of future PTSD diagnosis [54]. Patients will often report hyperarousal including irritability, poor sleep and excessive vigilance; nightmares or feelings of reliving trauma; avoidance of situations related to their diagnosis or treatment; and pervasive, often intrusive negative thoughts. However, many of these symptoms are shared by a diagnosis of MDD, requiring careful application of diagnostic criteria prior to treatment.

Mania is not generally associated with most neoplasms. As a result, the most likely cause of new-onset manic or hypomanic symptoms in cancer patients is medication-related, with corticosteroids being the most frequent culprit. Although steroids are not a core component of chemotherapy treatment for ovarian cancer patients, as they often are for those with lymphoma or myeloma, they are commonly used to address side effects including nausea. They are sometimes a key component of palliative care as well. The presence of corticosteroid-induced delirious mania or "steroid psychosis" is poorly studied, especially in cancer patients, and predictive factors are largely unknown [55, 56]. A dose-response curve is reported, with significantly higher risk at doses equivalent to 40 mg/day of prednisone or above [57]. One to two weeks of steroid treatment usually precede psychiatric phenomena [58]. Screening for symptoms in patients receiving more than 40 mg/day of prednisone daily should be part of any care regimen. While the best course of treatment remains unsettled, tapering the corticosteroids, when possible, is preferred management. Both antipsychotics and mood stabilizers have demonstrated efficacy in some instances [59, 60].

Psychological Distress & Demoralization

Demoralization had recently received considerable attention as a phenomenon in medical and psychiatric care. The demoralized patient loses her sense of efficacy [61]. It is a distinct condition from depression. Mehnart *et al.* studied 516 patients with advanced cancer and found that between 16% and 39% were seriously demoralized and 73% demonstrated moderate levels of demoralization [62]. Yet their key finding was that between 5% and 20% of patients who were seriously demoralized were *not* clinically depressed; that percentage rose to 60% among patients with moderate levels of demoralization [62]. In addition to demoralization, many patients often suffer existential concerns or crises as a result of a cancer diagnosis or prognosis. While these episodes may not manifest any formal psychiatric symptoms, they can none the less prove highly distressing as the patient confronts her own mortality, rethinks her life choices, or renegotiates her place in the world. As ovarian cancers often run in families, patients may experience guilt if they fear they have passed their condition on to their daughters [63]. Other patients may regret not having chosen prophylactic oophorectomy for themselves [23]. Since surgery is ablative, sense of self and feelings of attractiveness play a role in women's psychological distress [63]. All of these conditions require the care team to work with the patient to tap into appropriate social supports, which may range from group therapy to consultation with the chaplaincy, depending on the particular needs, background and wishes of individual patients.

Delirium

Cancer patients are at high risk of psychosocial stress, but they are also at high risk of delirium and other organic disorders of cognition [23]. The former often mimic the latter, and misdiagnosing organic illness as psychiatric may place the patient in severe jeopardy [64]. Hypoactive delirium, for example, may look like depression—but the two are treated differently [65]. To the untrained eye, agitated delirium may appear to be an anxiety disorder. Regular delirium screening should be a part of the evaluation of all hospitalized cancer patients [66]. Distinctive features of delirium are its waxing and waning quality, poor attention and concentration, and disorientation leading to short term memory impairment. Often asking a patient who is cognitively intact at baseline to say the months of the year backwards is a good bedside test and failure is sufficient evidence to generate a high suspicion of delirium. In cancer patients, treatment with opioids, benzodiazepines and steroids has been associated with higher levels of delirium [67]. Chemotherapy agents are also implicated. Low dose antipsychotics, rather than antidepressants or anxiolytics, are usually the treatment of choice. Most important, delirium is a syndrome that usually reflects underlying medication problems, such as infection or even organ failure, so further diagnostic workup is always indicated.

COMPLICATING FACTORS

Loss of Fertility

While the median age of diagnosis for ovarian cancers is roughly sixty years, five percent of diagnoses occur in women under thirty [68]. By ages 35-39, the incidence is 8.89 per 100,000 women and rises to 13.16 per 100,000 by ages 40-44 [69]. 9.9% of confirmed malignancies and 30.8% of borderline cases are found in women under forty [70]. For these patients, preservation of fertility may be a significant goal of treatment, while the loss of fertility may risk poor psychological outcomes. Options available to surgical patients with epithelial ovarian cancers often include "radical" treatments that are not fertility sparing (*e.g.* total abdominal hysterectomy or bilateral salpingo-oopherectomy) or conservative, fertility sparing operations [71]. Duffy and Allen observe that, "Even for persons who may have not planned to have children, the threat of infertility can result in a deep sense of loss and anger" [72]. Infertility is significantly associated with depression in the general population—both among women seeking medical advice and those who do not [73]. Domar *et al.* found that psychological distress, as measured by depression and anxiety, was similar in infertile women as in women who had suffered significant cardiac events or were battling cancer [74]. Canada and Stover report increased levels of fertility-related distress and intrusive thoughts among patients whose childbearing plans were interrupted by cancer [75]. A survey of Canadian women under 45 years by Fitch *et al.* found more than a third reported concerns over fertility to be a significant problem [52]. However, data specific to ovarian cancer is limited. Zagnolo *et al.* reported that women treated conservatively for ovarian cancer experienced increased psychological risk if they had fertility concerns, independent of whether they already had offspring [76]. Interestingly, Biselling *et al.* found no significant differences in levels of depression or anxiety among patients undergoing radical or conservative treatments. Biselling *et al.* also reported those patients receiving fertility-sparing surgery required more additional operations, suggesting that they may have deferred more radical interventions, likely at some risk, until family planning was complete [71].

Strong evidence suggests that both men and women wish for their providers to discuss with them the implications of both disease and treatment upon fertility [72]. Providers make a mistake in assuming that when fertility sparing poses a significant risk to maternal life or health, patients do not wish to engage in meaningful dialogue on the subject. Some providers may also be reluctant to discuss fertility implications with lesbians or same-sex female couples, based upon the false belief that these individuals do not wish to be informed [77]. Often overlooked is the physical location of treatment in the hospital setting, as patients with ovarian cancer are frequently treated on obstetrics and gynecology floors in close proximity to the mothers of newborns, creating a potential source of additional stress [77]. Premature menopause is also likely to be a serious concern for some patients [52]. At a minimum, providers should query all patients regarding their fertility concerns and discuss in greater depth the risks and treatment options for those who express interest in future childbearing. The rise of later-life motherhood as a result of artificial reproductive technologies suggest that even women in their fifties or older may wish to engage in such discussion.

Pain

Pain is the most distressing symptom for patients with advanced gynecological cancers [78]. In addition to actual pain, the fear of uncontrolled pain or future pain is likely to prove a significant stressor in its own right. Eight-five percent of women with advanced ovarian cancer reported pain during the final six months of life [79]. Portenoy *et al.* found that among women undergoing treatment for stage III or IV ovarian cancer, 68% reported pain interfered with daily activities, 62% with mood, 62% with work and 61% with "overall enjoyment of life" [46]. Providers remain widely ill-informed about analgesic tolerance, especially in the elderly, and a sizeable number still falsely believe that pain is an inevitable aspect of the final stages of terminal cancer [80].

Screening for pain should be a standard part of each clinical visit. Treatment should adopt a ladder-based approach: starting with non-opioid analgesics (such as acetaminophen and NSAIDS), progressing to weak opioids and then to stronger opioid-based medications. Provision should always be made for breakthrough pain. Referral to either palliative care services or a pain specialist is essential to help manage significant pain.

Fatigue

Fatigue is among the most significant concerns of women with an ovarian cancer diagnosis in both the pre- and post-diagnosis settings [81]. Prevalence rates for fatigue in cancer patients range from 61-90% [82]. Yet patients tend to underreport fatigue symptoms to their providers [83]. While oncologists believe that pain affects their patients to a greater degree than fatigue, Vogelzang *et al.* reported that patients themselves reported being affected by fatigue more than pain [84]. Vogelzang *et al.* also found that only 27% of patients reported that their providers offered any treatment or therapeutic guidance for fatigue [84]. Both patients and providers appear under-informed with regard to the treatment options for fatigue [84]. Screening for fatigue should be a standard part of each clinical visit.

The first step in addressing cancer-related fatigue is identifying the source [82]. Common causes of fatigue other than cancer should be ruled out including anemia and depression. Sleep hygiene should be emphasized. Some patients may benefit from the prescription of a stimulant like methylphenidate (Ritalin) or modafinil [85].

Cosmetic Issues

The treatment of ovarian cancer often involves both ablative surgery and chemotherapy, each of which may have significant impacts on self-image. Premature menopause associated with surgery may lead to significant doubts about self-identify, femininity and perceived attractiveness. Chemotherapy often results in hair loss, changes to skin and nails, and significant weight reduction. The underlying cancer may also cause fluctuations in appetite or sleep that results in significant changes to bodyweight. Kamlesh *et al.* report increased frequency of poor body image in women with gynecological cancers [86]. Interest in sex also decreases, although whether this relates to sense of self or physical symptoms or both remains unclear [86].

Caregivers

The relationship between patients and their primary caregivers is a crucial aspect of patient wellbeing. Strong social support is highly correlated with higher quality of life. The presence of an active caregiver may also facilitate compliance with medical care. Most caregivers assume the role unexpectedly and with limited preparation [87]. Caregivers report higher rates of depression and anxiety than the general population with anxiety levels among caregivers even higher than those suffered by patients [87]. Rates of distress are higher among spouses and partners than children and other caregivers [88]. At the same time, Fitch *et al.* reported that a majority of surveyed ovarian cancer patients over sixty-one reported a positive impact of the illness on their relationships with friends and family [51]. Yet while caregivers may feel privileged to look after their loved ones, they may also feel overwhelmed by the practical disruptions and burdens this care imposes [51]. What is clear is that the impact of her disease on her caregivers often plays a significant role in a patient's own considerations and distress. Older patients with gynecological cancers report the welfare of their partners to be a serious concern [87].

Caregiver burnout is a phenomenon that has received increased attention in both academic literature and the public consciousness in the past several decades [89].

Successful psychosocial management of cancer patients often necessitates attention to the psychosocial needs of caregivers. When appropriate, support groups can provide valuable benefits to caregivers. Respite, either in a formal setting or through the rotation of care, may prove necessary to rejuvenate primary care givers and renew social supports. Rather than ancillary aspects of treatment, these concerns are central to the wellbeing of nearly all patients.

TREATMENT

Anxiety and depression should not be viewed as inevitable consequences of cancer, even at its advanced stages [87]. Patients suffering from psychiatric illnesses related to cancer now have a wide range of treatment options readily available to them. These include antidepressants (*e.g.* selective serotonin reuptake inhibitors, selective norepinephrine reuptake inhibitors, tricyclics, and monoamine oxidase inhibitors), anxiolytics (both benzodiazepines and non-benzodiazepines) and off-label uses of second-generation antipsychotics. In addition, multiple modalities of therapy and psychosocial support have been shown to improve wellbeing and quality of life [29]. Any effective treatment plan should begin with management of symptoms stemming from the underlying cancer and side effects stemming from cancer treatment. Relief from pain, fatigue, nausea and similar stressors may reduce the need for pharmacological interventions.

Pharmacological Treatment - Depression

While numerous pharmacological treatment options exist for depression, no evidence categorically favors one medication over others. According to the Supportive Care Guidelines Group of Cancer Care Ontario's Program in Evidence-Based Care, "Current evidence does not support the relative superiority of one pharmacologic treatment over another, nor the superiority of pharmacologic treatment over psychosocial interventions" [90]. The SSRIs citalopram, escitalopram and sertraline are well tolerated and pose few drug-drug interactions [91]. Low dose mirtazapine may prove beneficial in patients struggling with sleep or appetite. Fatigue can be treated with stimulants including methylphenidate and modafinil.

Pharmacological Treatment – Anxiety

A wide range of pharmacologist treatments is available for cancer patients suffering from anxiety. Long-acting benzodiazepines, such as clonazepam, are highly effective, but also pose considerable risks including delirium and dependence; benzodiazepines may also worsen fatigue. Increasingly, psycho-oncologists favor low doses of the second-generation antipsychotics olanzapine and quetiapine, as these may also mitigate secondary symptoms including nausea

[92]. Again, sedation is a potential risk, although rare at lower doses. Long term anxiety may be treated with SSRIs, although it should be noted that fluoxetine, paroxetine and fluvoxetime may lower tamoxifen levels in patients (such as those with ovarian stromal tumors) on this regimen. Gabapentin may benefit some patients where these other agents are contraindicated.

Talk Therapy

Significant data from the general population favors the combination of pharmacological and talk-based therapies for the optimal treatment of depression, anxiety, PTSD and related disorders. Women suffering from ovarian cancer often wish for such psychosocial support. Among the older women surveyed by Fitch *et al.*, 54% reported a wish to talk to someone about the difficulties they faced regarding their cancer, a number that increased to 70% in those with recurrent disease [51]. For 34% a physician was their confidant, while 22% confided in a nurse [51]. One in five reported speaking to a mental health professional [51].

Psychosocial interventions have been tied to decreased psychological distress and improved quality of life in cancer patients [51]. Manualized therapies, such as Cognitive Behavior Therapy (CBT), offer systematic, concrete approaches to therapy. In CBT, the goal of the patient is to "change emotions by first changing thoughts and behaviors" [93]. Interpersonal therapy (IPT), which focuses on specific domains such as role transition and grief, is another manualized therapy with promising results in cancer patients [94]. Meaning Centered Therapy, which focuses on existential distress, improves patients' spiritual welfare, although gains in other domains (*e.g.* quality of life) are less persuasive [95]. Group based therapies have also shown potential in improving patients wellbeing, although not longevity. Supportive Expressive Group Therapy (SEGT) may help women cope with the advanced states of disease [96]. In addition, psychodynamic therapies may benefit a subset of cancer patients [97]. Yet considerable care should be taken when breaking down patients' defenses, often an integral part of psychodynamic treatments, as defenses and denial may prove essential forms of emotional protection during acute illness.

END OF LIFE ISSUES

Hope and optimism can prove valuable tools in battling the emotional and psychological effects of a cancer diagnosis. Unfortunately, in a disease with a high rate of lethality, many patients will not obtain the therapeutic outcomes they desire. In such cases, sensitive but candid preparation for the end stages of disease is an essential component in the relationship between the patient and her care team. Hospice use has increased significantly in recent years and older women with terminal ovarian cancer less likely to die in the hospital than a generation ago

[98]. Many patients may hold mistaken views about some end of life services, such as the belief that palliative care is incompatible with aggressive treatment or that all hospice care must occur in an inpatient setting [99]. Providing clear, easily understandable information will help patients make choices consistent with their own autonomy and care goals.

Palliative Care & Hospice

Although sometimes mistakenly thought of as an alternative to active treatment, palliative care is better conceived of as a holistic, interdisciplinary approach to symptom and comfort management that addresses both psychosocial and physical needs [100]. Co-management with oncological or medical providers is common [100]. Current guidelines recommend early incorporation of palliative care services into the therapeutic process [101]. Early initiation of palliative care has been tied to increased survival in some cancer patients [101]. The early introduction of palliative services has also been shown to reduce treatment costs significantly without compromising care [102]. Palliative care may best be thought of as an additional layer of support for each patient and should be integrated, whenever possible, into an overall care plan.

Hospice services can provide additional comfort and autonomy to those patients in the final states of their illness. Generally available when life expectancy falls below six months, such services are now often provided at home. Some patients may also choose to spend their final days in hospice facilities, which are increasingly covered by medical insurance. Both options remove vulnerable patients from the stressful, often disorienting setting of hospitals and intensive care units. However, the rise of hospice care has not witnessed a concomitant decline in end-of-life ICU admissions among ovarian cancer patients [102].

Aid in Dying

Aid in dying, often referred to by the misleading term "assisted suicide," is a deeply controversial issue. Leading ethicists and people of goodwill currently stand on either side of the debate. The practice is currently legal in the states of Oregon, Washington, California, Vermont and Montana, as well as the District of Columbia, Canada, Switzerland, The Netherlands, Belgium, Luxemburg, Columbia and—under very limited circumstances—Japan. Legislation is under consideration in several other states and the trend is toward increased legality. As a result, oncologists and mental health providers are likely to encounter patients requesting guidance regarding such options. Although the moral choices of individual patients and their providers are beyond the scope of this chapter, a few general observations may prove helpful. First, it is essential for clinical purposes to recognize aid in dying as a distinct phenomenon from suicidality. Patients seeking aid in dying are already dying of a terminal illness; many are merely seeking more control over the method, timing and location of their deaths. With that caveat, it is important for providers to identify patients suffering from significant psychiatric comorbidities, such as depression, who request aid in dying. Such patients may actually have treatable forms of suicidality and their capacity to choose to end their own lives may be diminished to the degree that nearly all mainstream ethicists and clinicians would seek to curtail their autonomy. Similarly, the reasons patients seek aid in dying should be explored thoroughly. A patient who fears pain may be given reassurances regarding pain control. In contrast, a patient whose concerns are rational and existential may benefit less from therapeutic interventions. Many patients who contemplate aid in dying never end their own live in this way, but nonetheless take solace in knowing that the option remains available as a last resort. Finally, physicians should be aware that providing information on aid in dying remains illegal in some states and that medical professionals who offer referrals or guidance may face criminal sanction.

CONCLUSIONS

Ovarian cancer is not merely a disease of the body, but a complex syndrome that affects the psychological and social wellbeing of its victims and their loved ones. Management of these aspects of patient welfare requires an interdisciplinary, team-based approach that includes medical and mental health professions. Clear communication among elements of the treatment team is essential for patient welfare. So is clear, compassionate communication with the patient herself during the entire course of care—from the presentation of initial symptoms through treatment regimens and, when necessary, the preparation for the final stages of disease. A collaborative approach between providers, patients and caregivers is likely to enhance quality of life and psychological health, helping patients to confront the ongoing challenges of their illness.

CONSENT FOR PUBLICATION

Not applicable.

CONFLICT OF INTEREST

The author confirms that this chapter contents have no conflict of interest.

ACKNOWLEDGEMENTS

Declared none.

REFERENCES

[1]   Cancer Statistics," National Cancer Institute. Available at . https://www.cancer.gov/about-cancer/understanding/statistics

[2]   Ovarian Cancer Statistics," Centers for Disease Control and Prevention. Available at:. https://www.cdc.gov/cancer/ovarian/statistics/index.htm

[3]   Borduka-Bevers D, Engquist K, *et al.* Depression, anxiety, and quality of life in patients with epithelial ovarian cancer. Gynecol Oncol 2000; 78: 302-8. P. 302

[4]   Cress RD, Chen YS, Morris CR, Petersen M, Leiserowitz GS. Characteristics of Long-Term Survivors of Epithelial Ovarian Cancer. Obstet Gynecol 2015; 126(3): 491-7.
[http://dx.doi.org/10.1097/AOG.0000000000000981] [PMID: 26244529]

[5]   Women's Health Research. Progress, Pitfalls, and Promise Institute of Medicine (US) Committee on Women's Health Research Washington (DC). US: National Academies Press 2010.

[6]   Geller SE, Adams MG, Carnes M. Adherence to federal guidelines for reporting of sex and race/ethnicity in clinical trials. J Womens Health (Larchmt) 2006; 15(10): 1123-31.
[http://dx.doi.org/10.1089/jwh.2006.15.1123] [PMID: 17199453]

[7]   Kim ESH, Carrigan TP, Menon V. Enrollment of women in National Heart, Lung, and Blood Institute-funded cardiovascular randomized controlled trials fails to meet current federal mandates for inclusion. J Am Coll Cardiol 2008; 52(8): 672-3.
[http://dx.doi.org/10.1016/j.jacc.2008.05.025] [PMID: 18702973]

[8]   Bird CE. Women and Health Research: Ethical and Legal Issues of Including Women in Clinical Studies Workshop and Commissioned Papers Institute of Medicine (US) Committee on the Ethical and Legal Issues Relating to the Inclusion of Women in Clinical Studies. Washington (DC): National Academies Press (US) 1999; 2.

[9]   Svensson CK. Representation of American blacks in clinical trials of new drugs. JAMA 1989; 261(2): 263-5.
[http://dx.doi.org/10.1001/jama.1989.03420020117041] [PMID: 2909024]

[10]   Sheikh A. Why are ethnic minorities under-represented in US research studies? PLoS Med 2006; 3(2)e49
[http://dx.doi.org/10.1371/journal.pmed.0030049] [PMID: 16370583]

[11]   Kunos CA. Commentary: Phase I Trial of Carboplatin and Gemcitabine Chemotherapy and Stereotactic Ablative Radiosurgery for the Palliative Treatment of Persistent or Recurrent Gynecologic Cancer. Front Oncol 2016; 6: 263.
[http://dx.doi.org/10.3389/fonc.2016.00263] [PMID: 28066719]

[12]   Congressional Record (Bound Edition). 2005; 151. Part 18

[13]   Gonçalves V, Jayson G, Tarrier N. A longitudinal investigation of psychological morbidity in patients with ovarian cancer. Br J Cancer 2008; 99(11): 1794-801.
[http://dx.doi.org/10.1038/sj.bjc.6604770] [PMID: 19002175]

[14]   Mitchell AJ, Chan M, Bhatti H, *et al.* Prevalence of depression, anxiety, and adjustment disorder in oncological, haematological, and palliative-care settings: a meta-analysis of 94 interview-based studies. Lancet Oncol 2011; 12(2): 160-74.
[http://dx.doi.org/10.1016/S1470-2045(11)70002-X] [PMID: 21251875]

[15]   Mehnert A, Brähler E, Faller H, *et al.* Four-week prevalence of mental disorders in patients with cancer across major tumor entities. J Clin Oncol 2014; 32(31): 3540-6.
[http://dx.doi.org/10.1200/JCO.2014.56.0086] [PMID: 25287821]

[16]   Mielcarek P, Nowicka-Sauer K, Kozaka J. Anxiety and depression in patients with advanced ovarian cancer: a prospective study. J Psychosom Obstet Gynaecol 2016; 37(2): 57-67.
[http://dx.doi.org/10.3109/0167482X.2016.1141891] [PMID: 26939616]

[17] Abbas FM, Sert MB. Cost, quality of life and outcome measures in ovarian cancer. Anticancer Drugs 1998; 9(10): 859-67.
[http://dx.doi.org/10.1097/00001813-199811000-00005] [PMID: 9890697]

[18] Naeim A, Reuben D, Ganz P. Management of Cancer in the Older Patient. Elsevier Health Sciences 2011.

[19] Appelbaum PS, Grisso T. Assessing patients' capacities to consent to treatment. N Engl J Med 1988; 319(25): 1635-8.
[http://dx.doi.org/10.1056/NEJM198812223192504] [PMID: 3200278]

[20] Buchanan AE, Brock DW. Deciding for Others: The Ethics of Surrogate Decision Making. Cambridge: Cambridge University Press 1989; p. 60.

[21] Fitch M, Deane K, Howell D, Gray RE. Women's experiences with ovarian cancer: reflections on being diagnosed. Can Oncol Nurs J 2002; 12(3): 152-68.
[http://dx.doi.org/10.5737/1181912x123152159] [PMID: 12271917]

[22] Elit LM, Levine MN, Gafni A, *et al.* Patients' preferences for therapy in advanced epithelial ovarian cancer: development, testing, and application of a bedside decision instrument. Gynecol Oncol 1996; 62(3): 329-35.
[http://dx.doi.org/10.1006/gyno.1996.0244] [PMID: 8812525]

[23] Ersek M, Ferrell BR, Dow KH, Melancon CH. Quality of life in women with ovarian cancer. West J Nurs Res 1997; 19(3): 334-50.
[http://dx.doi.org/10.1177/019394599701900305] [PMID: 9170991]

[24] McCabe MS, Wood WA, Goldberg RM. When the family requests withholding the diagnosis: who owns the truth? J Oncol Pract 2010; 6(2): 94-6.
[http://dx.doi.org/10.1200/JOP.091086] [PMID: 20592784]

[25] Zahedi F. The challenge of truth telling across cultures: a case study. J Med Ethics Hist Med 2011; 4: 11.
[PMID: 23908753]

[26] Opinion 8.082. AMA Journal of Ethics. Virtual Mentor 2012; 14(7): 555-6.

[27] Bonomo JB, Rinderknecht TN, Beiser EN. "It ain't easy being green," a case-based analysis of ethics and medical education on the wards. Med Health R I 2003; 86(9): 276-8.
[PMID: 14556410]

[28] Gonçalves V, Jayson G, Tarrier N. A longitudinal investigation of psychological disorders in patients prior and subsequent to a diagnosis of ovarian cancer. J Clin Psychol Med Settings 2010; 17(2): 167-73.
[http://dx.doi.org/10.1007/s10880-010-9196-1] [PMID: 20490630]

[29] Payne SA. A study of quality of life in cancer patients receiving palliative chemotherapy. Soc Sci Med 1992; 35(12): 1505-9.
[http://dx.doi.org/10.1016/0277-9536(92)90053-S] [PMID: 1283035]

[30] Hipkins J, Whitworth M, Tarrier N, Jayson G. Social support, anxiety and depression after chemotherapy for ovarian cancer: a prospective study. Br J Health Psychol 2004; 9(Pt 4): 569-81.
[http://dx.doi.org/10.1348/1359107042304542] [PMID: 15509362]

[31] Norton TR, Manne SL, Rubin S, *et al.* Ovarian cancer patients' psychological distress: the role of physical impairment, perceived unsupportive family and friend behaviors, perceived control, and self-esteem. Health Psychol 2005; 24(2): 143-52.
[http://dx.doi.org/10.1037/0278-6133.24.2.143] [PMID: 15755228]

[32] Kornblith AB, Thaler HT, Wong G, *et al.* Quality of life of women with ovarian cancer. Gynecol Oncol 1995; 59(2): 231-42.
[http://dx.doi.org/10.1006/gyno.1995.0014] [PMID: 7590479]

[33]   Okamura H, Watanabe T, Narabayashi M, *et al.* Psychological distress following first recurrence of disease in patients with breast cancer: prevalence and risk factors. Breast Cancer Res Treat 2000; 61(2): 131-7.
       [http://dx.doi.org/10.1023/A:1006491417791] [PMID: 10942098]

[34]   Casey P, Bailey S. Adjustment disorders: the state of the art. World Psychiatry 2011; 10(1): 11-8.
       [http://dx.doi.org/10.1002/j.2051-5545.2011.tb00003.x] [PMID: 21379346]

[35]   Sellick SM, Crooks DL. Depression and cancer: an appraisal of the literature for prevalence, detection, and practice guideline development for psychological interventions. Psychooncology 1999; 8(4): 315-33.
       [http://dx.doi.org/10.1002/(SICI)1099-1611(199907/08)8:4<315::AID-PON391>3.0.CO;2-G] [PMID: 10474850]

[36]   Evans M, Mottram P. Diagnosis of depression in elderly patients. Adv Psychiatr Treat 2000; 6(1): 49-56.
       [http://dx.doi.org/10.1192/apt.6.1.49]

[37]   Donovan HS, Hartenbach EM, Method MW. Patient-provider communication and perceived control for women experiencing multiple symptoms associated with ovarian cancer. Gynecol Oncol 2005; 99(2): 404-11.
       [http://dx.doi.org/10.1016/j.ygyno.2005.06.062] [PMID: 16112174]

[38]   Strömgren AS, Groenvold M, Pedersen L, Olsen AK, Spile M, Sjøgren P. Does the medical record cover the symptoms experienced by cancer patients receiving palliative care? A comparison of the record and patient self-rating. J Pain Symptom Manage 2001; 21(3): 189-96.
       [http://dx.doi.org/10.1016/S0885-3924(01)00264-0] [PMID: 11239737]

[39]   Rhondali W, Freyer G, Adam V, *et al.* Agreement for depression diagnosis between DSM-IV-TR criteria, three validated scales, oncologist assessment, and psychiatric clinical interview in elderly patients with advanced ovarian cancer. Clin Interv Aging 2015; 10: 1155-62.
       [PMID: 26203235]

[40]   Shankar A, Dracham C, Ghoshal S, Grover S. Prevalence of depression and anxiety disorder in cancer patients: An institutional experience. Indian J Cancer 2016; 53(3): 432-4.
       [PMID: 28244477]

[41]   Hung MS, Chen IC, Lee CP, *et al.* Incidence and risk factors of depression after diagnosis of lung cancer: A nationwide population-based study. Medicine (Baltimore) 2017; 96(19)e6864
       [http://dx.doi.org/10.1097/MD.0000000000006864] [PMID: 28489782]

[42]   Sood AK, Bhatty R, *et al.* Stress hormone-mediated invasion of ovarian cancer cells. Clin Cancer Res 2006; 15;12(2): 369-75.
       [http://dx.doi.org/10.1158/1078-0432.CCR-05-1698]

[43]   Thaker PH, Han LY, Kamat AA, *et al.* Chronic stress promotes tumor growth and angiogenesis in a mouse model of ovarian carcinoma. Nat Med 2006; 12(8): 939-44.
       [http://dx.doi.org/10.1038/nm1447] [PMID: 16862152]

[44]   Lutgendorf SK, DeGeest K, Sung CY, *et al.* Depression, social support, and beta-adrenergic transcription control in human ovarian cancer. Brain Behav Immun 2009; 23(2): 176-83.
       [http://dx.doi.org/10.1016/j.bbi.2008.04.155] [PMID: 18550328]

[45]   Huang T, Poole EM, Okereke OI, *et al.* Depression and risk of epithelial ovarian cancer: Results from two large prospective cohort studies. Gynecol Oncol 2015; 139(3): 481-6.
       [http://dx.doi.org/10.1016/j.ygyno.2015.10.004] [PMID: 26449316]

[46]   Portenoy RK, Thaler HT, Kornblith AB, *et al.* Symptom prevalence, characteristics and distress in a cancer population. Qual Life Res 1994; 3(3): 183-9.
       [http://dx.doi.org/10.1007/BF00435383] [PMID: 7920492]

[47]   Yeh YW, Chen CY, Kuo SC, Lin CK, Huang SY. Suicidal depression related to chemotherapy in a

patient with ovarian cancer. Psychosomatics 2012; 53(1): 98-100.
[http://dx.doi.org/10.1016/j.psym.2011.02.008] [PMID: 22221729]

[48]   Watts S, Prescott P. Depression and anxiety in ovarian cancer: a systematic review and meta-analysis of prevalence rates. BMJ Open 2015; 30;5(11)
[http://dx.doi.org/10.1136/bmjopen-2015-007618]

[49]   Sukegawa A, Miyagi E, Asai-Sato M, *et al.* Anxiety and prevalence of psychiatric disorders among patients awaiting surgery for suspected ovarian cancer. J Obstet Gynaecol Res 2008; 34(4): 543-51.
[http://dx.doi.org/10.1111/j.1447-0756.2008.00738.x] [PMID: 18937707]

[50]   Reid A, Ercolano E, Schwartz P, McCorkle R. The management of anxiety and knowledge of serum CA-125 after an ovarian cancer diagnosis. Clin J Oncol Nurs 2011; 15(6): 625-32.
[http://dx.doi.org/10.1188/11.CJON.625-632] [PMID: 22119973]

[51]   Fitch MI, Gray RE, Franssen E. Perspectives on living with ovarian cancer: older women's views. Oncol Nurs Forum 2001; 28(9): 1433-42.
[PMID: 11683313]

[52]   Fitch M, Gray RE, Franssen E. Perspectives on living with ovarian cancer: young women's views. Can Oncol Nurs J 2000; 10(3): 101-8.
[http://dx.doi.org/10.5737/1181912x103101108] [PMID: 11894277]

[53]   Matulonis UA, Kornblith A, Lee H, *et al.* Long-term adjustment of early-stage ovarian cancer survivors. Int J Gynecol Cancer 2008; 18(6): 1183-93.
[http://dx.doi.org/10.1111/j.1525-1438.2007.01167.x] [PMID: 18217977]

[54]   Gonçalves V, Jayson G, Tarrier N. A longitudinal investigation of posttraumatic stress disorder in patients with ovarian cancer. J Psychosom Res 2011; 70(5): 422-31.
[http://dx.doi.org/10.1016/j.jpsychores.2010.09.017] [PMID: 21511072]

[55]   Lewis DA, Smith RE. Steroid-induced psychiatric syndromes. A report of 14 cases and a review of the literature. J Affect Disord 1983; 5(4): 319-32.
[http://dx.doi.org/10.1016/0165-0327(83)90022-8] [PMID: 6319464]

[56]   Sirois F. Steroid psychosis: a review. Gen Hosp Psychiatry 2003; 25(1): 27-33.
[http://dx.doi.org/10.1016/S0163-8343(02)00241-4] [PMID: 12583925]

[57]   Casagrande Tango R. Psychiatric side effects of medications prescribed in internal medicine. Dialogues Clin Neurosci 2003; 5(2): 155-65.
[PMID: 22034468]

[58]   Stiefel FC, Breitbart WS, Holland JC. Corticosteroids in cancer: neuropsychiatric complications. Cancer Invest 1989; 7(5): 479-91.
[http://dx.doi.org/10.3109/07357908909041378] [PMID: 2695230]

[59]   Falk WE, Mahnke MW, Poskanzer DC. Lithium prophylaxis of corticotropin-induced psychosis. JAMA 1979; 241(10): 1011-2.
[http://dx.doi.org/10.1001/jama.1979.03290360027021] [PMID: 216818]

[60]   Kenna HA, Poon AW, de los Angeles CP, Koran LM. Psychiatric complications of treatment with corticosteroids: review with case report. Psychiatry Clin Neurosci 2011; 65(6): 549-60.
[http://dx.doi.org/10.1111/j.1440-1819.2011.02260.x] [PMID: 22003987]

[61]   Jacobsen JC, Maytal G, Stern TA. Demoralization in medical practice. Prim Care Companion J Clin Psychiatry 2007; 9(2): 139-43.
[http://dx.doi.org/10.4088/PCC.v09n0208] [PMID: 17607336]

[62]   Mehnert A, Vehling S, Höcker A, Lehmann C, Koch U. Demoralization and depression in patients with advanced cancer: validation of the German version of the demoralization scale. J Pain Symptom Manage 2011; 42(5): 768-76.
[http://dx.doi.org/10.1016/j.jpainsymman.2011.02.013] [PMID: 21592722]

[63]   Hurley KE, Miller SM, Costalas JW, Gillespie D, Daly MB. Anxiety/uncertainty reduction as a motivation for interest in prophylactic oophorectomy in women with a family history of ovarian cancer. J Womens Health Gend Based Med 2001; 10(2): 189-99.
[http://dx.doi.org/10.1089/152460901300039566] [PMID: 11268302]

[64]   Lawlor PG, Bush SH. Delirium in patients with cancer: assessment, impact, mechanisms and management. Nat Rev Clin Oncol 2015; 12(2): 77-92.
[http://dx.doi.org/10.1038/nrclinonc.2014.147] [PMID: 25178632]

[65]   Wada T, Wada M, Wada M, Onishi H. Characteristics, interventions, and outcomes of misdiagnosed delirium in cancer patients. Palliat Support Care 2010; 8(2): 125-31.
[http://dx.doi.org/10.1017/S1478951509990861] [PMID: 20307362]

[66]   Marchington KL, Carrier L, Lawlor PG. Delirium masquerading as depression. Palliat Support Care 2012; 10(1): 59-62.
[http://dx.doi.org/10.1017/S1478951511000599] [PMID: 22329938]

[67]   Gaudreau JD, Gagnon P, Roy MA, Harel F, Tremblay A. Association between psychoactive medications and delirium in hospitalized patients: a critical review. Psychosomatics 2005; 46(4): 302-16.
[http://dx.doi.org/10.1176/appi.psy.46.4.302] [PMID: 16000673]

[68]   Quirk JT, Natarajan N. Ovarian cancer incidence in the United States, 1992-1999. Gynecol Oncol 2005; 97(2): 519-23.
[http://dx.doi.org/10.1016/j.ygyno.2005.02.007] [PMID: 15863154]

[69]   Quirk JT, Natarajan N, Mettlin CJ. Age-specific ovarian cancer incidence rate patterns in the United States. Gynecol Oncol 2005; 99(1): 248-50.
[http://dx.doi.org/10.1016/j.ygyno.2005.06.052] [PMID: 16095676]

[70]   Heintz AP, Odicino F, Maisonneuve P, *et al.* Carcinoma of the ovary. FIGO 26th Annual Report on the Results of Treatment in Gynecological Cancer. Int J Gynaecol Obstet 2006; 95 (Suppl. 1): S161-92.
[http://dx.doi.org/10.1016/S0020-7292(06)60033-7] [PMID: 17161157]

[71]   Bisseling KC, Kondalsamy-Chennakesavan S, Bekkers RL, Janda M, Obermair A. Depression, anxiety and body image after treatment for invasive stage one epithelial ovarian cancer. Aust N Z J Obstet Gynaecol 2009; 49(6): 660-6.
[http://dx.doi.org/10.1111/j.1479-828X.2009.01074.x] [PMID: 20070719]

[72]   Duffy C, Allen S. Medical and psychosocial aspects of fertility after cancer. Cancer J 2009; 15(1): 27-33.
[http://dx.doi.org/10.1097/PPO.0b013e3181976602] [PMID: 19197170]

[73]   Herbert DL, Lucke JC, Dobson AJ. Depression: an emotional obstacle to seeking medical advice for infertility. Fertil Steril 2010; 94(5): 1817-21.
[http://dx.doi.org/10.1016/j.fertnstert.2009.10.062] [PMID: 20047740]

[74]   Domar AD, Zuttermeister PC, Friedman R. The psychological impact of infertility: a comparison with patients with other medical conditions. J Psychosom Obstet Gynaecol 1993; 14 (Suppl.): 45-52.
[PMID: 8142988]

[75]   Canada AL, Schover LR. The psychosocial impact of interrupted childbearing in long-term female cancer survivors. Psychooncology 2012; 21(2): 134-43.
[http://dx.doi.org/10.1002/pon.1875] [PMID: 22271533]

[76]   Zanagnolo V, Sartori E, Trussardi E, Pasinetti B, Maggino T. Preservation of ovarian function, reproductive ability and emotional attitudes in patients with malignant ovarian tumors. Eur J Obstet Gynecol Reprod Biol 2005; 123(2): 235-43.
[http://dx.doi.org/10.1016/j.ejogrb.2005.04.010] [PMID: 15921842]

[77]   Loscalzo MJ, Clark KL. The psychosocial context of cancer-related infertility. Cancer Treat Res 2007;

138: 180-90.
[http://dx.doi.org/10.1007/978-0-387-72293-1_13] [PMID: 18080665]

[78] Pathy S, Raheja SJ, Rakh S. Pain in advanced gynaecological maligancies: Institute of palliative care experience. Indian J Palliat Care 2008; 14: 89.
[http://dx.doi.org/10.4103/0973-1075.45451]

[79] Rolnick SJ, Jackson J, Nelson WW, *et al.* Pain management in the last six months of life among women who died of ovarian cancer. J Pain Symptom Manage 2007; 33(1): 24-31.
[http://dx.doi.org/10.1016/j.jpainsymman.2006.06.010] [PMID: 17196904]

[80] Elliott TE, Elliott BA. Physician attitudes and beliefs about use of morphine for cancer pain. J Pain Symptom Manage 1992; 7(3): 141-8.
[http://dx.doi.org/10.1016/S0885-3924(06)80005-9] [PMID: 16967581]

[81] Ferrell B, Smith S, Cullinane C, Melancon C. Symptom concerns of women with ovarian cancer. J Pain Symptom Manage 2003; 25(6): 528-38.
[http://dx.doi.org/10.1016/S0885-3924(03)00148-9] [PMID: 12782433]

[82] Passik SD, Kirsh KL, Donaghy K, *et al.* Patient-related barriers to fatigue communication: initial validation of the fatigue management barriers questionnaire. J Pain Symptom Manage 2002; 24(5): 481-93.
[http://dx.doi.org/10.1016/S0885-3924(02)00518-3] [PMID: 12547048]

[83] Scharf DH, Hartenbach EM, Method MW. Patient-provider communication and perceived control for women experiencing multiple symptoms associated with ovarian cancer. Gynecol Oncol 2005; 99: 404-11.

[84] Vogelzang NJ, Breitbart W, Cella D, *et al.* Patient, caregiver, and oncologist perceptions of cancer-related fatigue: results of a tripart assessment survey. The Fatigue Coalition. Semin Hematol 1997; 34(3) (Suppl. 2): 4-12.
[PMID: 9253778]

[85] Carroll JK, Kohli S, Mustian KM, Roscoe JA, Morrow GR. Pharmacologic treatment of cancer-related fatigue. Oncologist 2007; 12 (Suppl. 1): 43-51.
[http://dx.doi.org/10.1634/theoncologist.12-S1-43] [PMID: 17573455]

[86] Mishra K. Gynaecological malignancies from palliative care perspective. Indian J Palliat Care 2011; 17 (Suppl.): S45-51.
[http://dx.doi.org/10.4103/0973-1075.76243] [PMID: 21811372]

[87] Hartnett J, Thom B, Kline N. Caregiver Burden in End-Stage Ovarian Cancer. Clin J Oncol Nurs 2016; 20(2): 169-73.
[http://dx.doi.org/10.1188/16.CJON.169-173] [PMID: 26991710]

[88] Price MA, Butow PN, Costa DS, *et al.* Australian Ovarian Cancer Study Group; Australian Ovarian Cancer Study Group Quality of Life Study Investigators. Prevalence and predictors of anxiety and depression in women with invasive ovarian cancer and their caregivers. Med J Aust 2010; 193(5) (Suppl.): S52-7.
[PMID: 21542447]

[89] Myers Virtue S, Manne SL, Ozga M, *et al.* Cancer-related concerns among women with a new diagnosis of gynecological cancer: an exploration of age group differences. Int J Gynecol Cancer 2014; 24(1): 165-71.
[http://dx.doi.org/10.1097/IGC.0000000000000010] [PMID: 24346489]

[90] Traeger L, Greer JA, Fernandez-Robles C, Temel JS, Pirl WF. Evidence-based treatment of anxiety in patients with cancer. J Clin Oncol 2012; 30(11): 1197-205.
[http://dx.doi.org/10.1200/JCO.2011.39.5632] [PMID: 22412135]

[91] Rodin G, Katz M, Lloyd N, Green E, Mackay JA, Wong RK. Treatment of depression in cancer patients. Curr Oncol 2007; 14(5): 180-8.

[http://dx.doi.org/10.3747/co.2007.146] [PMID: 17938701]

[92]   Li M, Fitzgerald P, Rodin G. Evidence-based treatment of depression in patients with cancer. J Clin Oncol 2012; 30(11): 1187-96.
[http://dx.doi.org/10.1200/JCO.2011.39.7372] [PMID: 22412144]

[93]   Daniels S. Cognitive Behavior Therapy for Patients With Cancer. J Adv Pract Oncol 2015; 6(1): 54-6.
[PMID: 26413374]

[94]   Donnelly JM, Kornblith AB, Fleishman S, *et al.* A pilot study of interpersonal psychotherapy by telephone with cancer patients and their partners. Psychooncology 2000; 9(1): 44-56.
[http://dx.doi.org/10.1002/(SICI)1099-1611(200001/02)9:1<44::AID-PON431>3.0.CO;2-V] [PMID: 10668059]

[95]   Breitbart W, Rosenfeld B, Pessin H, Applebaum A, Kulikowski J, Lichtenthal WG. Meaning-centered group psychotherapy: an effective intervention for improving psychological well-being in patients with advanced cancer. J Clin Oncol 2015; 33(7): 749-54.
[http://dx.doi.org/10.1200/JCO.2014.57.2198] [PMID: 25646186]

[96]   Walker LM, Bischoff TF, Robinson JW. Supportive expressive group therapy for women with advanced ovarian cancer. Int J Group Psychother 2010; 60(3): 407-27.
[http://dx.doi.org/10.1521/ijgp.2010.60.3.407] [PMID: 20590436]

[97]   Straker N. Psychodynamic psychotherapy for cancer patients. J Psychother Pract Res 1997; 7(1): 1-9.
[PMID: 9407471]

[98]   Wright AA, Hatfield LA, Earle CC, Keating NL. End-of-life care for older patients with ovarian cancer is intensive despite high rates of hospice use. J Clin Oncol 2014; 32(31): 3534-9.
[http://dx.doi.org/10.1200/JCO.2014.55.5383] [PMID: 25287831]

[99]   Hui D, Mori M, Parsons HA, *et al.* The lack of standard definitions in the supportive and palliative oncology literature. J Pain Symptom Manage 2012; 43(3): 582-92.
[http://dx.doi.org/10.1016/j.jpainsymman.2011.04.016] [PMID: 22104619]

[100]   Hardiman L. The Case for Early Palliative Care in the Treatment of Ovarian Cancer. J Adv Pract Oncol 2014; 5(4): 290-3.
[PMID: 26110073]

[101]   Bakitas MA, Tosteson TD, Li Z, *et al.* Early Versus Delayed Initiation of Concurrent Palliative Oncology Care: Patient Outcomes in the ENABLE III Randomized Controlled Trial. J Clin Oncol 2015; 33(13): 1438-45.
[http://dx.doi.org/10.1200/JCO.2014.58.6362] [PMID: 25800768]

[102]   Lowery WJ, Lowery AW, Barnett JC, *et al.* Cost-effectiveness of early palliative care intervention in recurrent platinum-resistant ovarian cancer. Gynecol Oncol 2013; 130(3): 426-30.
[http://dx.doi.org/10.1016/j.ygyno.2013.06.011] [PMID: 23769759]

CHAPTER 6

Role of Belief in Healing: Placebo Effect, Nocebo Effect, and The Mind-Body Interaction

Tamara Kalir*

The Icahn School of Medicine at Mount Sinai, USA

Abstract: This chapter explores the role of belief in healing, beginning with a brief review of western medicine's changing foundations - initially religious and later scientific. The chapter relates to disease in general and is inclusive of ovarian cancer. Disease in ancient times was attributed to Divine cause; religious leaders served as physicians and belief played a prominent role in healing. Groundbreaking nineteenth- and twentieth-century scientific discoveries, which offered physical explanations for disease and fostered the development of companion therapies, diminished appreciation of the importance of belief in the healing process. Beginning around the mid- twentieth century and continuing to this day, scientific studies have investigated treatment outcomes in relation to the beliefs of patients and healers. The power of the placebo and nocebo are discussed, and studies and comments by both conventional and 'alternative' modern-day healers illustrate a renewed appreciation of the importance of belief in the healing process.

Keywords: Belief, Church, Chakra, Faith, Fleming, Galen, Hippocrates, Intuitive, Koch, Mind-body, Medieval, Miracle, Nocebo, New Testament, Osler, Old Testament, Old Testament, Osler, Placebo, Pope, Priest, Pasteur, Qur'an, Rabbi.

ANCIENT & MEDIEVAL TIMES: RELIGION-BASED MEDICINE

In ancient times, people related illness to divinity. The Book of Leviticus in the Old Testament, written around 1450 B.C [1], details how the God of Abraham chose the ancient Hebrew priests to protect the health of the Israelites during their desert trek to the Promised Land [2]. God told Moses and Aaron to instruct the priests regarding the proper procedure to follow when anyone in the camp developed a skin disease described as a rash. Translated from the Hebrew as "tzara'at," commentators believe this term refers to either leprosy or some other type of skin infection. The affected individual was to be brought to either Aaron or his sons, the priests. An infectious process was diagnosed if the hair on the

---

* **Corresponding author Tamara Kalir:**The Icahn School of Medicine at Mount Sinai, USA; E-mail: Tamara.Kalir@mountsinai.org

Tamara L. Kalir (Ed.)

lesion had turned white and the lesion appeared more than skin deep. The person was pronounced ceremonially unclean and was isolated from the camp. If the hair had not turned white or the lesion did not appear skin deep, the person was placed in isolation for seven days. The priest was to re-examine the person after seven days and if the lesion was unchanged, he/she was placed in isolation another seven days after which he/she was again examined. If the lesion had faded upon re-examination after the seven-day period, the priest could diagnose a rash and pronounce the person clean. The person would wash their clothes and after evening, re-join the camp. If however the lesion had spread on the skin, the priest would then diagnose an infectious disease and the person would have to be quarantined and dwell outside the camp. The person diagnosed with a skin infection would have to tear their garments, allow their hair to grow, cover their face with a garment and call out, "defiled, defiled" so people in the camp would know to avoid them. When the lesion disappeared, they were to be re-examined by one of the priests to be declared clean; bathe, wash their clothes and then re-enter the camp after nightfall.

The Book of Exodus of the Old Testament, written around 500 B.C [3], tells how the God of Abraham also said to the Israelites in the desert [4]:

"If you will listen to the voice of the Lord your God, and obey it, and do what is right, then I will not make you suffer the diseases I sent on the Egyptians, for I am the Lord who heals you."

Given the sacredness of the Old Testament to Judeo-Christians, the association of illness with Divinity and Divine decree persisted through much of western history, in spite of attempts to dismiss it. Around 400 B.C., the Greek physician Hippocrates put forth the novel idea that disease is a result of natural causes, and not due to superstition or the gods [5]:

"It is thus with regard to the disease called Sacred: it appears to me to be nowise more divine nor more sacred than other diseases, but has a natural cause from the originates like other affections. Men regard its nature and cause as divine from ignorance and wonder…" and "natural forces within us are the true healers of disease" [6].

Hippocrates' philosophy was consistent with that of the ancient Greeks of his time, who sought to explain things in a non-religious way. Nonetheless the intertwining of disease and religion persisted and developed further such that in Anglo-Saxon times, around 410 – 1066 A.D [7]. it was believed that sickness was sent by God as a result of some sin committed by the ill person. The focus was more on caring for the sick person's soul rather than trying to cure the person, as the idea was that a certain amount of suffering was necessary to cleanse the sick person's soul of its sin. However, a simultaneous belief was that if a cure was available, it was not only prudent but right even in the eyes of God to attempt a cure. Similarly to Old Testament-times physicians were most often religious people - monks who studied in the existing medical schools at the time.

WESTERN MEDIEVAL PHYSICIANS' TRAINING: MEDICINE & THE PRIESTHOOD

In contrast to modern western medicine where training is scientifically-based, the program of medicine in Anglo-Saxon times was under Church jurisdiction and individuals (men) trained for the priesthood. Training lasted from six to nine years, and consisted firstly of a basic three-year curriculum of grammar, rhetoric and logic called the trivium. After completing this, the student would move on to a four-year quadrivium of astronomy, geometry, music and algebra [8]. Physicians drew up astrological charts to aid both in working out suitable treatments and predicting the course of their patients' ailments. Interestingly, music was believed to be conducive to health and doctors might also sing [7, 9].

Due to a lack of scientific advancement, Galen's theory of the four humors, formulated during his lifetime in A.D. 129-216 was still prevalent one thousand years later [10]. In his theory, are four basic elements of which the human body is made: earth, fire, water and air, which combine to form the humors: blood, phlegm, black bile and yellow bile. Every individual had an excess of one or another, making them sanguine, phlegmatic, choleric or melancholy. Illness occurred when the humors became unbalanced.

TREATING DISEASE IN WESTERN ANCIENT TIMES: FANCIFUL THERAPIES

To re-adjust the unbalanced humors and restore well-being, a physician could prescribe a suitable diet and life-style changes. Alternatively, enemas could be employed, or bleeding the patient. Also popular were counter spells, incantations, potions, inciting the soul to return to the body, and songs. Exemplified below are treatments for fever which, by modern standards seem fanciful at best [11, 12]:

"First make an amulet of wafers, then sing a charm, first in the patient's left ear, then the right and, finally, over the top of the head while hanging the amulet around the patient's neck."

"Take a small fresh jar to a river and say to the river: 'River, O river, please loan me a jar full of water for a guest who is visiting me.' Fill the jar with water from the river. Then spin the jar seven times around your head and pour the water over your back while saying: 'River, O river, please take back the water you gave to me, for the guest who visited me came and left on the same day.'"

Whooping cough (pertussis), an illness which today is vaccine-preventable and treatable by antibiotics, was treated in Anglo-Saxon times by the following, also fanciful method [13]:

"Take a caterpillar, wrap it in a small bag of muslin, and hang the bag around the neck of the affected child. The caterpillar will die and the child will be cured. Or pour a bowl of milk and get a ferret to lap from the bowl. After the child drinks the rest of the milk, she will recover."

Because of lacking knowledge of the scientific basis of disease, western medieval physicians focused on treating the whole person, body and soul. If the treatment had no physical effect, the patient might still experience relief when they and the healer believed in the treatment. The power of belief was held in high esteem in ancient times, and will soon be discussed in more detail under the placebo effect.

Still, some treatments were more practical and may be recognized by the modern reader. For example Moses Maimonides, a medieval Torah (Jewish religious) scholar and physician [14] used various remedies familiar today from holistic practices including: hydrotherapy, specific food combinations, exercise, pleasant surroundings, meditation, seasonal fruits, and the direction the bed faces; akin to feng shui.

SEPARATION OF MEDICINE AND RELIGION: TRANSFER OF WESTERN MEDICAL PRACTICE FROM PRIESTS TO THE LAITY

Three historical events served to separate western medicine from religion: i) Pope Innocent III's edict of 1215 A.D., ii) Descartes writings in the 1600's A.D., and, iii) the discoveries of Drs. Koch and Pasteur in the 1800's A.D.

In 1215 A.D., an important occurrence initiated the transfer of medical practice from the clergy to the public, and began paving the way for the association of medicine with science. Pope Innocent III's new edict stated that clerics were forbidden to spill blood [15]. This edict divested monks and priests of their ability to cauterize and make incisions, and thrust the practice of surgery into the hands of laymen and women. To briefly digress, women were barred from universities in medieval times however, they could work as surgeons because this practice required an apprenticeship rather than university training [16]. Further, because men were prohibited from the birthing quarters, women were at the front of the ranks in midwifery. The only requirement was a parish priest's note of good character to enable the midwife to act in the role of priest and baptize an infant who died or was stillborn during the birthing process [7]. Also of note, because of the close association of crafting medicinal mixtures with cooking, women were known to create herbal and medicinal remedies.

The practice of medieval lay-medicine evolved into three groups: i) physicians, ii) surgeons/barber surgeons, and iii) apothecaries. Physicians were university-trained and concerned with the patient's internal disposition. Surgeons and barber-surgeons, trained *via* an apprenticeship, dealt with bleedings, lancing, and setting broken bones. Apothecaries, also trained *via* an apprenticeship, learned the secrets of concocting medicines, ointments, and other remedies. For concoctions, dosages were largely due to guesswork as strengths of active ingredients were not regulated; hence a small error could prove lethal to the patient. Below is an example of a medieval anesthetic solution [17]:

"To make a drink that men call dwale, to make a man sleep during an operation. Take the gall of a boar, three spoonfuls of the juice of hemlock and three spoonfuls of wild bryony, lettuce, opium poppy, henbane and vinegar. Mix them well together and then let the man sit by a good fire and make him drink of the potion until he falls asleep. Then he may safely be operated upon."

Without the regulatory and oversight mechanisms that we have today, individuals operating independently and at their own discretion could resort to charlatanism. As would be expected, concerns were voiced by physicians and surgeons to ensure the medicines they were prescribing and the devices they were using were of the highest quality. An early but aborted attempt at a quality cooperative was the College of Physicians and Surgeons in the City of London, formed in 1423 A.D. Power struggles between the different guilds brought the College demise after only one year of operation, but demonstrated the willingness of the groups to be seen as true professionals with high standards of patient care [17].

Along with the lay-peoples' struggles, a gap persisted between science and medicine. Despite the fact that the first dissections and autopsies were carried out in 335 B.C [18], they were not accepted. Due to taboos regarding desecration of the human body and beliefs that the soul remained entrapped within the body after death, human dissection was abandoned for the next 1800 years. Then along came Descartes, who was perhaps the first to suggest that the body did not need the mind to function [19, 20]. Descartes' revolutionary ideas were instrumental in furthering the schism between religion and medicine and promoting medicine's association with science. In 1637 Descartes proposed a method based on doubt, analysis, synthesis and verification, which gave rise to the scientific method [21]. Descartes' mind-body separation influenced medical science to look toward natural causes of disease rather than supernatural. This separation downplayed the importance of anything that could not be observed and measured [21].

Descartes contribution, important as it was, would reveal a flip side later on in history. As stated by Dr. Candace Pert in her book Molecules of Emotion [20]:

"If psychological contributions to physical health and disease are viewed with suspicion, the suggestion that the soul - the literal translation of psyche - might matter is considered downright absurd. For now we are getting into the mystical realm, where scientists have been officially forbidden to tread ever since the seventeenth century. It was then that Rene Descartes, the philosopher and founding father of modern medicine, was forced to make a turf deal with the Pope in order to get the human bodies he needed for dissection. Descartes agreed he would not have anything to do with the soul, the mind or the emotions - those aspects of human experience under the virtually exclusive jurisdiction of the church at the time - if he could claim the physical realm as his own. Alas, this bargain set the tone and directions of Western science over the next two centuries, dividing human experience into two distinct and separate spheres that could never overlap, creating the unbalanced situation that is mainstream science as we know it today."

A NEW PARADIGM - GERM THEORY OF DISEASE, ANTIBIOTICS AND SCIENCE-BASED MEDICINE

While the germ theory [22] was first proposed by Girolamo Fracastoro in 1546 and further developed by Marcus von Plenciz in 1762, it was not accepted. Rather, Galen's 'miasma' theory [23] predominated among doctors of the time. The miasma theory held that diseases including cholera, Chlamydia infection, and the Black Death were caused by miasma, a form of 'bad air' emitted by rotting organic matter. The miasma theory was finally successfully challenged first by the revolutionary experiments of Dr. Louis Pasteur [24] in the 1850's and further by the work of Dr. Robert Koch in the 1880's [25]. Drs. Pasteur and Koch both demonstrated the relationship between germs and disease, and the medical and scientific communities were finally persuaded to accept the germ theory of disease. Then in 1928 Dr. Alexander Fleming [26] discovered penicillin, the first antibiotic that could be used in the treatment of germ-initiated disease. With the emergence and finally acceptance of the germ theory of disease and subsequent discovery of antibiotic drugs, a whole new world opened for doctors: a new world that could question the contribution of belief and its role in the healing process.

SCIENTIFIC STUDY OF BELIEF: THOUGHTS, PLACEBO AND NOCEBO POWER

While many ancient and medieval treatments contained healing substances we have scientifically identified, it seems other treatments if they worked at all, may have been successful as a result of belief, or the placebo effect. The placebo effect as defined in the American Heritage Dictionary is: "a beneficial effect in a patient following a particular treatment that arises from the patient's expectations concerning the treatment rather than from the treatment itself" [27]. The Merriam-Webster Dictionary [28] defines it as: "improvement in the condition of a patient that occurs in response to treatment but cannot be considered due to the specific treatment used." Equally powerful is the nocebo effect. Wikipedia defines the nocebo effect [29], "when a patient anticipates a side effect of a medication, they can suffer that effect even if the medication is actually an inert substance. Both placebo and nocebo effects are presumably psychogenic, but they can induce measurable changes in the body and the brain."

The placebo effect has been extensively studied and written about by a cardiologist named Dr. Herbert Benson, who founded the Mind/Body Medical Institute at Deaconess Hospital in Boston. He terms the placebo effect 'remembered wellness', as he feels the term 'placebo' has a pejorative connotation with use of such terms as 'sugar pill' or 'dummy pill' [19]. He believes the term 'remembered wellness' is a more accurate phrase for the patient's role in the healing process, echoing Hippocrates' statement that healing results from natural forces within.

In an interesting paper, Dr. Benson contrasted his findings with an earlier report by Dr. Henry Beecher of the Massachusetts General Hospital, who touted a 30% success rate attributable to the placebo effect [30]. Dr. Benson however found much higher levels in a study on alleviation of angina pectoris [31]. In this report, Dr. Benson along with his colleague Dr. McCallie studied treatments of angina which today are considered misguided, such as injections of cobra venom, or removal of the thyroid gland or partial pancreatectomy. They found that when these treatments were initially enthusiastically introduced by physicians, i.e., when the physicians believed in the treatments, they were effective 70 to 90% of the time whereas later when physicians began to doubt their efficacy, the effectiveness dropped to the same 30% levels published by Dr. Beecher. Similarly in 1993, Dr. Alan Roberts of the Scripps Clinic and Research Foundation published a retrospective study of various treatments, both medical and surgical that were once thought to be successful but later debunked for common conditions such as: bronchial asthma, Herpes cold sores, and duodenal ulcers. He found a 70% response rate and reported that "under conditions of heightened expectations the power of the placebo effect far exceeds that commonly reported in the literature" [32].

To investigate this further, Dr. K.B. Thomas performed an interesting study of two hundred patients with symptoms not attributed to any particular cause. For one group the physician told them with confidence the treatment they would receive (which was vitamins) would alleviate their symptoms within two weeks whereas for the other group, their physician told them no specific cause was identified and therefore they would either receive no treatment or a treatment (again vitamins) for which the physician was uncertain as to its providing symptom relief. In the final analysis, 64% of the patients who received 'good news' improved within two weeks compared with 39% of those who received negative feedback [33].

A study by Kaplan & Greenfield explored the placebo effect *via* the influence of patients' expectations on outcome. They found that in a 15 minute encounter a patient has with their doctor, the patient is likely to ask up to but not more than four questions, one of which is practical such as validating their parking. To improve the encounter the researchers coached patients with chronic illnesses to first reliably attend their appointments and then to plan out prior to their appointment, the questions they wanted to ask their doctor. They found that coached patients overall felt more satisfied with their experience and developed fewer illness-related lifestyle limitations than did un-coached patients. And diabetic patients had lower follow-up glucose levels [34].

Another, equally interesting study involved patients who received either a cholesterol-lowering drug or a placebo after having a heart attack [35]. These men were followed for five years and, in comparing compliant with noncompliant **placebo-takers** it was found that death occurred in 28% of poor adheres compared with only 15% of compliant patients. Hence, not taking the placebo resulted in an increased death rate, and patients who believed in the placebo had better survival than patients who did not.

The placebo's opposite is the nocebo effect, or power of negative thinking. Dr. Herbert Basedow in 1925 [36] recounts the power of the nocebo *via* the method of voodoo:

"The man who discovers that he is being boned is, indeed, a pitiable sight. He stands aghast, with his eyes staring at the treacherous pointer, and with his hands lifted as though to ward off the lethal medium, which he imagines is pouring into his body. His cheeks blanch and his eyes become glassy, and the expression of his face becomes horribly distorted...He attempts to shriek but usually the sound chokes in his throat, and all that one might see is a froth at his mouth. His body begins to tremble and the muscles twist involuntarily. He sways backwards and falls to the ground, and after a short time appears to be in a swoon; but soon after he writhes as if in mortal agony, and covering his face with his hands, beings to moan...His death is only a matter of comparatively short time."

Another example of the power of the mind negatively impacting the body is through dreams, as mentioned by Dr. Menninger von Lerchenthal of Vienna in the late 1700s, in which sudden death resulted from extreme fright as recounted in composer Joseph Haydn's diary [37]:

"On the 26th of March at the concert of Mr. Bartholemon (London) there was an English clergyman who while hearing my Andante sank into the deepest melancholy because of the fact that on the previous night he had dreamed of such an Andante which announced his death. He immediately left [our] company, went to bed, and today I heard through Mr. Bartholemon that this clergyman had died."

Similarly, Dr. George Engel described feelings of hopelessness and helplessness, which he termed the "giving up-given up complex" resulting in sudden death, familiar to us when we describe widows and widowers as 'dying of a broken heart' [38]. Dr. Engel also concluded, based on a study in which he re-created the psychological status of one hundred sudden deaths from unusual circumstances recounted in newspaper clippings, that a person's sense of powerlessness and inability to cope with life often led to their death and, that one's attitude to the circumstances of life determines one's fate [39].

In another example of the power of negative thinking on the body, Dr. L.J. Saul [40] wrote about a man who was torn between remaining in an intolerable home situation *versus* moving to a new town and leaving behind what he felt were his responsibilities. He boarded a train to the make the move to the new town. At a train stop roughly halfway between his old home and new, he disembarked and was pacing the platform in great indecision. As the train was leaving the man remained undecided as to how to proceed, collapsed on the train platform and died. His medical records indicated no significant or life-threatening illnesses.

The above studies demonstrate the power of our belief and thinking on our well-being. What is the relation between thinking and belief? A Google query brings up the following [41]: "a belief is a thought that you make real, or accept as true". Undoubtedly our emotions and feelings are intertwined with our thoughts and beliefs. To illustrate this, more recent studies by Dr. Jensen *et al.* [42] demonstrated the influence of our thinking and beliefs on how we feel (our perceptions), *via* patients' responses to thermal pain stimuli. They found that both conscious and nonconscious brain-processing pathways are involved. In two different experiments, subjects were asked to rate a thermal pain stimulus on their arm on a scale of 0 (no pain) to 100 (worst imaginable pain). In the first experiment the subjects were exposed to a computer screen which showed a clearly-visible image of a male face demonstrating either high- or low-pain. Subjects were significantly more likely to rate their pain as high after having been exposed to the high-pain image, and similarly, subjects were significantly more likely to rate their pain as low after having been exposed to the low-pain image, **for the same thermal stimulus for all subjects**. In a second experiment using different subjects, the high-pain, low-pain images were masked by virtue of being presented as a rapid exposure-image, and interestingly the findings were similar to those seen with the clearly visible images. These findings support the notion of the powerful influence of our thinking on our bodies perceptions. Both conscious cues in the form of explanations and instructions, and unconscious cues from the patient-clinician interaction appeared to be involved in activating the perceived pain in these experimental subjects.

The aforementioned studies illustrate the tremendous power of the mind, both our own minds and that of our healers, to impact our health and well-being. Interestingly and perhaps unexpectedly, the great breakthroughs of 20th- and 21st-century medical science, such as sequencing the human genome and discovering the molecular basis of disease, have enabled practitioners of modern medicine to become largely physically-focused, relegating aspects of mind-body healing to others. How important is this mind-body connection to modern-day healing? Let us explore the evidence.

SCIENTIFIC STUDY OF BELIEF: BELIEF AFFECTS PHYSIOLOGY

Studies in the past have concluded that the majority of causes that bring patients to medical clinics are of unknown origin and likely either the result of 'psychosocial' factors, or stress [19, 43]. Dr. Herbert Benson [19] opined that practitioners are focused on physical derangement and in cases where nothing can be found, the patient may either be reassured or dismissed by the doctor, possibly culminating in two very different results: assurance in the former situation, and possibly some level of frustration in the latter because the patient's beliefs were not addressed. Drs. Weisman and Hackett [44] demonstrated that patient's beliefs and expectations play a powerful role in outcome. They performed a three-year study of patients who were scheduled for surgery, and found that of the six hundred patients in the study who were unusually apprehensive about their surgery, only five were convinced they would die while on the operating table. Most of the apprehensive patients survived their surgery, compared with none of the patients who were convinced they would die!

Another study demonstrating the power of belief was published by Drs. Butler and Steptoe [45] who reported the results of a placebo trial in asthmatics. Both groups of patients received inert, distilled water. However the first group was told they were receiving a chest-constricting chemical and the second believed they were getting a powerful new bronchodilator agent. The first group experienced significant deterioration in their breathing ability, while the second group had no such experience, even though both groups received the same treatment.

In another equally interesting study, Drs. Ikemi and Nakagawa [46] demonstrated the influence of our beliefs on our bodies. In Japan, lacquer and wax trees are similar to poison ivy in the United States; a source of potential skin allergic reactions. These investigators studied fifty-seven high school boys who were tested for sensitivity to allergic items. The boys filled out questionnaires about their past history with allergens, and provided family histories. For those who reported marked allergic reactions to the lacquer trees, they were blindfolded and one arm was brushed with lacquer tree leaves while being told these were from chestnut trees, and the other arm was brushed with chestnut tree leaves while being told they were lacquer tree leaves. Within minutes, the arms which the boys believed had been brushed by lacquer tree leaves showed reactions including bumps, itching and burning, while the arms believed to have been brushed by chestnut leaves in most cases did not manifest any reaction. The conclusion was that patient reactions are a function of a combination of susceptibility to toxin, amount of toxin, the power of suggestion and a patient's belief; where in 51% of cases, suggestion/belief was the most powerful factor. This study supports the belief–physiology, or mind-body connection. That our perceptions become our reality or, as some sages have said, "as above, so below" (*i.e.*, as you think, so you are) alludes to the interconnectedness of the metaphysical and the physical realms [47]. Perhaps most succinctly said long-ago by an 18th century leader, Rabbi Yisro'el Ba'al Shem Tov [12]:

"Where your thought is, is precisely where you are – all of yourself is there."

From the potions and procedures of primitive medicines physicians and surgeons not subjected to clinical trials and hence of scientifically unproven efficacy; for which the majority of treatments may have done more harm than good, it is reasonable to conclude that cures for some medieval patients were likely the result of the healing power of the placebo - the power of their belief [48].

The great discovery of microbes as the cause of disease [49] and the success of antibiotic treatments would predictably diminish the appreciation of belief's role in the healing process. And the continued remarkable breakthroughs in medical science: the discovery of cancer susceptibility genes (BRCA, APC, and MMR), tumor genotyping and targeted drug therapies, stem cell transplantation, and *in vitro* fertilization strengthen the appearance of a schism between the mind and body, and enable medical doctors to focus on science and tangible physical treatments. But inevitably, there are cases which medical science cannot cure. What then? A patient will seek an alternative practitioner or other individual they believe can help them; someone in whom they can have faith.

FAITH, BELIEF & THE MIND-BODY INTERACTION

What is the relationship between belief and faith? According to Merriam-Webster Dictionary [50] belief is "a state or habit of mind in which trust or confidence is placed in some person or thing; something that is accepted, considered to be true; conviction of the truth of some statement or the reality of some being or phenomenon especially when based on examination of the evidence." Faith is "allegiance to duty or a person; belief and trust in and loyalty to God; something that is believed especially with strong conviction." The dictionary uses the term 'belief' to define 'faith.' Author Gregg Braden clarifies this further [51] writing that, "[Faith] is defined in The American Heritage Dictionary as belief that does not rest on logical proof or material evidence."

What is the evidence that faith can influence health and well being? For Westerners, the word 'faith' has religious overtones and the most familiar accounts occur in our Holy Bible. In the New Testament [52] Mark 5:25 recounts an incident in which a woman who bled for twelve years was healed when she touched Christ's cloak. Jesus turned around when he felt her touch and said, "Daughter, thy faith hath made thee whole; go in peace." In Luke 18:42 [53] Jesus restores sight to a blind man, saying "Receive thy sight; thy faith hath saved thee," and after cleansing lepers says, "Arise, go thy way; thy faith hath made thee whole." Dr. J.S. Levin in 1994 has written [54]:

"The mere belief that religion or God is health enhancing may be enough to produce salutatory effects. That is, significant associations between measures of religion and health ... may in part present evidence akin to the placebo effect. Various scriptures promise health and healing to the faithful, and the physiological effects of expectant beliefs such as this are now being documented by mind-body researchers."

The Holy Qur'an also says [55] "And I heal the blind and the leprous, and bring the dead to life with Allah's permission and I inform you of what you should eat and what you should store in your houses; most surely there is a sign in this for you if you are believers."

On a more secular note in 1910 Dr. William Osler, among the fathers of modern American medicine, wrote on the subject of faith while at Johns Hopkins University [56]: "Faith in St. John's Hopkins, as we used to call him, an atmosphere of optimism, and cheerful nurses, worked just the same sort of cures as did Aesculapeus [Roman god of medicine and healing] at Epidaurus."

More recently in 1995, Dr. Oxman reported a three-fold greater likelihood for survival among heart disease patients who underwent open-heart surgery, aged fifty-five and older, who received a sense of peace and comfort from their religious beliefs, when compared with their non-religious cohort [57]. In another study, Dr. Matthews and colleagues found that religious beliefs positively correlated with better quality of life and improved survival for cancer and heart disease patients who also showed lower blood pressure levels and decreased use of drugs, cigarettes and alcohol, and reduced levels of anger, depression and anxiety [58]. Matthews *et al.* [58], also found that people who were part of a religious group were more likely to report greater self-esteem, feelings of well being, marital- and life-satisfaction, and altruism than people who considered themselves non-religious. Dr. Levin reported that "epidemiological studies suggest that social support, a sense of belonging, and fellowship engendered by religion serve to buffer the adverse effects of stress and anger, perhaps *via* psycho-neuro-immunologic pathways", speculating that religious involvement "may trigger a multi-factorial sequence of biological processes leading to better health." [59 - 61]. Dr. Pressman followed thirty elderly women recovering from surgery for a broken hip, and found that those who considered themselves religious were less likely to be depressed and showed a better recovery by virtue of their ability to walk significantly farther than non-believers [62]. Dr. Spiegel and colleagues found, after ten years of following patients treated for breast cancer, those who participated in support groups lived on average eighteen months longer than those who did not and, those who participated in both social activities and religious groups had a tenfold increase in survival [63].

Faith, similarly to the placebo cannot be scientifically explained. Alternative religious healers too, employ ways yet to be understood. Rabbi Laibl Wolf speaks of the healing powers of those Kabbalists who are publicly accessible and receive people seeking their help [14]:

"Many people turn to these "miracle workers" for healing, and each Kabbalist has his [or her] individual modality. Often the ordinary and commonplace advice he [she] gives obscures the true source of the healing. For example, some Kabbalists advise eating a particular fruit or lighting a candle. What is not evident to the recipient of this advice is that the Kabbalist is actually focusing G[o]dly spiritual energy. The fruit or candle becomes the physical conduit through which spiritual energy can flow. Were the fruit to remain uneaten or the candle untouched, the Kabbalist's blessing would have no effect. This is called 'building a keili' (a container to hold the blessing). There are Kabbalists who 'read mezuzot' (small cases placed on doorposts of Jewish homes which contain scriptural verses from Deuteronomy). These Kabbalists can perceive all aspects of a person's life through the mezuzah and offer advice based on what they find. Others recognize the soul through the person's name and that of the mother. Yet others will simply ask you to open a page of Psalms. Many Hasidic rebbes hide the miraculous in the ordinary. The late Lubavitcher Rebbe... often camouflaged his miraculous gifts in 'ordinary' advice. He might advise a suffering individual to a see a particular doctor or to undertake a specific home therapy. Somehow his advice resulted in the spontaneous remission of serious illness. At other times the Rebbe simply intimated that the person would be healed - and that was enough. And at yet other times he instructed the person 'to make a l'chaim' (to have an alcoholic drink, usually a shot of vodka, and wish the person l'chaim - 'to life'), and it would affect a cure. Or he would take the person's Hebrew name and the name of his or her mother to the graveside of his saintly father-in-law (his spiritual predecessor), seeking heavenly intervention. The famous Kabbalist of the Middle East known as Baba Sali, who died only a few decades ago, affected miraculous cures of seriously ill hospitalized patients. Under the watchful eye of doctors he instructed the patient to sip a little water. The doctors' responses of amazement and awe are on record."

Placebo effect and/or faith? And how does each element contribute to the end result? We cannot answer these questions but as Dr. H. Benson [19] pointed out, the old medical treatments for angina: cobra venom, removal of the thyroid gland or pancreas; all remedies of no scientific merit had a 70-90% success rate when physicians believed in them! When doctors doubted the value of these treatments, their effectiveness dropped 30-40%. These findings demonstrate the placebo effect being twice as potent "under conditions of heightened expectation," and highlight the power of the healer's belief on the patient's ability to heal.

THOUGHTS, EMOTIONS AND THE MIND-BODY INTERACTION

Dr. Candace Pert, in her book Molecules of Emotion [20] points out that emotion is linked with physiology; an emotion generates molecule(s) that enable cell-to-cell communication that diffuse throughout the entire body, a true psycho-somatic phenomenon. Dr. Pert also says that the mind-body schism that has existed for so long in the western world is currently dissolving due to a paradigm shift that will have major implications for health, disease, and healing. She believes we are moving into a more holistic view of health and disease and that emotions are a key element in linking the mind and body [20]:

"the molecules of emotion run every system in our body, and [20] this communication system is in effect a demonstration of the body-mind's intelligence, an intelligence wise enough to seek wellness, and one that can potentially keep us healthy and disease-free without the modern high tech medical intervention we now rely on...".

Dr. Pert's comments parallel those of Rabbi Wolf – who stated that our minds, emotions, and bodies appear to be interconnected with and influence each other.

Taking this one step further, in Jewish thought performance of a good deed, termed a mitzvah "taps into diffused emotions and reorients them so that the result is wellness and good health" [14].

Scientific studies have shown that our emotions and feelings can influence the chemistry in our own bodies and, changing our feelings can in turn change the chemistry! To illustrate, Dr. Rein and colleagues in 1995 reported their study on salivary immunoglobulin A (S-IgA), for which they found that positive emotions were associated with a significant increase in S-Ig A levels, and anger was associated with decreased S-Ig A levels [64]. Earlier in 1993, Dr. Rein and colleagues made the equally intriguing observation that emotions can change the shape of DNA molecules [65]! Comparing individuals who were able to emotionally self-manage with control subjects who had no prior specialized training, they found that "individuals trained in generating focused feelings of deep love...were able to intentionally cause a change in the conformation of the DNA." If one can extrapolate from this finding in one cell - to every cell in a person's body - imagine the tremendous impact of emotions on a person's physical state!

The aforementioned cases and studies serve as testament to the mind-body interplay and role of belief in wellness and well being. Luckily, it seems this holistic view of the mind-body duality has been catching on in modern medicine. In 2006 Vicki Brower wrote of [66]:

"mounting evidence for the role of the mind in disease and healing leading to a greater acceptance of mind-body medicine. The common sense notion that 'too much stress makes you sick' might hold more than a grain of truth. The second of two large-scale epidemiological and medical studies among civil servants in the UK, known as the Whitehall studies [67], found that workers in low-level jobs, in which they have high stress and little autonomy, have more than twice the risk of developing metabolic syndrome - a precursor of heart disease and diabetes - compared with employees in high-level jobs... Stress is defined as a high level of demand, a low level of control and little support from co-workers or supervisors. By measuring heart rate, and cortisol and adrenaline levels, researchers also found that stress affects the autonomic nervous system and neuroendocrine function...Although the understanding that emotions affect physical health date as far back as the second-century physician Galen and the medieval physician and philosopher Moses Maimonides, modern medicine has largely continued to treat the mind and body as two separate entities. In the past 30 years, however, research into the link between health and emotions, behavior, social and economic status and personality has moved both research and treatment from the fringe of biomedical science into the mainstream."

Professor Oakley Ray has said that "according to the mind-body or bio-psychosocial paradigm, which supersedes the older biomedical model, there is no real division between mind and body because of networks of communication that exist between the brain and neurological, endocrine and immune systems [68]." Vicki Brower has also said [66] that several factors have been responsible for the growth of mind-body research and treatment: "patients' increasing interest in self-care, wellness and alternative medicine, and their concomitant dissatisfaction with the success of allopathic medicine in preventing and treating chronic illnesses. The consumer demand for and use of complementary and alternative medicine has also prompted the US government to become involved. In 1992, under pressure from consumers and with the help of Ohio Congressman Tom Harkin, an alternative medicine enthusiast, Congress mandated the National Institutes of Health (NIH, Bethesda, MD, USA) to open an Office of Alternative Medicine and gave it a US \$2 million budget... when OAM was founded, more than one-third of Americans said that they used relaxation techniques and imagery, biofeedback and hypnosis, and more than 50% used prayer as a complementary or alternative therapy."

Further supporting mind-body interplay, Dr. Deepak Chopra [69] has said:

"We know from many scientific studies that whatever you anticipate happening with your health is much more likely to occur. Doctors sometimes ridicule this as the placebo effect, but the placebo effect is a testimony to the power of intention. When a doctor and a patient believe in a treatment, the positive results can be as high as 100 percent, even if the treatment is later found to have no pharmacological effect. If patients with asthma are given salt water and told it will help their breathing, they will breathe more easily due to the placebo effect. Given the same salt water with the suggestion that their breathing will worsen, they experience the expected deterioration. This is called the nocebo effect. In every condition imaginable – from high blood pressure to cancer, from stomach ulcers to anginal heart pain – your expectations can make the difference between health and illness, life and death. We can summarize this principle in one line: What you believe you become."

As we have seen, positive thinking contributes to well being, whereas negative thinking has the opposite effect both on ourselves and on those about whom we are thinking - Dr. Benson's placebo and nocebo effects. Let us examine this thinking-power further, *via* examples from doctors, alternative healers and writers.

ALTERNATIVE HEALINGS AND THE MIND-BODY INTERACTION

Author Gregg Braden recounts what Western medicine may consider a 'miracle healing,' illustrating the complex interplay between mind-body and the power of belief and suggestion [51]:

"While studying at a specialized clinic outside of Beijing, our instructor had documented on video the effects of an ancient healing art based on techniques of movement, breath, thought, and feeling. He began by preparing us for what we were about to see. The video would show a phenomenon from Asian traditions that Western science could not explain. Anomalous experiences of this kind are often classified as miracles. For people who had turned to this clinic as a last resort, the choice of love, specialized movement, and the development of life force (ch'i) over medicine and surgery was the answer to their prayers..."

Braden goes on to describe such a healing that he viewed on a videotaped recording made at the Huaxia Zhineng Qigong Clinic and Training Center in Qinhuangdao, China, a center known as the 'medicineless hospital'. The video showed a woman patient, loosely clothed but with her abdomen exposed, awake and conscious, lying on her back. Her stomach glistened due to the prior application of a preparatory gel. A nurse practitioner, seated next to the patient waved an ultrasound wand across the woman's stomach. Directly behind the woman stood three male practitioners dressed in white. The men were focused on her upper body and one of them began moving his hands above the woman's face and chest. The video then showed the ultrasound image of the woman's urinary bladder, which contained a roughly 3-inch diameter tumor. While the camera zoomed in on the tumor, then three men could be heard chanting, repeating a single word that can be loosely translated in English as 'already accomplished' or 'already gone.' The cancerous tumor could be seen to begin to quiver and then, within a matter of seconds, began to fade from view. In a couple of minutes it was completely gone. The camera backed away and the patient appeared relieved, and the three male practitioners and nurse could be seen conferring amongst themselves and appeared pleased with their result.

Braden gives another account in the following miracle healing [51]:

"...I had noticed [an] elderly gentleman... and a woman I assumed to be his wife, threading their way through a small crowd of people onto the sidewalk in front of the reception area. Together they had just passed through the swinging doors into the hot, thick air of a summer night in coastal Georgia. His stainless-steel walker preceded each step, securing a stable position from which he could shuffle through his next movement. Suddenly the rhythm changed. Unexpectedly, he had reached a curb that dropped six inches or so, to the surface at street level. In slow motion, I watched as his walker rocked with uncertainty, tipped, then crashed onto the asphalt... 'Help us! Please, someone help us!' [screamed the man's wife]......Already kneeling at the fallen man's side, ..[and] cradling his head in her lap, was another woman. A zigzag trail of red glistened along the base of the man's head, just below his ear. Gently she tilted his body in the overhead light, searching for the source of blood...Without saying a word, the woman touched the broken tissue, then began to stroke the wound as if she were petting a tiny animal. I looked into her face. Her eyes were closed as she tilted her head upward toward the sky...Later that evening, some of the onlookers said that they had sensed a kind of sacredness in that moment. Some went so far as to suspect that a holy act was occurring...There, in the poorly lit parking lot of this little restaurant, I witnessed what modern science would consider a miracle. In full view of a dozen or so witnesses, as the woman silently stroked the tear in the man's flesh, it began to disappear. Within moments his wound had healed without any trace of the injury from his fall just moments earlier. Someone in the restaurant had called 911, and the paramedics arrived within moments...Still cradling the man's head and shoulders, the woman made room for the EMT. We watched as he examined the bloodstains on the man's shirt. Expertly the technician traced them to the back of the fallen man's head, then to the place just below his ear. Just as the woman had done moments earlier, the paramedic carefully separated the folds of skin where blood had pooled. To the amazement of the paramedics and the awe of the onlookers, there was no wound. The blood seemed to have just appeared at a point on the elderly man's neck, run its course, and spilled onto the collar of his shirt. There was no trace of wound, opening, or scar. Still wet on the man's skin, the blood appeared to have no source! The questions flashed into my mind as I watched: How was this possible? In the presence of a science so advanced that it can peer into the world of an atom and build machines that travel to the edge of our galaxy, why does the same science consider the healing that I had just witnessed a miracle?"

Shakti Gawain [70], a pioneer in the world consciousness movement, has said:

"People get sick because they believe on an inner level that illness is an appropriate or inevitable response to some situation or circumstance, because it in some way seems to solve a problem for them or gets them something that they need, or because it is a desperate solution to some unresolved and unbearable inner conflict.

Some examples of this are: the person who becomes ill because he has been 'exposed' to a communicable disease (and thus believes it is inevitable or highly likely); the person who dies of the same disease a parent or other member of her family had (because she has unconsciously programmed herself to follow the same pattern); the person who gets sick or has an accident in order to get out of work (either there's something he can't confront at work, or he won't allow himself the necessary relaxation and quiet time unless he is sick); the person who gets sick in order to get love and attention (this was how she was able to get her parents' love as a child); the person who represses his feelings all his life and eventually dies of cancer (he cannot resolve the conflict between the pressure of his stored-up emotions and the belief that it's not okay for him to express those emotions…so he eventually kills himself as a solution).

I do not mean to imply by these examples that I believe all illness is a simple problem with a pat explanation. As with all our problems, there are often many complex factors. I do intend to illustrate the fact that illness is a result of emotional, mental, and spiritual factors as well as physical ones, and that illness may be an attempt to find a solution to a problem we are having inside ourselves or in our lives. If we are willing to recognize and look deeply into our feelings and beliefs, we can often find healing on all levels."

Dr. Larry Dossey, a proponent for holistic practice in medicine, has said [71]:

"I used to believe that we must choose between science and reason on one hand, and spirituality on the other, in how we lead our lives. Now I consider this a false choice. We can recover the sense of sacredness, not just in science, but perhaps in every area of life."

Dr. Reginald Cherry, a Christian physician whose unique approach combines traditional medicine with alternative medicine and prayer, shared the following case history [72]:

"Jonathan Collins, a distinguished businessman, came to the clinic for a medical evaluation, and during the course of his exam I noted a nodule on his prostate gland. His PSA blood level (a test for prostate cancer) was normal, but the PSA level is normal in a small percentage of men who, in fact, do have prostate cancer. This nodule was particularly ominous as prostate cancer is the most common malignancy in older men and is particularly prominent in men of Afro-American descent.

As Jonathan and I prayed about his pathway to healing concerning this nodule, the Spirit of God led us in a direction contrary to conventional medical treatment. Though the traditional approach is to do an ultrasound-guided biopsy of nodules this size, we felt directed to do nothing in this situation except pray. I prayed the prayer of agreement with Jonathan, speaking directly to this nodule according to Mark 11:23, commanding it to shrink and disappear. I further spoke to his immune system to become activated and attack any abnormal cells that might be present in his prostate. I felt the Lord gave us another specific directive – that Jonathan was to return to the clinic in three months for a repeat evaluation and examination of the prostate.

When he returned three months later, the nodule, the location of which I carefully noted in the right lobe of his prostate, was totally gone! His prostate gland was normal.

Our God is not a god of foolishness. When a supernatural healing occurs, it can be documented and will stand up to medical scrutiny. While we do not have to have scientific evidence that God is a healer, documenting medical healing such as this gives glory to God, and confirmed testimonies like this give hope to others and stir faith in God as our Healer. Medical experts might say, 'Well, this was just a spontaneous remission, or just an area of inflammation.' I say that a spontaneous remission such as this, which at last check had lasted for more than two years, is a healing!"

Medical intuitive Caroline Myss has said [73]:

"… if people got to the 'root' cause of their emotional or psychological stress, then their illness was 90 percent healed. The rest would take good nutrition, a handful of the right vitamins, and daily exercise. I also learned through doing medical intuitive readings that there are as many different stress patterns as there are personalities. But what all people share is the need to purge themselves of their wounds, emotional traumas, and the memories of hard times or abusive relationships. Regrets also need resolution, as healing requires that we look at whom we have injured, not just who has injured us. I learned that forgiveness was essential and that the inability to forgive is as painful as the wound itself. Yet, in spite of that, forgiveness remains the greatest hurdle of all for most people…"

"…Then I encountered the work of Teresa of Avila… which drew me into the domain of healing as a mystical experience. The piece I had been missing was the power of grace. Since absorbing 'mystical reasoning' into my consciousness, and teaching the work of Teresa and now John of the Cross, I have seen people heal completely and permanently… Some of the healings were instant and others occurred over months, but none of these people have experienced a return of their diseases. Let me state clearly that their healings have nothing to do with Catholicism. This is not a treatise on healing through Catholic teachings. Further, most of these people were not Catholic and did not suddenly convert. The addition of 'mystical reasoning' was a missing piece that I consider to be 'cosmic' or 'spiritually archetypal' rather than related to any particular religion – a universal truth that has filtered into all the major world traditions in some way, much like the teaching 'thou shalt not kill'''.

"Once mystical reasoning was put on my radar, and in particular the work of

Teresa and John of the Cross, I realized that most people conduct their healing process in the 'active night' of the dark night. During the active night, we identify our hurts, what was done to us, our regrets, our stress patterns, all the things that are wrong. Perhaps we repair some of our relationships or try to make good on some of our regrets, but rarely do those efforts reach the source of why we really suffer or cause others to suffer. For all the determination we put forth in identifying past wounds, the identification process ends up being only an exercise in crime solving unless we complete the healing with forgiveness. Identifying a wound does not heal the wound. Healing must include getting to the source of why we struggle with forgiveness, why we want to hurt others, or why we hold on to our wounds hoping to make others feel guilty. This is where we encounter our true 'inner demons,' which John of the Cross referred to as the seven deadly sins in the passive stage of the dark night of the soul."

Intuitive consultant and counselor Cyndi Dale has described a 32-center energy system involving the chakras, remarkably harmonizing the psycho-spiritual with the physical in her segment entitled 'Living as a Shaman' [74]:

"A shaman's purpose is to walk in both the spiritual and physical worlds. Since ancient times, communities all over the world selected representatives to link the spiritual and physical planes for the benefit of all. In The Celtic Shaman, John Matthews describes a shaman as "one whose work is so integrated into everyday life that the 'join' does not show". The shaman's job was to help individuals heal physical and spiritual issues, and assist the community in doing the same. To do this, the shaman had to negotiate the revolving doors between the two dimensions.

Our energy systems are designed to enable each of us to be our own shamans. Our in-body chakras have front and back sides. The center points in the spine act like portals connecting our conscious and unconscious, our spiritual and tangible selves. We really are wheels of light, spinning in the stillness of our own being. As shamans for ourselves, it is our responsibility to keep the doorways between both worlds open at all times. By doing this, we can receive the 'other-world' messages we need to heal and to manifest, and we can project the reality-based energies necessary to move through the world.

Our shaman self is the one capable of stretching to the stars, often *via* our uppermost energy points. This capability would be worthless to our here-and-now self if we could not ground these energies into practical reality. How can our kundalini help us pay the bills? How can the feeling of peace soothe a difficult relationship? Conversely, how can having a disease teach us about faith or grace? Whether we work these questions through our spine, our feelings, our thoughts, or anything else, work them through we must."

THE MIND - BODY CONNECTION

More recently, Drs. Sternberg and Gold have written [75]:

"For centuries, taking the cure at a mountain sanatorium or a hot-springs spa was the only available treatment for many chronic diseases. New understanding of the communication between the brain and immune system provides a physiological explanation of why such cures sometimes worked. Disruption of this communication network leads to an increase in susceptibility to disease and can worsen the course of the illness. Restoration of this communication system, whether through pharmacological agents or the relaxing effects of a spa, can be the first step on the road to recovery… There is growing evidence that our view of ourselves and others, our style of handling stresses, and our genetic makeup can affect the immune system. Similarly, there is good evidence that diseases associated with chronic inflammation significantly affect one's mood or level of anxiety. Finally, these findings suggest that classification of illnesses into medical and psychiatric specialties, and the boundaries that have demarcated mind and body, are artificial."

Interestingly, the Jewish Likuttei Ha'MaHaRaN, No. 268 written in the 1800's, alludes to the mind-body connection [12]:

"You are here by default. Yet it would be a good idea to make a conscious commitment to being here, to being in life. The more conscious your commitment to being here, the deeper your soul will manifest in your being. The less the life commitment, the less the soul becomes manifested in the body, and the more vulnerable the body then becomes to death – toward which illness is believed to be a momentum."

CONCLUSION

We reviewed a number of studies demonstrating the powerful influence of our thoughts and beliefs on our wellbeing and healing ability: the placebo-nocebo effects, and the mind-body connection. Ancient healers may have had a relatively more complete hold on the reins of healing and wellbeing - enabled by an environment of scientific ignorance. Modern physicians who utilize sophisticated scientific knowledge and applied technologies to focus on physical healing, run the risk of ignoring the mind - relegating this important component of well-being to alternative practitioners learned in other modalities. Modern medicine will continue to search for scientific breakthroughs including the realm of the mind-body. In fact very recently, Dr. Tamar Ben-Shaanan and colleagues at the Technion (Israeli Institute of Technology) reported an apparent connection between mental states and cancer progression in mice [76]. Their exciting work suggests that positive emotions may help combat cancer! Have we now come full circle, or perhaps spiraled forward is the better word choice?

Around 400 B.C., Plato had said, "the great error in the treatment of the human body is that physicians are ignorant of the whole. For the part can never be well unless the whole is well" [77]. And around 1000 A.D., the Persian physician Avicenna said, "the imagination of man can act not only on his own body but even others and very distant bodies. It can fascinate and modify them; make them ill, or restore them to health" [78].

While our focus in medicine may have changed from religion-based to science-based, the recognition of the mind-body interaction has persisted. Will we moderns eventually find a molecular explanation for belief? Or, will belief be incorporated into an ideal treatment of the future when teams of experts work together to achieve cures? The answers to these questions will undoubtedly revolutionize the field of medicine. Luckily though, today's physician armed with complex scientific explanations and sophisticated technological treatments, retains the power of belief; the power of simple, faithful optimism in their ability to connect with, and help their patient achieve a healing.

CONSENT FOR PUBLICATION

Not applicable.

CONFLICT OF INTEREST

The author confirms that this chapter contents have no conflict of interest.

ACKNOWLEDGEMENTS

Declared none.

REFERENCES

[1]   Google online. Quora>What-year-was-Leviticus-written.

[2]   Leviticus, 13:1. Life Application Study Bible, New International Version. Wheaton, Illinois: Tyndale House Publishers, Inc 1997; pp. 185-6.

[3]   Google online. Wikipedia>wiki>Book_of_Exodus

[4]   Exodus, 15:25. The Living Bible, Paraphrased, A Thought-for-Thought Translation,. Wheaton, Illinois: Tyndale House Publishers, Inc 1971; pp. 185-6.

[5]   Yapijakis C. Hippocrates of Kos, the father of clinical medicine, and Asclepiades of Bithynia, the father of molecular medicine. Review. In Vivo 2009; 23(4): 507-14.
        [PMID: 19567383]

[6]   Byrne R. The Magic. New York: Atria Books 2012; p. 154.

[7]   Mount T. Medieval Medicine: Its Mysteries & Science. Gloucestershire: Amberley Publishing 2015;

pp. 15-, 37-38, 75, 89-90, 114, 143-144.

[8]   French R. Medicine Before Science. Cambridge: Cambridge University Press 2003; p. 62.
[http://dx.doi.org/10.1017/CBO9780511614989]

[9]   Robbins R, Ed. Secular Lyrics of the Fourteenth and Fifteenth Centuries. Oxford: Oxford University Press 1952; pp. 95-6.

[10]   Ancient Civilizations – Rome. Claudius Galen. Toothillschool.co.uk. Toot Hill School > uk>files>dept>hist. viewed online.

[11]   Pollington S. Leechcraft: Early English Charms, Plantlore and Healing. London: Anglo-Saxon Books 2000; pp. 454-5.

[12]   Winkler G. Kabbalah 365. Daily Fruit from the Tree of Life. Kansas City: Andrews McMeel Publishing 2004; 39: p. 231.

[13]   Moses B A. Look Inside a Tudor Medicine Chest. London: Hodder Wayland 1997; 17: p. 21.

[14]   Wolf L. Rabbi. Practical Kabbalah. A guide to Jewish wisdom for everyday life. New York: Three Rivers Press 1999; 119: pp. 44-7.

[15]   Papal Encyclicals Online. Your guide to online Papal and other official documents of the Catholic Church. Fourth Lateran Council: 1215. Constitutions. 18. Clerics to dissociate from shedding blood. http://www.papalencyclicals.net/Councils/ecum12-2.html

[16]   Wyman AL. The surgeoness: the female practitioner of surgery 1400-1800. Med Hist 1984; 28(1): 22-41.
[http://dx.doi.org/10.1017/S0025727300035298] [PMID: 6387334]

[17]   Beck RT. The Cutting Edge - Early History of the Surgeons of London. London: Lund Humphrey 1974; p. 135.

[18]   Bay NS, Bay B-H. Greek anatomist herophilus: the father of anatomy. Anat Cell Biol 2010; 43(4): 280-3.
[http://dx.doi.org/10.5115/acb.2010.43.4.280] [PMID: 21267401]

[19]   Benson H. Timeless Healing. The Power and Biology of Belief. New York: Fireside Book, Simon & Schuster 1996; p. 20-21, 30, 39-45, 49-50, 67.

[20]   Pert CB. Molecules of emotion The science behind mind-body medicine. New York: Scribner and Sons 1997; pp. 41-3.

[21]   González Hernández A, Domínguez Rodríguez MV, Fabre Pi O, Cubero González A. Descartes' influence on the development of the anatomoclinical method. Neurologia 2010; 25(6): 374-7.
[PMID: 20738957]

[22]   Germ theory of disease. Wikipedia [Online] en.m.wikipedia.org'germ theory'

[23]   Miasma theory. Wikipedia [Online] en.m.wikipedia.org'miasma theory'

[24]   Louis Pasteur. Wikipedia [Online] en.m.wikipedia.org'Pasteur'

[25]   Robert Koch. Wikipedia [Online] en.m.wikipedia.org'Robert Koch'

[26]   Alexander Fleming. Wikipedia [Online] en.m.wikipedia.org'Alexander Fleming'

[27]   The American Heritage Dictionary of the English Language. 3rd ed. Boston: Houghton Mifflin Company 1996; p. 1382.

[28]   Merriam-Webster Dictionary. [App for i-phone] Merriam-Webster, Inc. 2017: 'placebo effect'

[29]   Nocebo effect. Wikipedia [Online] en.m.wikipedia.org'nocebo'

[30]   Beecher HK. The powerful placebo. J Am Med Assoc 1955; 159(17): 1602-6.
[http://dx.doi.org/10.1001/jama.1955.02960340022006] [PMID: 13271123]

[31] Benson H, McCallie DP Jr. Angina pectoris and the placebo effect. N Engl J Med 1979; 300(25): 1424-9.
[http://dx.doi.org/10.1056/NEJM197906213002508] [PMID: 35750]

[32] Roberts AH, Kewman DG, Mercer L, Howell M. The power of nonspecific effects in healing. Implications for psychosocial and biological treatments. Clin Psychol Rev 1993; 13: 375-91.
[http://dx.doi.org/10.1016/0272-7358(93)90010-J]

[33] Thomas KB. General practice consultations: is there any point in being positive? Br Med J (Clin Res Ed) 1987; 294(6581): 1200-2.
[http://dx.doi.org/10.1136/bmj.294.6581.1200] [PMID: 3109581]

[34] Kaplan S, Greenfield S. Enlarging patient responsibility. Forum. Risk Management Foundation of the Harvard Medical Institutions 1993; 14: 9-11.

[35] Coronary Drug Project Research Group. Influence of adherence to treatment and response of cholesterol on mortality in the coronary drug project. N Engl J Med 1980; 303(18): 1038-41.
[http://dx.doi.org/10.1056/NEJM198010303031804] [PMID: 6999345]

[36] Basedow H. The Australian aboriginal, Adelaide: F. W. Preece, 1925. As quoted in Cannon, WB, 'Voodoo' death.'. Am Anthropol 1942; 44: 169-81.

[37] Menninger Von Lerchenthal E. Death from psychic causes. Bull Menninger Clin 1948; 12(1): 31-6.
[PMID: 18920466]

[38] Engel GL. A life setting conducive to illness. The giving-up--given-up complex. Bull Menninger Clin 1968; 32(6): 355-65.
[PMID: 5757975]

[39] Engel GL. Sudden and rapid death during psychological stress. Folklore or folk wisdom? Ann Intern Med 1971; 74(5): 771-82.
[http://dx.doi.org/10.7326/0003-4819-74-5-771] [PMID: 5559442]

[40] Saul LJ. Sudden death at impasse. Psychoanal Forum 1966; 1: pp. 88-9.

[41] Google. www.mindreality.com difference between thought and belief

[42] Jensen KB, Kaptchuk TJ, Kirsch I, *et al.* Nonconscious activation of placebo and nocebo pain responses. Proc Natl Acad Sci USA 2012; 109(39): 15959-64.
[http://dx.doi.org/10.1073/pnas.1202056109] [PMID: 23019380]

[43] Kroenke K, Mangelsdorff AD. Common symptoms in ambulatory care: incidence, evaluation, therapy, and outcome. Am J Med 1989; 86(3): 262-6.
[http://dx.doi.org/10.1016/0002-9343(89)90293-3] [PMID: 2919607]

[44] Weisman AD, Hackett TP. Predilection to death. Death and dying as a psychiatric problem. Psychosom Med 1961; 23: 232-56.
[http://dx.doi.org/10.1097/00006842-196105000-00005] [PMID: 13784028]

[45] Butler C, Steptoe A. Placebo responses: an experimental study of psychophysiological processes in asthmatic volunteers. Br J Clin Psychol 1986; 25(Pt 3): 173-83.
[http://dx.doi.org/10.1111/j.2044-8260.1986.tb00693.x] [PMID: 3768575]

[46] Ikemi Y, Nakagawa S. A psychosomatic study of contagious dermatitis. Kyushu J Med Sci 1962; 13: 335-50.

[47] Berg, Kabbalist Rav PS The power of you. Los Angeles: Kabbalah Centre International 2004; p. 66.

[48] Shapiro AK. A contribution to a history of the placebo effect. Behav Sci Notes 1960; 5: 109-35.
[http://dx.doi.org/10.1002/bs.3830050202]

[49] Rosenberg C. The therapeutic revolution. In: Leavitt J, Number R, Eds. Sickness and Health in America: Readings in the History of Medicine and Public Health. Madison: University of Wisconsin Press 1985.

[50]   Merriam-Webster Dictionary. [App for i-phone] Merriam-Webster, Inc. 2017; "belief"

[51]   Braden G. The Isaiah effect Decoding the lost science of prayer and prophecy. New York: Three Rivers Press 2000; 172: pp. 31-3.

[52]   The Holy Bible Old and New Testaments in The King James Version. Nashville TN: Nelson 1983; p. Mark 5:25.

[53]   The Holy Bible Old and New Testaments in The King James Version. Nashville TN: Nelson 1983; p. Luke 18:42.

[54]   Levin JS. Religion and health: is there an association, is it valid, and is it causal? Soc Sci Med 1994; 38(11): 1475-82.
        [http://dx.doi.org/10.1016/0277-9536(94)90109-0] [PMID: 8036527]

[55]   Holy Qur'an. Shakir MH, Ed. New York: Tahrike Tarsile Qur'an 1982.

[56]   Osler W. The faith that heals. BMJ 1910; 1(2581): 1470-2.
        [http://dx.doi.org/10.1136/bmj.1.2581.1470] [PMID: 20765152]

[57]   Oxman TE, Freeman DH Jr, Manheimer ED. Lack of social participation or religious strength and comfort as risk factors for death after cardiac surgery in the elderly. Psychosom Med 1995; 57(1): 5-15.
        [http://dx.doi.org/10.1097/00006842-199501000-00002] [PMID: 7732159]

[58]   Matthews DA, Larson DB, Barry CP. The faith factor: an annotated bibliography of clinical research on spiritual subjects. John Templeton Foundation 1993; Vol. 1.

[59]   Levin JS, Schiller PL. Is there a religious factor in health? J Relig Health 1987; 26(1): 9-36.
        [http://dx.doi.org/10.1007/BF01533291] [PMID: 24301836]

[60]   Levin JS, Vanderpool HY. Is frequent religious attendance really conducive to better health? Toward an epidemiology of religion. Soc Sci Med 1987; 24(7): 589-600.
        [http://dx.doi.org/10.1016/0277-9536(87)90063-3] [PMID: 3589753]

[61]   Levin JS. Religion and health: is there an association, is it valid, and is it causal? Soc Sci Med 1994; 38(11): 1475-82.
        [http://dx.doi.org/10.1016/0277-9536(94)90109-0] [PMID: 8036527]

[62]   Pressman P, Lyons JS, Larson DB, Strain JJ. Religious belief, depression, and ambulation status in elderly women with broken hips. Am J Psychiatry 1990; 147(6): 758-60.
        [http://dx.doi.org/10.1176/ajp.147.6.758] [PMID: 2343920]

[63]   Spiegel D, Bloom JR, Kraemer HC, Gottheil E. Effect of psychosocial treatment on survival of patients with metastatic breast cancer. Lancet 1989; 2(8668): 888-91.
        [http://dx.doi.org/10.1016/S0140-6736(89)91551-1] [PMID: 2571815]

[64]   Rein G, Atkinson M, McCraty R. The physiological and psychological effects of compassion and anger. J Adv Med 1995; 8(2): 87-103.

[65]   Rein G, McCraty R. Modulation of DNA by coherent heart frequencies. Proceedings of the Third Annual Conference of The International Society for the Study of Subtle Energies and Energy Medicine Monterey. California. 1993; p. 2.

[66]   Brower V. Mind-body research moves towards the mainstream. EMBO Rep 2006; 7(4): 358-61.
        [http://dx.doi.org/10.1038/sj.embor.7400671] [PMID: 16585935]

[67]   Chandola T, Brunner E, Marmot M. Chronic stress at work and the metabolic syndrome: prospective study. BMJ 2006; 332(7540): 521-5.
        [http://dx.doi.org/10.1136/bmj.38693.435301.80] [PMID: 16428252]

[68]   Ray O. The revolutionary health science of psychoendoneuroimmunology: a new paradigm for understanding health and treating illness. Ann N Y Acad Sci 2004; 1032: 35-51.
        [http://dx.doi.org/10.1196/annals.1314.004] [PMID: 15677394]

[69]   Chopra D, Simon D. Grow Younger, Live Longer. New York: Harmony Books 2001; p. 26.

[70]   Gawain S. Creative Visualization: Use the Power of Your Imagination to Create What You Want in Your Life. San Rafael, California: New World Library 1995; pp. 93-5.

[71]   Dossey L. [Online, 2018]. larrydosseymd.com

[72]   Cherry R. Healing Prayer, God's divine intervention in medicine, faith, and prayer. Nashville: Thomas Nelson Publishers 1999; pp. 134-5.

[73]   Myss C. Defy Gravity Healing Beyond the Bounds of Reason. New York City: Hay House, Inc. 2009; pp. 88-, 90-91.

[74]   Dale C. New Chakra Healing The Revolutionary 32-Center Energy System. St. Paul, MN: Llewellyn Publications 1996; pp. 277-8.

[75]   Sternberg E, Gold P. The mind-body interaction in disease. On Being with Krista Tippett. 2015. Online: Onbeing.org

[76]   Ben-Shaanan TL, Schiller M, Azulay-Debby H, *et al.* Modulation of anti-tumor immunity by the brain's reward system. Nat Commun 2018; 9(1): 2723.
[http://dx.doi.org/10.1038/s41467-018-05283-5] [PMID: 30006573]

[77]   Allen DE, Bird L, Herrman R. The Ministry of Medicine in the Care of the Whole Person An International Symposium. Downer's Grove, IL; InterVarsity Press 1980; p. 231.

[78]   Dossey L. Healing Words: The Power of Prayer and the Practice of Medicine. San Francisco: Harper 1993; pp. 37-8.

SUBJECT INDEX

A

Abdominal cavity 3, 4, 5
Abnormalities, chromosomal 113, 114
Activation of CdC2-Cyclin 139
Adenofibroma 52, 84, 95
Adjuvant chemotherapy 7, 14, 18, 154
Agents, first-line platinum 19
Aid in dying 148, 163, 164
Alvocidib in ovarian carcinoma 140
Analyses 130, 132, 136 137, 140, 141, 144
  core 136, 137
  original 140, 141
  secondary 130, 132, 140, 144
Angiogenesis inhibitors 22, 25, 26
Antibody–drug conjugates 31
Antidepressants 156, 157, 161
Apothecaries 176
Appelbaum 151
Appetite 154, 160, 161
Apprenticeship 175, 176
Arms 16, 17, 18, 21, 23, 25, 180, 182
  concurrent 25
  dose-dense IV therapy 17
  reference 25
Atypia 53, 72, 75, 85, 95, 98, 112, 131
  severe 72, 85, 98
Atypical mitoses 67, 72
Atypical proliferative clear cell tumors
  (APCCT) 95, 97
Atypical proliferative endometrioid tumor
  (APET) 85, 86, 88
Atypical proliferative mucinous tumor
  (APMT) 76, 77, 78, 79, 80, 81, 83
Atypical proliferative serous tumor (APST)
  53, 54, 55, 56, 57, 77

B

Back-to-back glands 88, 89, 90, 91, 92
Bartholemon 180
Benign clear cell tumors 94
Benign ovarian endometrioid neoplasms 83

Benzodiazepines 157, 161
Borderline 7, 46, 48, 109, 110
Borderline brenner tumors 111
Borderline tumors 7, 48, 53, 74, 83, 108, 110,
  116
Bowel obstruction 23, 24
Bowel resection 2, 3, 10
BRAF mutations 49, 63, 66, 110, 116
BRCA 27, 46, 47, 48, 50, 114, 117, 182
  defects in 117
BRCA1, carriers of 11
BRCA1 mutations 10, 47
BRCA2 germline mutations 130, 131
BRCA2 mutation 2, 10, 11, 12, 47
BRCA genes, wild-type 117
BRCA mutations 1, 10, 11, 27, 28, 49, 53
Breast cancer 10, 11, 66, 184
Brenner tumors 76, 81, 108, 110, 111
  malignant 108, 111
British columbia ovarian cancer research 12

C

Cancer 2, 3, 7, 8, 11, 12, 22, 23, 47, 48, 49,
  51, 52, 74, 106, 111, 113, 115, 116, 143,
  148, 149, 150, 152, 153, 158, 160, 161,
  162, 184, 187, 190, 194
  disease-associated colorectal 106
  hereditary breast/ovarian 47
  low grade endometrioid 115
  non-ovarian 8
  primary 2, 3, 8, 51
  primary ovarian mucinous 74
  prostate 190
  underlying 160, 161
Cancer antigen (CA) 3, 27
Cancer cells, ovarian 117, 118, 119, 120
Cancer diagnosis 148, 150, 152, 153, 154,
  155, 157, 159, 162
  ovarian 154, 159
The cancer genome atlas (TCGA) 108, 114,
  118, 131
Cancer therapies, ovarian 149
Cancer treatment 20, 155, 160